Tony Siadak



# Using Antibodies

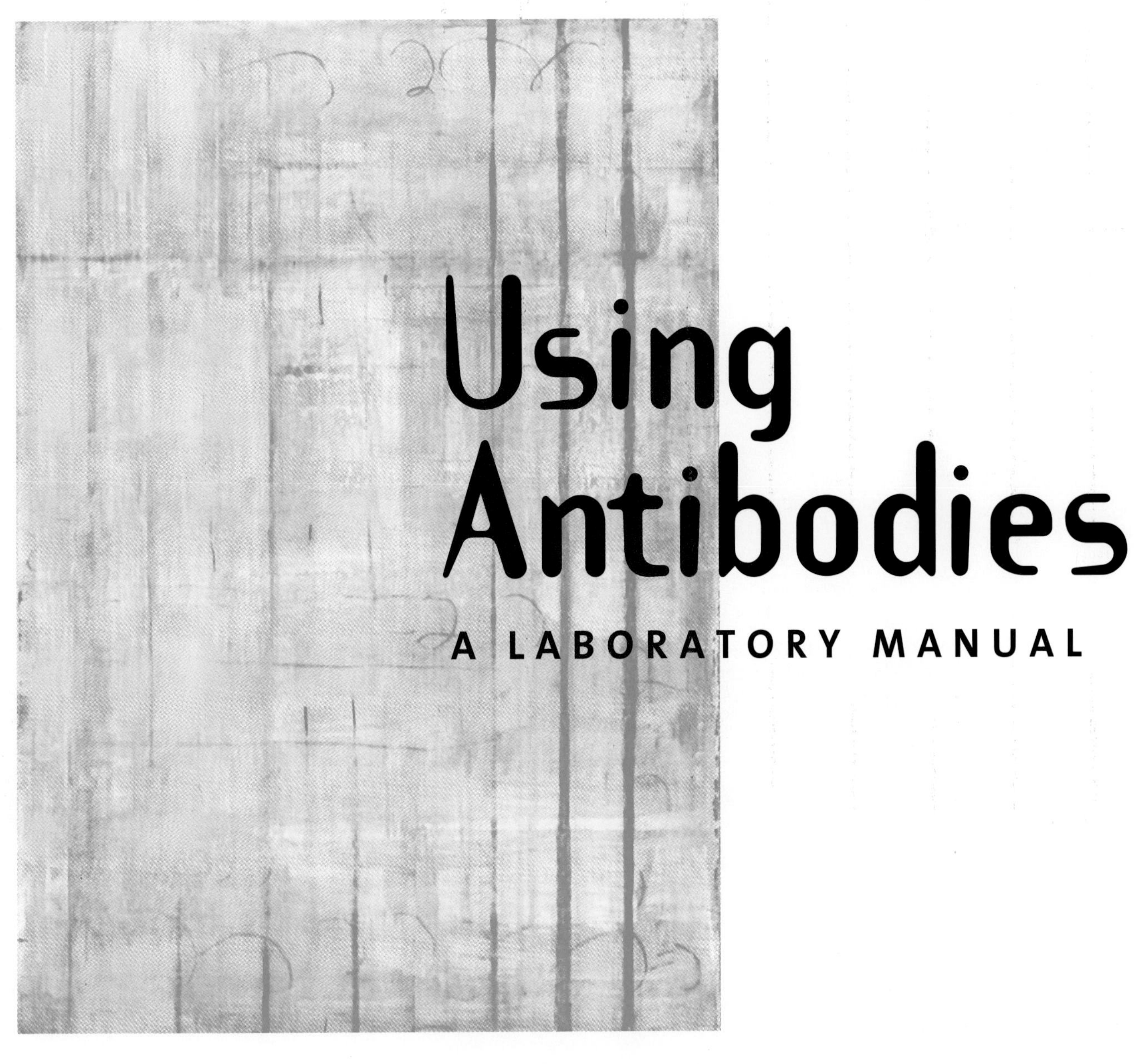

# Using Antibodies

## A LABORATORY MANUAL


**Ed Harlow**

MASSACHUSETTS GENERAL HOSPITAL CANCER CENTER

HARVARD MEDICAL SCHOOL

**David Lane**

DUNDEE UNIVERSITY



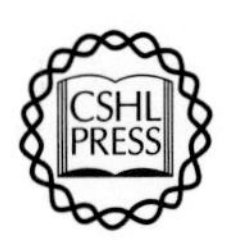

COLD SPRING HARBOR LABORATORY PRESS

Cold Spring Harbor, New York

**Using Antibodies: A Laboratory Manual**



**Design by H C & L Design; Berg Design**
*Developmental Editor* Judy Cuddihy
*Assistant Developmental Editor* Tracy Kuhlman
*Project Coordinators* Inez Sialiano and Mary Cozza
*Production Editor* Patricia Barker

**Library of Congress Cataloging-in-Publication Data**

Harlow, Edward.
Using antibodies : a laboratory manual / Ed Harlow, David Lane.
p. cm.
Includes bibliographical references and index.
ISBN 0-87969-543-9 (cloth : alk. paper). —ISBN 0-87969-544-7
(paper : alk. paper)
1. Immunoglobulins—Laboratory manuals. 2. Immunochemistry—
Laboratory manuals. I. Lane, David, 1952– . II. Title.
QR186.7.H37 1998
616.07′98—dc21 98-42802
CIP



Procedures for the humane treatment of animals must be observed at all times. Check with the local animal facility for guidelines.

Certain experimental procedures in this manual may be the subject of national or local legislation or agency restrictions. Users of this manual are responsible for obtaining the relevant permissions, certificates, or licenses in these cases. Neither the authors of this manual nor Cold Spring Harbor Laboratory assume any responsibility for failure of a user to do so.



All Cold Spring Harbor Laboratory Press publications may be ordered directly from Cold Spring Harbor Laboratory Press, 10 Skyline Drive, Plainview, New York 11803-2500. Phone: 1-800-843-4388 in Continental U.S. and Canada. All other locations: (516) 349-1930. Fax: (516) 349-1946. E-mail: cshpress@cshl.org. For a complete catalog of all Cold Spring Harbor Laboratory Press publications , visit our World Wide Web site: http://www.cshl.org.

# Dedication

*In memory of my father (11/22/17–8/16/98)*
*EH*

*To Birgitte, Amelia, and Oliver*
*DL*

# Theory

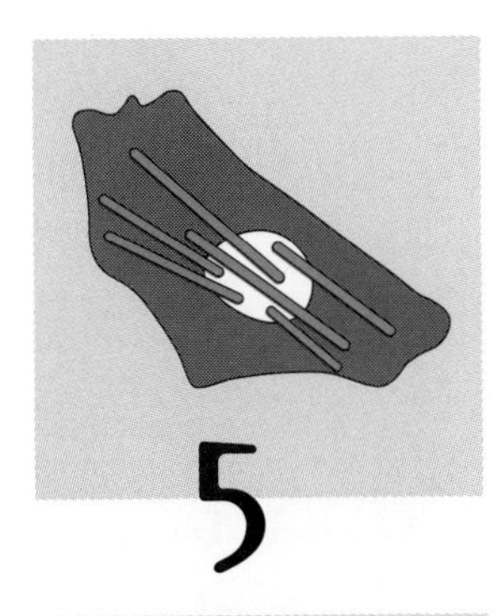

5

## Staining Cells

*Immunostaining can be used to pinpoint the subcellular localization of a protein antigen, to follow its changing cellular address as cells respond to stimuli, or to compare its locale to other proteins in the same cell. With careful controls, you may also be able to get an idea of how much protein is present in the cell. In this book, the immunostaining procedures have been separated into two major variations based on the source of the cells to be examined. In this chapter, staining cells growing in tissue culture is discussed.*

101

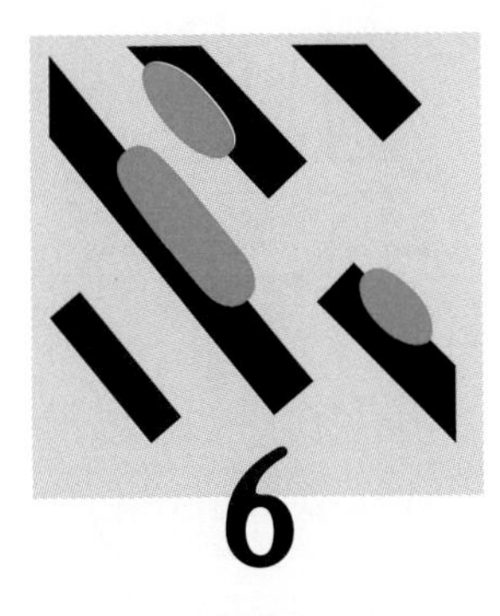

6

## Staining Tissues

*Immunostaining of tissues of whole organisms can be used to examine the localization of antigens in physiological settings. Using these methods, you can follow an antigen's distribution during development, mark the location of a particular cell type in a multicellular in vivo setting, or determine the presence of an antigen in a diseased tissue. The protocols normally require multiple steps over several days as well as extensive knowledge of the architecture of the tissues being studied. These procedures demand methods to preserve the structure of tissues, which unfortunately are often damaging to the antigens.*

151

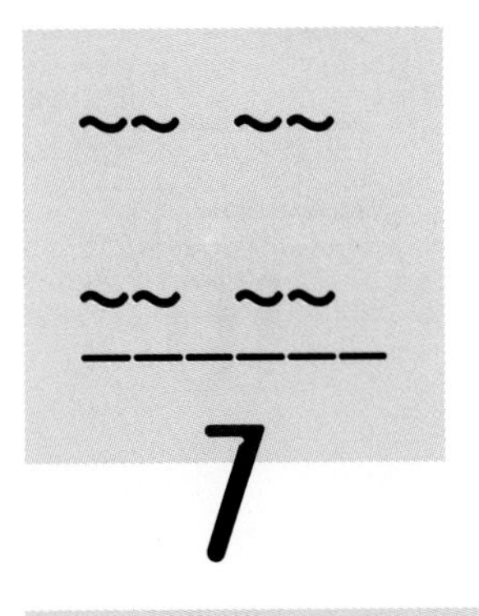

7

## Immunoprecipitation

*Immunoprecipitation allows the partial purification of antigens, normally proteins, from complex mixtures of soluble molecules. The antigens can be purified up to 10,000-fold by simple and rapid methods that collect the proteins on inert beads. The technique takes about a day and can be combined with any other method that can utilize immobilized proteins as a starting material.*

221

8

## Immunoblotting

*Immunoblotting provides a reliable method to check any sample for the presence of protein antigen. The assay identifies the protein on the basis of both its interaction with a specific antibody and its relative molecular weight. Immunoblotting can be used to determine other characteristics of your antigen, such as the relative abundance of the antigen or association with other well-characterized antigens. It is also a useful method to characterize new antibody preparations. Immunoblotting involves multiple simple steps that take about a day to complete.*

267

# Practice

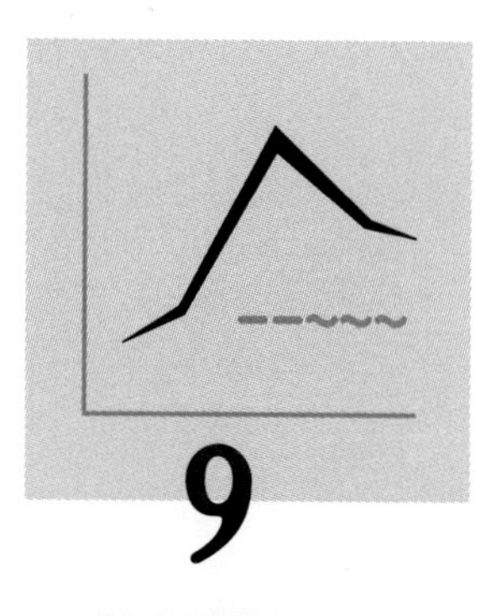


## Immunoaffinity Purification

*Immunoaffinity purification takes advantage of the high binding affinity and specificity of an antibody for its antigen to allow large quantities of antigen to be isolated in native or near-native states. Not all antibodies are suitable for immunoaffinity purifications, but when a good antibody is available, the procedure is quick and reliable. The procedure can be scaled to any size, takes not more than a half-day to perform, and can achieve levels of purification unmatched by other methods of chromatography.*



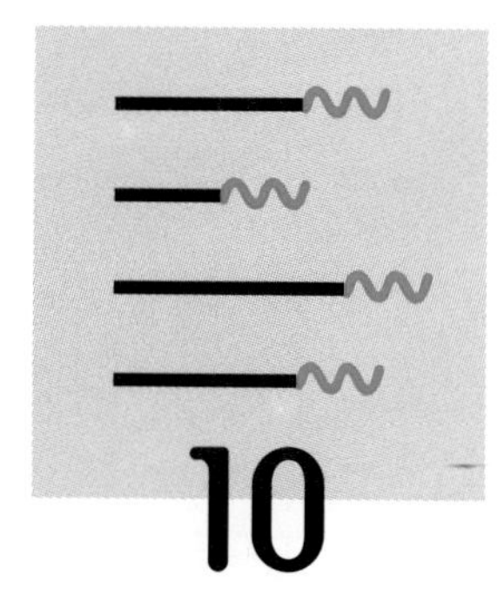


## Tagging Proteins

*Proteins can be tagged using recombinant DNA techniques to allow their ready purification and their specific detection in different host cell systems. These include tags designed to help specifically with detection (such as green fluorescent protein tags) or with purification (such as the His tags and glutathione-S-transferase tags). Epitope tags—short peptide sequences to which strong and specific antibodies have already been produced—can be used for detection and purification using all of the immunological methods described in this book. This chapter describes the different available tag systems, their advantages and disadvantages, and how to choose the right tag for your experiment.*



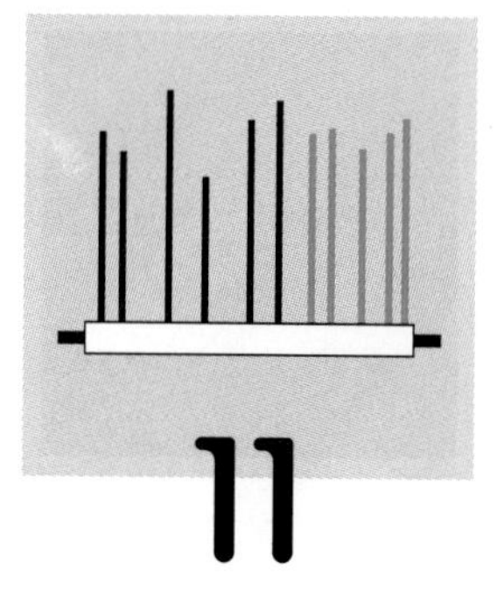


## Epitope Mapping

*Determining the binding sites (epitopes) for monoclonal and polyclonal antigens on protein antigens often provides extremely useful information that greatly extends the power of immunochemical analysis. Epitope mapping is used to examine the specificity of the immune response or to distinguish between different antibodies.*



## Appendixes

*Appendix I contains information about Electrophoresis; Protein Techniques are covered in Appendix II; and Appendix III provides General Information.*



Practice

Useful Info

## Preface

It has been almost exactly a decade since the first edition of *Antibodies: A Laboratory Manual* came out. The first edition was published on one of the last few days of 1988, and this one will hit the streets early in December, 1998. Both of us were gratified and relieved that *Antibodies* gathered so much praise, and we have been particularly heartened by the unsolicited comments from strangers letting us know that they had tried something new and found that they got through it without too many emotional or physical scars.

Among these kind comments, however, were some criticisms and more than a couple of grumbles. We've been collecting those suggestions over the years, and when we began the process of tackling a second edition, we set out to catalog them more thoroughly. We asked Gerard Evan, Deborah French, Kevin Johnson, and Jennifer Rabinowitz to criticize the manual and make suggestions. They kindly sat down and read the book—a task in itself for a manual that wasn't designed with plot development in mind. Their comments were very helpful. There have been many specific gripes and suggestions, but the recurring requests fell into two main pleas—fix the binding and add your own advice to the book. We've tried to do this. Here are some of the changes from the first round of *Antibodies.*

First, we've gotten rid of that comb binding. But to be fair, there isn't much in the way of innovative new bindings for books like this one. For this round we've settled on two options. There is a standard sewn hardcover version and a wire-O hardbound binding for the commonly used lab copies. This binding should allow the book to lay flat on the bench, and it should stand up to heavy lab use. We realize that this still is not a perfect solution, but we think it's the best available; we're sure we'll hear if this isn't the case.

The second major change is that this book covers only about one-half of the information found in the first edition. As we began to assemble the material for the second edition, we realized immediately that a single volume would only be possible if we deleted whole subject areas and put out an enormously thick tome. Our discussions quickly led to what we hope is a useful compromise. Antibody work falls roughly into two sections. One is found here in *Using Antibodies,* where we've tried to cover all of the commonly used immunochemical methods. The rest of the antibody methods will be found in the next volume, *Making Antibodies,* which we will address after this volume is out. This division of labors is not flawless, but it allows us sufficient space to tackle the needed subjects without arbitrary and confusing separations between closely related methods.

The other major change is that this edition contains considerably more advice. In the first edition we tried to be encyclopedic, presenting many different versions of each method. (You probably will still find this first edition useful as a resource for alternative approaches.) However, in the second edition, we've taken a different tack. If we believed that there was sufficient reason to recommend one method over another, then we have presented just the preferred method, which might be more reliable, cheaper, or more widely used than another. Experienced workers may find that their favorite variations aren't presented. Our advice here would be to continue to use methods that are working for you. We have tried to give enough information about the chosen methods to enable a beginner to pick up the book and get the method to work. This shouldn't be a hindrance to experienced workers using other variations. In addition to listing fewer methods, we have included extensive notes to help point out difficult steps, potential shortcuts, or small variations. We have viewed these as a way to include all of the comments that we might give to someone in our own lab starting on a method for the first time or to someone troubleshooting a problem. These comments are found in the beginning of each technique or in the side bars that are placed throughout the text.

There are several other changes in the book. We have designed various new devices to help readers navigate through the book and move through each technique. Each chapter has an icon that is an abstraction of a classic figure relating either to the development of the technique itself or to the development of this area. This icon is used in all of the running heads as a pointer to get readers to the right place as quickly as possible. We also have added locators in each technique to direct workers to the next or previous steps of the method. The idea for these locators came from looking at public transportation maps; each step is represented as another stop on the railway "technique" map. Again, we hope that these will help readers navigate through the steps of a technique. The other new device is the inclusion of shortened techniques for all of the major methods in the book. These are the methods presented without much explanation, and they are meant to be used after workers are comfortable with the method. These method sheets have been dubbed "Portable Protocols" and are found at the end of each chapter in the book and also as separate laminated cards that can be used at the bench. Additional copies of these protocols will be available as separate items.

The audience for this book is much the same as for the first version. We have written this for the experienced molecular biologist who has not had much experience with immunochemical methods. We hope that experienced immunologists, pathologists, and others will find the book helpful, but we have not tried to include all of the methods that they might use routinely. We have tried to keep the discussions as general as possible about all types of antigens, but in practice this manual deals primarily with protein antigens. It is meant to be used as a standard methods manual for those who need to move from the world of cloning to the world of protein analysis.

The most important function of this preface is to thank all the people who helped make this book possible. There is one person who deserves our most deeply felt thanks. This is our editor, Judy Cuddihy. Judy has been leader, problem-solver, creative force, and good friend throughout this process. It is completely true that this book could not have been done without her. At several times during this project she was the only one who could calm the waters and keep the work proceeding. Judy now has survived both editions working with us, a true sign of friendship and perhaps a dash of hardheadedness to boot.

Many others made major contributions as well. Tracy Kuhlman was our editorial assistant, putting up with round after round of maddening queries from both of us.

She did a remarkable job of feeding us a stream of needed information and then reading and correcting our misplaced facts and notions. Portions of the book were read and critiqued by Peter Hall, Andi McClatchey, Shiv Pillai, and Sander van den Heuvel. We thank them for lending us their expert eyes.

Throughout this process, John Inglis was our ringleader and friend. He got us interested in this project again, and he and his staff at CSHL Press did a remarkable job of not only getting the book out, but also putting up with us when we were at our authorial worst. Thanks here go especially to Denise Weiss, Pat Barker, Inez Sialiano, Mary Cozza, and Jan Argentine.

Finally, we thank all of our colleagues who provided or directed us to new techniques or variations on the old ones. One of the nicest things about doing this book has been the interaction with our colleagues.

As with the last round, we hope it's fun,

**EH** and **DPL**

## Preface to Antibodies: A Laboratory Manual

This manual was inspired by "the cloning manual," *Molecular Cloning: A Laboratory Manual* by Tom Maniatis, Ed Fritsch, and Joe Sambrook, a book that did so much to expand the community of scientists using molecular biology methods. The great joy of that manual was and is the confidence it gives to beginners and the way it tempts all workers to try new approaches. At present, many of the methods of modern immunochemistry seem beyond the reach of nonimmunologists, and one of the goals of *Antibodies* is to make these methods accessible to a wider group. We hope that this manual is judged by how well it succeeds in breaking this barrier.

*Antibodies* has a long and complex genesis. The original ideas for an immunology manual were developed with Ron McKay, Steve Blose, and Jim Lin. Some portions of those early plans remain in this version, and we would like to thank Ron, Steve, and Jim for their contributions. Version 2, the eventual precursor to this book, was conceived in a naive burst of enthusiasm in the summer of 1986. In those early days, we talked of pooling our lab protocols and finishing quickly. As we worked and talked to our colleagues, two things became clear. First, there seemed to be a genuine need for a practical guide to immunochemical methods for the nonimmunologist (which was encouraging), and second, the gap between modern immunology and the backgrounds of most molecular biologists was larger than we had thought. This meant that more background information was needed if the book were to help a reasonable cross section of scientists (which was less encouraging).

The final version of *Antibodies* contains four introductory chapters that summarize the key features of the immune response, the structures of the antibody molecule, the activities of antibodies, and the mechanism of the antibody response. These summaries are designed to be an up-to-date consensus, and they will no doubt excite some ire among immunologists by their oversimplifications and omissions, but we hope that the nonspecialist will find them a helpful framework for the ideas and techniques presented in later chapters. The bulk of the book contains protocols for raising, purifying, and labeling monoclonal and polyclonal antibodies, as well as chapters describing ways of using antibodies to study antigens. Two biases are clear: we have concentrated on protein antigens, and we have excluded several of the classical methods of immunochemistry. In their place, we have concentrated on protocols for cell staining, immunoprecipitation, immunoblotting, immunoaffinity purification, and immunoassay, as these are the techniques most commonly required by the nonimmunologist.

The actual origin of a protocol is often hard to determine, and although we have given appropriate references wherever possible, there are many sins of omission. The methods have been derived mostly from those used in our labs or those of our close associates. Clearly, few protocols are definitive, and this is particularly true where so much depends on the individual qualities of a particular antibody. We have included both general notes on the procedures themselves plus more personalized comments. These are distinguished by different types of "boxes" in the text. The phrase "some workers find. . ." is used either when we could not reach an agreement among ourselves or when friends assured us the effect was significant but neither of us had any direct experience with it. We have attempted to give a clear explanation of the theoretical and practical basis of the techniques to provide an effective guide when problems arise.

For further general information, *Handbook of Experimental Immunology* edited by Weir, Herzenberg, Blackwell, and Herzenberg (1986) is the best source of technical advice, and *Monoclonal Antibodies: Principles and Practice* by Goding (1987) and *Hybridoma Technology in the Biosciences and Medicine* edited by Springer (1985) are excellent sources of information on monoclonal antibodies. More specific references are listed in the appropriate sections. For new protocols, the reader should scan the pages of the *Journal of Immunological Methods* and *Analytical Biochemistry.*

Many, many people helped us with these protocols, and our job has often been one of collation, checking, and interpretation. We would like to thank Joan Brugge and her lab (Michael DeMarco, Adele Filson, Lawrence Fox, Andy Golden, Joan Levy, Sally Lynch, Susan Nemeth, John Schmidt, and Susan Schuh) who used an early version of the manual and were immensely helpful, both in finding fault and in making powerful suggestions for improvement. Several members of our own labs, Carmelita Bautista, Karen Buchkovich, Margaret Falkowski, Julian Gannon, Richard Iggo, Margaret Raybuck, and Carmella Stephens, used the manual on a day-to-day basis and were very definite and precise in their criticisms!

The manual was read in its entirety by Lionel Crawford, Larry Banks, Mike Krangel, Margaret Raybuck, and David Chiswell and his colleagues at Amersham. Their many comments helped us resolve difficult decisions about content and presentation. Chapters 1–4 were read and critiqued by Winship Herr, Richard Iggo, and John Inglis. Steve Dilworth, Ann Harris, and Bob Knowles sorted out Chapters 6–9 and 15, and Jean Beggs and Birgitte Lane helped enormously to get Chapters 10–14 into shape. The appendices were read and amended by Carl Anderson and Mark Zoller. In addition to these main readers, many others kindly helped with specific sections. Advice on yeast came from John Kilmartin, Jean Beggs, Paul Nurse, and David Beach. Advice from Susan Alpert on cell staining was invaluable, as were Rebbeca Rowehl's and Jacqueline Bortzner's comments on Chapters 6 and 7. Ian Mohr forced us to get the immunoassay chapter into intelligible form, Seth Grant helped on Chapter 12, and Ella Wetzel read and reviewed an early version of Chapter 11. All these people helped to make this a better book. Usually, we took their advice, and we hope they will forgive us for those times that we didn't.

Special personal thanks to Birgitte Lane, Nicky Williamson, Gordon Peters, Brenda Marriot, Frank Fitzjohn, and Marilyn Goodwin who helped by getting us onto planes at the right time, by finding us places to sleep and write, and by fending off a wide range of tempting distractions. Somehow they managed still to be nice, even when we were at our most crabby. The excellent art work is by Mike Ockler, and looking at Carl Molno's suggestions for cover art was a wonderful break. Jim Pflugrath provided the computer graphics. Christy Kuret, Michele Ferguson, Inez Sialiano, and Susan Schaefer provided invaluable editorial assistance. The book was designed by Emily Harste (despite our interference), and Nancy Ford and Annette Kirk provided overall supervision and kind support throughout the work.

A final and special thanks to Judy Cuddihy, our editor, whose patient advice, encouragement, and fine judgement kept us going through the best and worst of times.

Hope it's fun,

**EH** and **DL**

---

## Cover

The cover image (for printed case) is "Rio Ledger III" (oil on canvas, 35" × 26") by abstract expressionist Robert Kelly. A resident of both Santa Fe, New Mexico, and New York City, Kelly was born in 1956 and is a graduate of Harvard University. His work has been shown in numerous one-person and group exhibitions throughout the world and is represented in several museum collections, including the Brooklyn Museum and the Museum of Fine Arts in Santa Fe. Kelly's paintings hang in many prestigious corporate and private art collections.

## Fonts

abcdefgh
HIJKLM
opqrstuv
W X Y Z

Minion, the text font for *Using Antibodies,* is an Adobe Original typeface designed in 1990 by Robert Slimbach. Its style is based on the classical typefaces of the late Renaissance period designed by such masters as Aldus Manutius and Claude Garamonde. We chose this typeface because its easy readability makes it perfect for use at the bench. Adobe Systems Incorporated began producing fonts and software in 1982 and was instrumental in launching the "desktop publishing" revolution.

abcdefgh
HIJKLMN
opqrstuv
W X Y Z

Template Gothic, the display font used in this manual, is an Emigre typeface designed by Barry Deck in 1990. In contrast to the elegance and ancient heritage of Minion, this very vernacular typeface celebrates type that is not perfect and that has been distorted by photomechanical reproduction. The designer's inspiration for this typeface was a sign created with lettering templates that was hanging in the laundromat that he used. Emigre, Inc., was founded in 1984. It was one of the first independent type foundries to create typefaces that center around personal computer technology and is recognized as a leader in producing innovative typeface design.

# Antibody Structure and Function

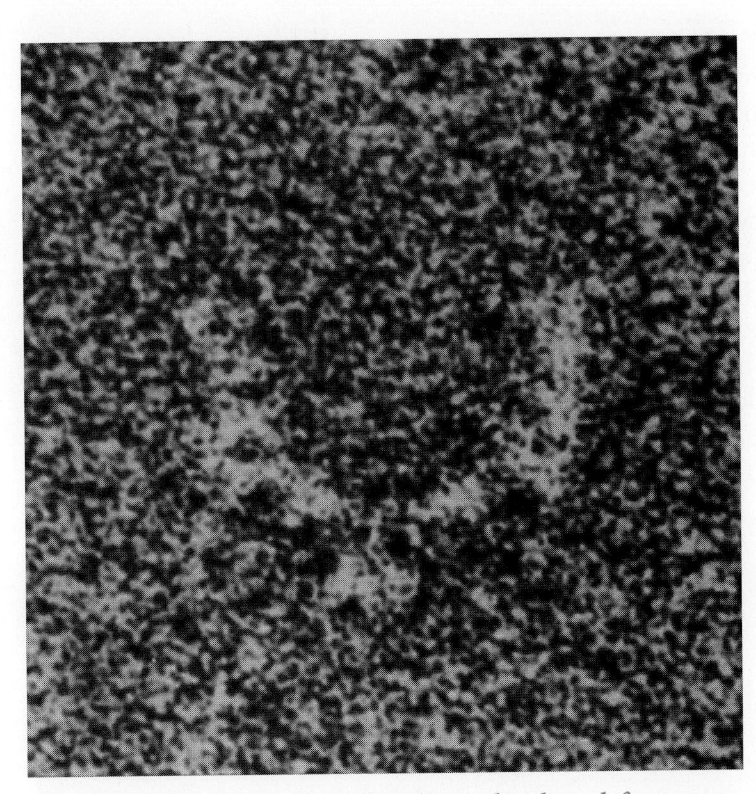

From Wrigley N.G., Brown E.B., and Skehel J.J. 1983. Electron microscopic evidence for the axial rotation and inter-domain flexibility of the Fab regions of immunoglobulin G. *J. Mol. Biol.* **169:** 771–774. (Reprinted with permission [copyright Academic Press].)

Fig. 1. Three different configurations of a single type of complex with 1 IgG (HC19) molecule binding 2 HAs.... Magnification 250,000 ×. [*Note from authors*: For clarity, only one image of 45 in original figure is displayed.]

Many different approaches have been important in bringing our current understanding of antibody structure and function to its current detailed level. As a result, we probably know as much or more about the biology of antibodies than we do for any other protein in mammalian biology. This information base has been developed from many diverse fields. Early protein biochemistry showed how the antibody molecule could be proteolytically cleaved into different functional domains. Protein sequencing of homogeneous antibody preparations, which came from patients or animals with rare immune diseases, led to our first glimpse of antibody diversity. The origin of this diversity and the understanding of its generation came from elegant genetic and molecular biology studies. These molecular biology studies gave us the tools to investigate the details of functional domains and provided the genetic targets for altering the mouse genes to test theories of antibody regulation and function. Cell biological studies have shown how and where the antibodies were synthesized and transported. And finally, the structure of the antibodies has been revealed by cryo-electron microscopy work like that shown here and by detailed X-ray crystallographic analysis. This collection of work has led to a spectacularly sophisticated view of how antibodies function, and this knowledge allows workers to use antibodies as one of the most important tools for modern biological research.

Antibodies are host proteins produced in response to the presence of foreign molecules, organisms, or other agents in the body. Antibodies are synthesized predominantly by plasma cells, terminally differentiated cells of the B-lymphocyte lineage, and circulate throughout the blood and lymph, where they bind to the antigens. Once formed, the antibody–antigen complexes are removed from circulation mostly through phagocytosis by macrophages. This antibody response is one of the key mechanisms that a host organism uses to protect against the action of foreign molecules or organisms.

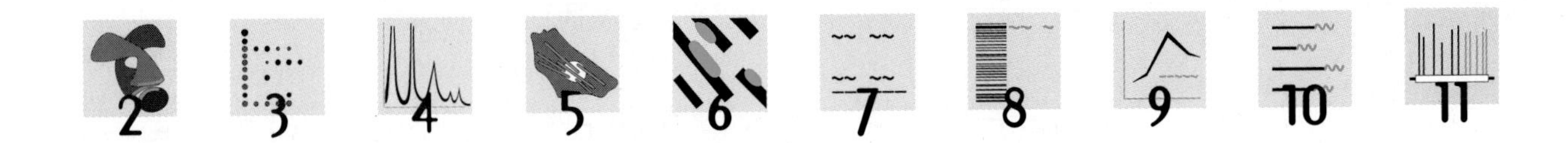


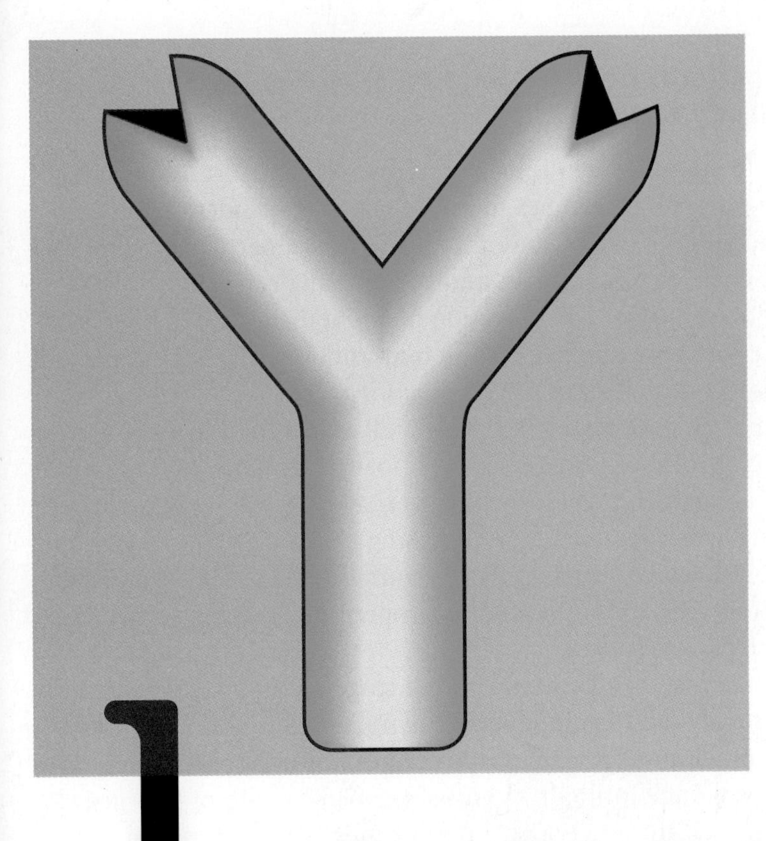

# 1 Antibody Structure and Function

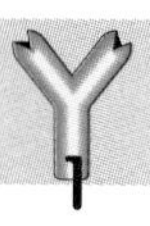



## Antibodies are useful reagents that can bind with high affinity to chosen antigens

Researchers have learned to manipulate the antibody response to produce a wide range of useful affinity reagents. For example, specific antibodies can be used to determine the precise subcellular location of an antigen, to isolate an individual antigen from a complex mixture of competing molecules, to find other macromolecules that interact with the antigen, and even to determine the exact concentration of the antigen. These types of methods have made antibodies one of the most useful reagents for studying molecules of interest.

To produce specific antibodies, a selected antigen is injected into a laboratory animal and serum samples are collected. The serum then becomes a source of antibodies that can bind specifically to the antigen under study. In most cases, antibodies bind with sufficient affinity that they can be used as specific reagents to study their cognate antigens.

## Serum contains a collection of antibodies that bind to the antigen on different epitopes

The antibody-binding site on an antigen is known as an *epitope*. Most often, an animal will produce a large group of antibodies that recognize independent epitopes on the antigen. Each individual type of antibody that recognizes a particular epitope is produced by a different clone of plasma cells, and each plasma cell can secrete antibodies that bind to only one epitope. The collection of antibodies in serum is synthesized by the concerted effort of a number of different antibody-producing plasma cells. Therefore, serum is a good source of *polyclonal antibodies*.

In 1975, Köhler and Milstein introduced the first version of a method to make monoclonal antibodies. Precursors of the plasma cells were isolated and fused with immortal cells of the B-cell lineage, which previously had been selected to no longer secrete antibodies. The resultant *hybridoma* cells could be single-cell cloned and then expanded as individual clones, which secrete only one antibody type. All of these antibodies are identical, with specific and easily studied properties of antigen recognition, and are known as *monoclonal antibodies*.

Polyclonal antibodies are the most commonly used reagents for immunochemical techniques. They are normally used as crude serum samples and in this form are fine for most purposes. For some more specialized techniques, the antibodies need to be purified prior to use. Polyclonal antibodies can be purified by one of two general methods. They can be purified from the other proteins in serum to prepare a collection of all antibodies. Alternatively, the antibodies that recognize the antigen under study can be purified to remove not only the other proteins in the serum, but also all but the specific antibodies.

Monoclonal antibodies already have a defined specificity for the antigen under study, so they have this advantage to start. They are commonly used as tissue culture supernatants that are harvested as spent media from growing the hybridomas. To obtain large quantities, monoclonal antibodies are often collected by growing the hybridoma cells as tumors in syngeneic mice. Here the antibodies are secreted into an ascitic fluid, which can be collected easily from the tumor-bearing mice. This gives a very high titer preparation of monoclonal antibodies. For specialized needs, the mono-

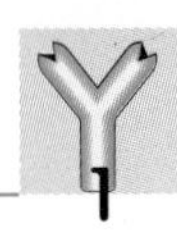

***What is the difference between an antigen and an immunogen?***

*These terms are closely related and often are used as synonyms. Antigen and immunogen are two classifications of molecules that describe different ways a molecule can be recognized by the immune system. An immunogen is any substance foreign to the host that provokes an immune response. An antigen is a substance that is bound by an antibody or a T-cell receptor. In the process of developing an immune response, the terms "immunogen" and "antigen" can be considered identical, because one essential step in inducing immunity is that the molecule must be bound by an antibody or a T-cell receptor. However, when discussing an immunochemical technique that relies on antibodies, the correct term should be antigen.*

clonal antibodies can be purified from either tissue culture supernatants or ascites. Table 1.1 lists the possible sources of antibodies and their characteristics.

Table 1.1 *Commonly used sources of antibodies*

| Antibody source | Antibody type | Total antibody concentration | Specific antibody concentration | Contaminating antibodies |
|---|---|---|---|---|
| Serum | Polyclonal | 10 mg/ml | Normally less than 0.5 mg/ml | Other serum antibodies |
| Tissue culture supernatant with 10% FBS | Monoclonal | 1 mg/ml | 0.05 mg/ml | Calf antibodies |
| Ascites | Monoclonal | 1–10 mg/ml | 0.9–9 mg/ml | Mouse antibodies |

## Antibodies are composed of antigen-binding and cell-binding regions

Antibodies are secreted glycoproteins that perform two key functional roles. To be effective, they must have regions that bind to foreign antigens and to specialized cells of the immune system. These functions are carried out by different structural regions of the antibody. Structurally, antibodies are composed of one or more copies of a characteristic unit that can be visualized as forming a Y shape (Fig. 1.1). Many of the important structural features of antibodies are easiest to discuss by considering immunoglobulin G (IgG) antibodies, which contain only one structural Y unit and are also the most abundant immunoglobulin in serum.

IgG molecules have three protein regions, and Figure 1.2 shows how these are organized. Two of the regions are identical and form the arms of the Y. Each arm contains a site that can bind to an antigen, making IgG molecules bivalent. The third region forms the base, or tail, of the Y, and this region is important in certain aspects of the immune response, including the interaction with macrophages or the activation of complement.

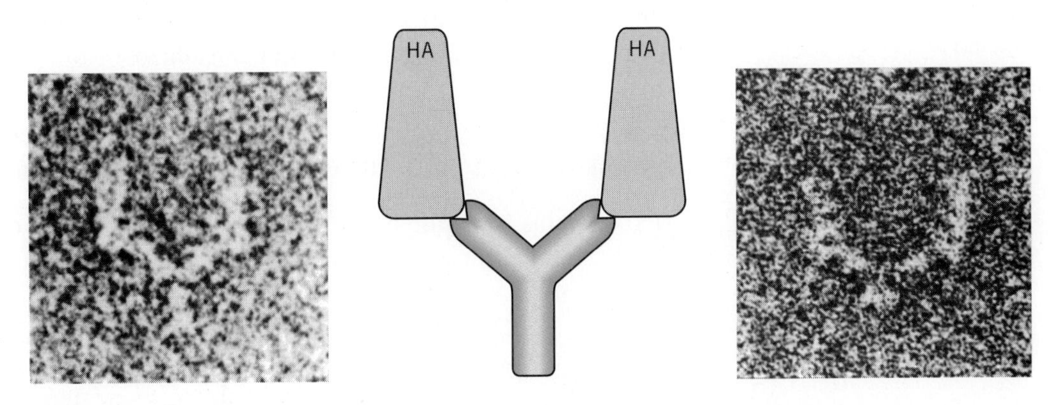


Figure 1.1
Two influenza hemagglutinin (HA) molecules bound by an IgG molecule. (Adapted, with permission, from Wrigley et al. 1983 [copyright Academic Press].)

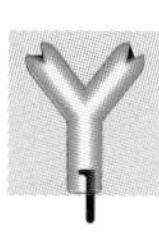


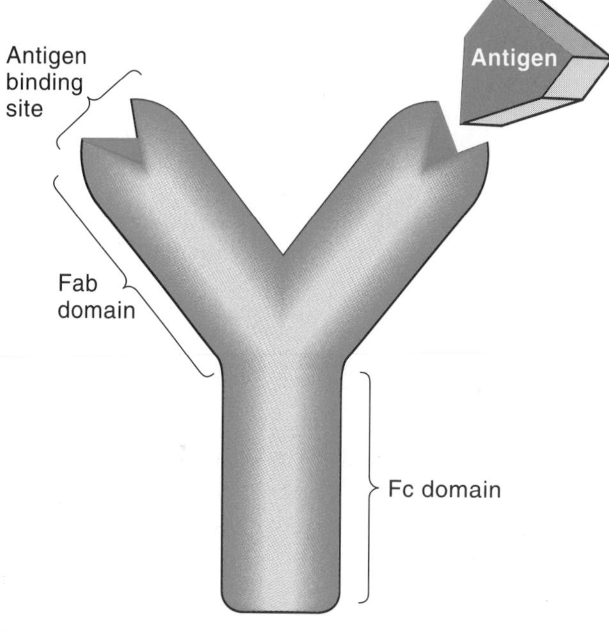


Figure 1.2
Antibody domains.

***What's the difference between an immunoglobulin and an antibody?***

*These terms arose from different subdisciplines of immunology but describe the same class of proteins. Although they have some preferred usages, they are synonymous. Immunoglobulin is a slightly more formal term, giving rise to the gene names, and this name should always be used to describe the various subclasses of this family (immunoglobulin G, IgG, etc.). The term "antibody" is used more colloquially, and it is derived from the ability to bind to an antigen. It is not widely used to describe the generation of an immune response nor to discuss the genetics of the immunoglobulin gene family or their rearrangements. It is more commonly used when describing the use of antibodies in immunochemical methods.*

The connector between the antigen-binding region and the immune cell-binding region is called the hinge. This segment allows lateral and rotational movement of the two antigen-binding domains. In practice, this movement allows the binding regions freedom to interact with a large number of different antigen conformations (Fig. 1.3), and thus greatly increases the utility of antibodies as antigen-binding reagents by expanding the stereochemistry of antigen recognition.

The three regions of the Y may be separated from each other by cleavage with the protease papain. The two regions that carry the antigen-binding sites are known as Fab fragments (named for the *f*ragment having the *a*ntigen *b*inding site), and the protein region that is involved in immune regulation, the tail region of the molecule, is termed the Fc fragment (for the *f*ragment that *c*rystallizes).

## IgG proteins are composed of two copies of a heavy-chain polypeptide and two copies of the light-chain polypeptides

Each Y contains four polypeptides—two identical copies of a polypeptide known as the heavy chain and two identical copies of a polypeptide called the light chain.

The two heavy-chain polypeptides in the Y structure of IgGs are identical and are approximately 55,000 daltons. The two light chains are also identical and are about 25,000 daltons (Fig. 1.4). One light chain associates with the amino-terminal region of one heavy chain to form an antigen-binding domain. The carboxy-terminal regions of the two heavy chains fold together to make the Fc domain. The four polypeptide chains are held together by covalent disulfide bridges and noncovalent bonds.

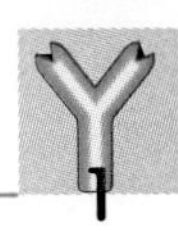

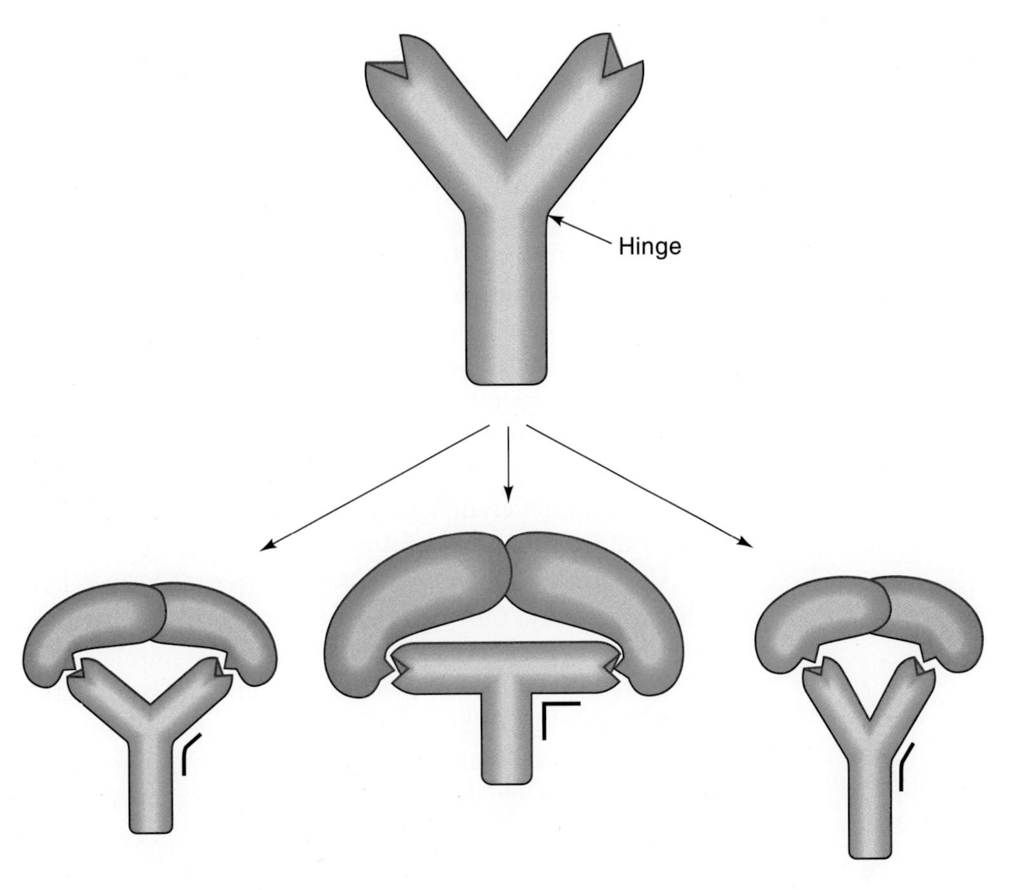


*The hinge is a short peptide sequence that links the Fab and Fc regions and provides a flexible linker between the major functional regions of the antibody. Hinge sequences are highly enriched in proline, serine, and threonine, with the degree of flexibility correlating with the length of the hinge region. The hinge is the site of the major disulfide linkages between the heavy chains and is also the part of the molecule most susceptible to proteolysis.*

**Figure 1.3**
Hinge and flexibility.

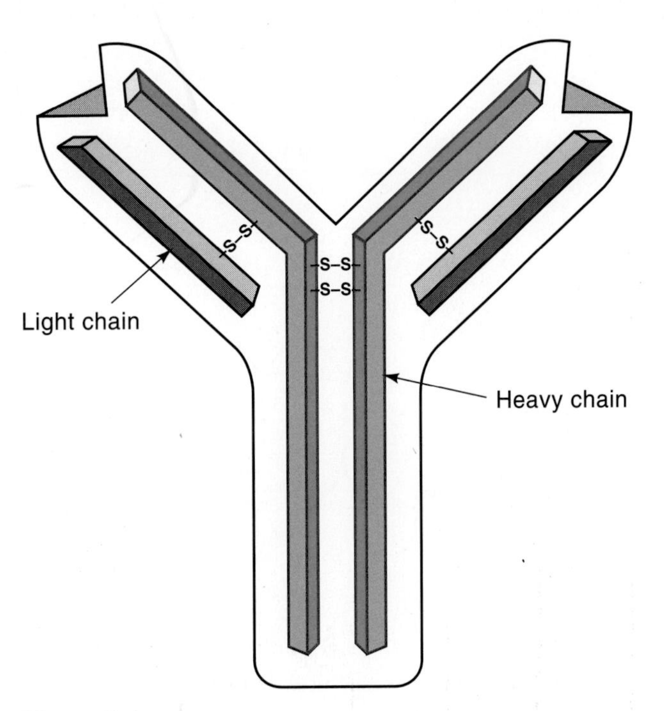


**Figure 1.4**
Heavy and light chains combine to form an antibody.

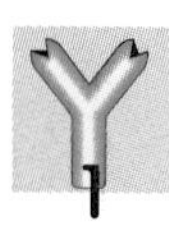



## In addition to the IgG molecules, serum contains other classes of antibody molecules

Antibodies are divided into five classes, IgG, IgM, IgA, IgE, and IgD, on the basis of the type of heavy-chain polypeptide they contain. Where IgG molecules have heavy chains known as γ-chains, IgMs have μ-chains, IgAs have α-chains, IgEs have ϵ-chains, and IgDs have δ-chains. The differences in the heavy-chain polypeptides allow these proteins to function in different types of immune responses and at particular stages of the maturation of the immune response. The protein sequences responsible for these differences are found primarily in the Fc fragment. Different classes of antibodies may also vary in the number of Y-like units that join to form the complete protein. IgM antibodies, for example, have five Y-shaped units. Because each Y unit has two antigen-binding sites, IgMs have 10 identical antigen-binding sites. The sites for association between the different Y units are also found in the Fc region. Table 1.2 summarizes many of the properties of these antibody classes.

Although there are five different types of heavy chains, there are only two light chains, κ and λ. One light chain always associates with one heavy chain, so the total number of light chains will always equal the number of heavy chains. Because the basic structural Y unit has two heavy chains and two light chains, IgMs, which have five Y-units, have 10 light chains and 10 heavy chains. However, any one antibody molecule has only one type of light chain and one type of heavy chain. There are no restrictions on which types of heavy or light chains can form antibodies, so antibodies of all classes (i.e., with different heavy chains) can contain either κ or λ light chains.

Table 1.2 *Classes of antibodies*

| Characteristics | IgG | IgM | IgA | IgE | IgD |
|---|---|---|---|---|---|
| Heavy chain | γ | μ | α | ϵ | δ |
| Light chain | κ or λ | κ or λ | κ or λ | κ or λ | κ or λ |
| Molecular formula | $\gamma_2\kappa_2$ or $\gamma_2\lambda_2$ | $(\mu_2\kappa_2)_5$ or $(\mu_2\lambda_2)_5$ | $(\alpha_2\kappa_2)_n$ [a] or $(\alpha_2\lambda_2)_n$ | $\epsilon_2\kappa_2$ or $\epsilon_2\lambda_2$ | $\delta_2\kappa_2$ or $\delta_2\lambda_2$ |
| Y structure | | | | | |
| Valency | 2 | 10 | 2, 4, or 6 | 2 | 2 |
| Concentration in serum | 8–16 mg/ml | 0.5–2 mg/ml | 1–4 mg/ml | 10–400 ng/ml | 0–0.4 mg/ml |
| Function | Secondary response | Primary response | Protects mucous membranes | Protects against parasites (?) | ? |

[a] $n$ = 1, 2, or 3.

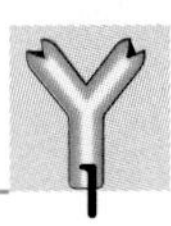

## Comparison of the primary amino acid sequences of light chains reveals a constant and a variable region

*An exception to the one light chain, one heavy chain rule is found in camels and sharks, whose antibodies have no light chain.*

Light chains are approximately 220 amino acids long and can be divided into two regions, or domains, each about 110 amino acids in length (Fig. 1.5). When sequences from a number of light chains were first compared, it was found that the amino-terminal half was heterogeneous. This region is known as the variable (V) region. The carboxy-terminal half is known as the constant (C) region, and amino acid sequencing studies have shown that there are only two types of constant regions, one for κ light chains and one for λ light chains. In the mouse, the gene for the κ light chain is located on chromosome 6, and the λ gene is found on chromosome 16. In humans, the κ light chain is on chromosome 2 and λ on 22.

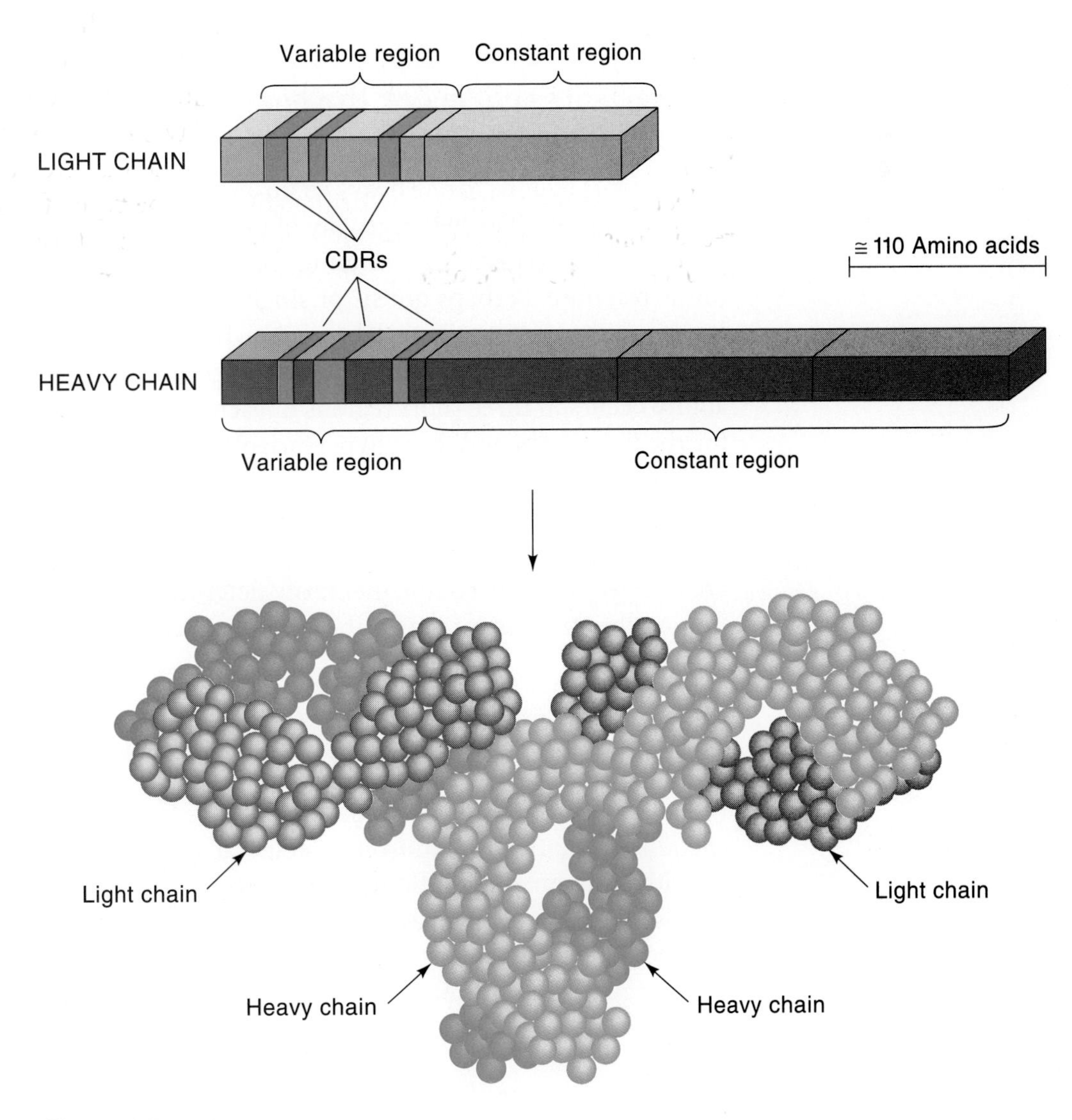


Figure 1.5
Light- and heavy-chain structure. (Adapted from Silverton et al. 1977.)

## Comparison of the sequences of heavy chains also reveals variable and constant regions

The IgG heavy chains are approximately 440 amino acids long and are also divided into variable and constant regions (Fig. 1.5). Like the light chains, sequencing studies showed that the amino-terminal domains had highly variable primary amino acid sequences, whereas the carboxy-terminal domains were constant structures. However, IgG heavy chains contain one variable region and three constant regions. Like the light chain, each of these four regions is about 110 amino acids in length. Heavy chains from different classes may have additional constant regions. For example, μ-chains from IgMs have one variable region but four constant regions. The sequences of the IgG heavy chains have also shown that there are four subclasses of γ-chains. In the mouse, these subclasses of IgG antibodies are known as $IgG_1$, $IgG_{2a}$, $IgG_{2b}$, and $IgG_3$. The coding region for the heavy-chain polypeptides is found on chromosome 12 in the mouse and on chromosome 14 in humans.

## The variable regions of the heavy and light chains form the antigen-binding site

The variable regions of one heavy chain and one light chain combine to form one antigen-binding site. The heterogeneity of the variable regions provides the structural basis for the large repertoire of binding sites used by an animal to mount an effective immune response. Perhaps not surprisingly, the sequence heterogeneity does not occur randomly throughout the variable region, but is concentrated in hypervariable regions of 5–10 amino acids that form the sites of contact with the antigen. Most of the variability occurs in three short regions of each chain, giving three hypervariable regions for the light chain and three hypervariable regions for the heavy chain. These hypervariable regions form the majority of contact residues for the binding of the antibody to the antigen and are located on short amino acid loops extending into the region that interacts with the antigen. Because they are the actual binding site for the antigen, they are referred to as the complementarity determining regions or CDRs. More information on the structure of the antibody–antigen complex is found in Chapter 2.

## Multiple genetic mechanisms provide immense diversity at the antigen-binding site

For an animal to be able to respond to a wide variety of different and previously unencountered antigens, it must have at its call an extremely large repertoire of antibodies with different antigen-binding sites. Each antibody is secreted by a unique clone of B cells or their progeny plasma cells. Therefore, the diversity of antigen-binding sites is a measure of the ability to produce a large number of different B-cell clones, each secreting a different antibody with a specific antigen-binding site. Animals have

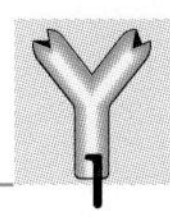

evolved an elaborate and spectacularly inventive series of methods to generate large numbers of B cells that can synthesize antibodies with different binding sites. Although it is not essential to know the molecular details for the methods of generating diversity to be able to use antibodies in the lab, some knowledge of the range of differences in the hypervariable regions is helpful.

The heterogeneity in the variable regions of both light and heavy chains is due to four main sources: (1) the use of multiple coding segments, each specifying a portion of the antigen-binding site; (2) a slightly inaccurate homologous recombination process that both realigns the various coding regions to create the final antibody sequence and adds random nucleotides to the recombination joints to create novel diversity; (3) the generation of mutations in the coding regions themselves; and (4) the random association of the different heavy and light chains each undergoing the three types of changes listed above. It has been estimated that animals are able to produce as many as $10^{12}$ different antigen-binding domains. Understanding the molecular mechanisms that generate this immense variation in antigen-binding sites has been one of the most exciting and important fields in modern biology. We have included an extensive reading list at the end of this chapter to allow interested nonspecialists the opportunity to explore these research fields in more depth.

Since each of these different antibodies is secreted by only one clone of B cells, the differentiation of B cells and their progenitors allows them to specialize on the generation of antibodies with a limited focus. During each round of exposure to a particular antigen, B cells that produce antibodies specific for an epitope on that antigen are selected through engaging an antigen receptor which is an antibody that has been modified for transport to the plasma membrane. These stimulated B cells undergo proliferation based on how well their surface antibodies bind to the antigen, and during the proliferation process introduce further variation that leads to more refinement of the antigen-binding site. At the next round of antigen exposure, the cells that have created antibodies with higher antigen-binding affinities are selected and are further stimulated for proliferation and diversification. This iterative process allows a heightened response that can produce more and better-quality antibodies in reply to the presence of a foreign antigen. For lab researchers this provides the opportunity to generate a strong antibody response to an antigen and the availability of useful reagents.

## Additional recombination events are used to generate the different classes and subclasses of antibodies

One fascinating aspect of the maturation of an immune response has been the discovery of a second set of recombination events that involve the heavy-chain constant regions. These rearrangements do not affect the variable region and do not alter the antigen-binding domain. They do not contribute to the diversity of binding sites, but instead allow the replacement of one heavy-chain constant region with another. The rearrangement occurs downstream from the variable region. Aligned here in germline DNA is a tandem array of the heavy-chain constant region genes: μ-chain (IgM),

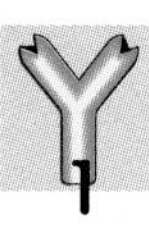


δ-chain (IgD), and then the various γ-chain genes. In essence, these rearrangements move the same antigen-binding site onto different antibody classes and subclasses. This process is known as class switching and is one of the characteristic events of the maturation of the antibody response. Because the different classes and subclasses determine many of the functional properties of antibodies—for example, whether they will appear in serum or mucous secretions—this class switching creates an important mechanism for controlling where and how the antigen-binding site will be used.

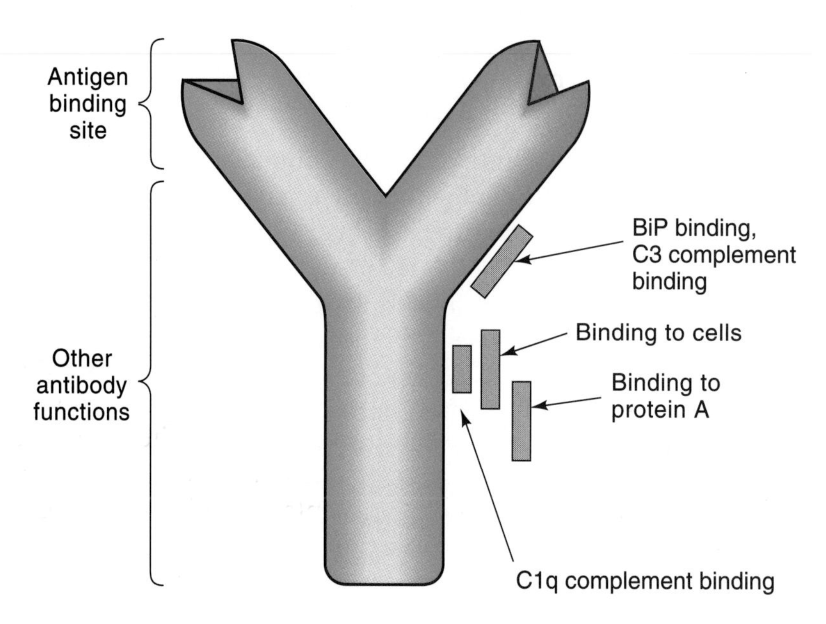


Figure 1.6
Functional domains in immunoglobulin constant regions. Linear models of each heavy chain marked with binding domains.

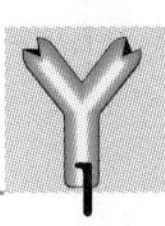

## Variable domains provide antigen binding and specificity; constant domains determine how the antibody will function

The constant domains of all the immunoglobulin classes and subclasses provide a series of binding sites that allow for antibody and antigen processing during a normal immune response. Figure 1.6 shows the location of several of the more important functional domains in the constant regions. Not all immunoglobulin classes and subclasses contain each of these domains, and the presence of the specific domains in the different classes and subclasses lets each immunoglobulin with a different heavy-chain constant region specialize in particular tasks during the immune response.

Each of the key functional domains is important in the generation of the immune response. These domains promote such functions as the binding to BiP, a chaperone that facilitates endoplasmic reticulum entry and association between heavy and light chains. There are domains that allow interaction with Fc receptors on effector cells. This interaction of antibody bound with antigen to this FcR promotes phagocytosis when bound to macrophages and granulocytes or antibody-dependent cellular cytotoxicity when bound to lymphocytes and natural killer cells. There are important domains for the binding and activation of the complement cascade, a key pathway in the lysis of invading foreign cells.

For the purposes of modern immunochemical techniques, the constant domains also provide an important site for interaction with key secondary reagents. Since these regions are distal to the antigen-combining sites, they offer a site to interact with the antibody without disturbing the antibody–antigen interaction. This is the region where protein A and protein G interact with the antibodies and where the epitopes of the most effective secondary antibodies bind.

## References


Köhler G. and Milstein C. 1975. Continuous cultures of fused cells secreting antibody of predefined specificity. *Nature* **256:** 495–497.

Silverton E.W., Navia M.A., and Davies D.R. 1977. Three-dimensional structure of an intact human immunoglobulin. *Proc. Natl. Acad. Sci.* **74:** 5140–5144.

Wrigley N.G., Brown E.B., and Skehel J.J. 1983. Electron microscopic evidence for axial rotation and inter-domain flexibility of the Fab regions of immunoglobulin G. *J. Mol. Biol.* **169:** 771–774.


## Further readings

### Structural studies of antibodies


Al-Lazikani B., Lesk A.M., and Chothia C. 1997. Standard conformations for the canonical structures of immunoglobulins. *J. Mol. Biol.* **273:** 927–948.

Amit A.G., Mariuzza R.A., Phillips S.E., and Poljak R.J. 1985. Three-dimensional structure of an antigen-antibody complex at 6 Å resolution. *Nature* **313:** 156–158.

Amzel L.M. and Poljak R.J. 1979. Three-dimensional structure of immunoglobulins. *Annu. Rev. Biochem.* **48:** 961–997.

Amzel L.M., Poljak R.J., Saul F., Varga J.M., and Richards F.F. 1974. The three dimensional structure of a combining region-ligand complex of immunoglobulin NEW at 3.5-Å resolution. *Proc. Natl. Acad. Sci.* **71:** 1427–1430.

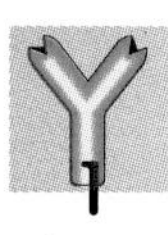



Bentley G.A. 1996. The crystal structures of complexes formed between lysozyme and antibody fragments. *Exper. Suppl.* **75:** 301–319.

Bhat T.N., Bentley G.A., Fischmann T.O., Boulot G., and Poljak R.J. 1990. Small rearrangements in structures of Fv and Fab fragments of antibody D1.3 on antigen binding. *Nature* **347:** 483–485.

Capra J.D. 1971. Hypervariable region of human immunoglobulin heavy chains. *Nat. New Biol.* **230:** 61–63.

Carayannopoloulos L. and Capra J.D. 1993. Immunoglobulins: Structure and function. In *Fundamental immunology* (ed. W.E. Paul), pp. 283–314. Raven Press, New York.

Davies D.R. and Cohen G.H. 1996. Interactions of protein antigens with antibodies. *Proc. Natl. Acad. Sci.* **93:** 7–12.

Davies D.R. and Metzger H. 1983. Structural basis of antibody function. *Annu. Rev. Biochem.* **1:** 87–117.

Derrick J.P. and Wigley D.B. 1992. Crystal structure of a streptococcal protein G domain bound to an Fab fragment. *Nature* **359:** 752–754.

Edelman G.M. 1959. Dissociation of gamma globulin. *J. Am. Chem. Soc.* **81:** 3155–3156.

Edelman G.M., Cunningham B.A., Gall W.E., Gottlieb P.D., Rutishauser U., and Waxdal M.J. 1969. The covalent structure of an entire gG1 immunoglobulin molecule. *Biochemistry* **63:** 78–85.

Fields B.A., Goldbaum F.A., Ysern X., Poljak R.J., and Mariuzza R.A. 1995. Molecular basis of antigen mimicry by anti-idiotope. *Nature* **374:** 739–742.

Gally J.A. 1973. Structure of immunoglobulins. In *The antigens* (ed. M. Sela), vol. 1, pp. 162–298. Academic Press, New York.

Givol D. 1991. The minimal antigen-binding fragment of antibodies-Fv fragment. *Mol. Immunol.* **28:** 1379–1386.

Herron J.N., He X.M., Ballard D.W., Blier P.R., Pace P.E., Bothwell A.L., Voss E.W. Jr., and Edmundson A.B. 1991. An autoantibody to single-stranded DAN: Comparison of the three-dimensional structures of the unliganded Fab and a deoxy nucleotide-Fab complex. *Proteins* **11:** 159–175.

Hilschmann N. and Craig L.C. 1965. Amino acid sequence studies with Bence-Jones proteins. *Biochemistry* **53:** 1403–1409.

Jeske D.J. and Capra J.D. 1984. Immunoglobulins: Structure and function. In *Fundamental immunology* (ed. W.E. Paul), pp. 131–165. Raven Press, New York.

Kato K., Lian L.Y., Barsukov I.L., Derrick J.P., Kim H., Tanaka R., Yoshino A., Shiraishi M., Shimada I., Arata Y. et al. 1995. Model for the complex between protein G and an antibody Fc fragment in solution. *Structure* **3:** 79–85.

Kehoe J.M. and Capra J.D. 1971. Localization of two additional hypervariable regions in immunoglobulin heavy chains. *Proc. Natl. Acad. Sci.* **68:** 2019–2021.

Lesk A.M. and Chothia C. 1988. Elbow motion in the immunoglobulin involves a molecular ball-and-socket joint. *Nature* **335:** 188–190.

MacCallum R.M., Martin A.C., and Thornton J.M. 1996. Antibody-antigen interactions: Contact analysis and binding site topography. *J. Mol. Biol.* **262:** 732–745.

Pascual V. and Capra J.D. 1991. Human immunoglobulin heavy-chain variable region genes: Organization, polymorphism, and expression. *Adv. Immunol.* **49:** 1–74.

Poljack R.J., Amzel L.M., Avey H.P., Chen B.L., Phizackerley R.P., and Saul F. 1973. Three-dimensional structure of the Fab′ fragment of a human immunoglobulin at 2.8-Å resolution. *Proc. Natl. Acad. Sci.* **70:** 3305–3310.

Porter R.R. 1959. Hydrolysis of rabbit gamma globulin and antibodies with crystalline papain. *Biochem. J.* **73:** 119–126.

Rini J.M., Schulze-Gahment U., and Wilson I.A. 1992. Structural evidence for induced fit as a mechanism for antibody-antigen recognition. *Science* **255:** 959–965.

Schiffer M., Girling R.L., Ely K.R., and Edmundson A.B. 1973. Structure of a λ-type Bence-Jones protein at 3.5-Å resolution. *Biochemistry* **12:** 4620–4631.

Segal D.M., Padlan E.A., Cohen G.H., Rudikoff S., Potter M., and Davies D.R. 1974. The three-dimensional structure of a phosphorylcholine-binding mouse immunoglobulin Fab and the nature of the antigen binding site. *Proc. Natl. Acad. Sci.* **71:** 4298–4302.

Stanfield R.L., Fieser T.M., Lerner R.A., and Wilson I.A. 1990. Crystal structure of an antibody to a peptide and its complex with peptide antigen at 2.8Å. *Science* **248:** 712–719.

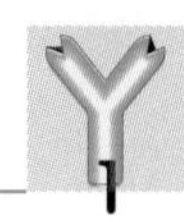

Titani K., Whitley E. Jr., Avogardo L., and Putnam F.W. 1965. Immunoglobulin structure: Partial amino acid sequence of a Bence-Jones protein. *Science* **149:** 1090–1092.

Wade H. and Scanlan T.S. 1997. The structural and functional basis of antibody catalysis. *Annu. Rev. Biophys. Biomol. Struct.* **26:** 461–493.

Wedemayer G.J., Patten P.A., Wang L.H., Schultz P.G., and Stevens R.C. 1997. Structural insights into the evolution of an antibody combining site. *Science* **276:** 1665–1669.

Wu T.T. and Kabat E.A. 1970. An analysis of variable regions of Bence-Jones proteins and myeloma light chains and their implications of antibody complementarity. *J. Exp. Med.* **132:** 211.

## General reviews on antibody genes and diversity

Alt F.W., Blackwell T.K., and Yancopoulos G.D. 1987. Development of the primary antibody repertoire. *Science.* **238:** 1079–1087.

Berman J.E. and Alt F.W. 1990. Human heavy chain variable region diversity, organization, and expression. *Int. Rev. Immunol.* **5:** 203–214.

Cook G.P. and Tomlinson I.M. 1995. The human immunoglobulin VH repertoire. *Immunol. Today* **16:** 237–242.

Fanning L.J., Connor A.M., and Wu G.E. 1996. Development of the immunoglobulin repertoire. *Clin. Immunol. Immunopathol.* **79:** 1–14.

Hood L., Campbell J.H., and Elgin S.C.R. 1975. The organization, expression and evolution of antibody genes and other multigene families. *Annu. Rev. Genet.* **9:** 305–353.

Litman G.W., Rast J.P., Shamblott M.J., Haire R.N., Hulst M., Roess W., Litman R.T., Hinds-Frey K.R., Zilch A., and Amemiya C.T. 1993. Phylogenetic diversification of immunoglobulin genes and the antibody repertoire. *Mol. Biol. Evol.* **10:** 60–72.

Matsuda F. and Honjo T. 1996. Organization of the human immunoglobulin heavy-chain locus. *Adv. Immunol.* **62:** 1–29.

Max E.E. 1993. Immunoglobulins: Molecular geneties. In *Fundamental immunology* (ed. W.E. Paul), pp. 315–382. Raven Press, New York.

Tonegawa S. 1983. Somatic generation of antibody diversity. *Nature* **302:** 575–581.

## Recombination in immunoglobulin genes

Dreyer W.J. and Bennett J.C. 1965. The molecular basis of antibody formation: A paradox. *Biochemistry* **54:** 864–869.

Hozumi N. and Tonegawa S. 1976. Evidence for somatic rearrangement of immunoglobulin genes coding for variable and constant regions. *Proc. Natl. Acad. Sci.* **73:** 3628–3632.

Lieber M. 1996. Immunoglobulin diversity: Rearranging by cutting and repairing. *Curr. Biol.* **6:** 134–136.

Papavasiliou F., Casellas R., Suh H., Qin X.F., Besmer E., Pelanda R., Nemazee D., K. Rajewsky D., and Nussenzweig M.C. 1997. V(D)J recombination in mature B cells: A mechanism for altering antibody responses. *Science* **278:** 298–301.

Schatz D.G. 1997. V(D)J recombination moves in vitro. *Semin. Immunol.* **9:** 149–159.

Tonegawa S., Hozumi N., Matthyssens G., and Schuller R. 1977. Somatic changes in the content and context of immunoglobulin genes. *Cold Spring Harbor Symp. Quant. Biol.* **41:** 877–889.

## VJ and VDJ joining

Brack C., Hirama M., Lenhard-Schuller R., and Tonegawa S. 1978. A complete immunoglobulin gene is created by somatic recombination. *Cell* **15:** 1–14.

Davis M.M., Calame K., Early P.W., Livant D.L., Joho R., Weissman I.L., and Hood L. 1980. An immunoglobulin heavy-chain gene is formed by at least two recombinational events. *Nature* **283:** 733–739.

Early P., Huang H., Davis M., Calame K., and Hood L. 1980. An immunoglobulin heavy chain variable region gene is generated from three segments of DNA: VH, D and JH. *Cell* **19:** 981–992.

Max E.E., Seidman J.G., and Leder P. 1979. Sequences of five potential recombination sites encoded close to an immunoglobulin κ constant region gene. *Proc. Natl. Acad. Sci.* **76:** 3450–3454.

Okazaki K., Davis D.D., and Sakano H. 1987. T cell receptor β gene sequences in the circular DNA of thymocyte nuclei: Direct evidence for intramolecular DNA deletion in V-D-J joining. *Cell* **49:** 477–485.

Sakano H., Hüppi K., Heinrich G., and Tonegawa S. 1979. Sequences at the somatic recombination sites of immunoglobulin light-chain genes. *Nature* **280:** 288–294.

Sakano H., Maki R., Kurosawa Y., Roeder W., and Tonegawa S. 1980. Two types of somatic recombination are necessary for the generation of complete immunoglobulin heavy-chain genes. *Nature* **286:** 676–683.

Seidman J.G. and Leder P. 1978. The arrangement and rearrangement of antibody genes. *Nature* **276:** 790–795.

Seidman J.G., Max E.E., and Leder P. 1979. A κ-immunoglobulin gene is formed by site-specific recombination without further somatic mutation. *Nature* **280:** 370–375.

## *Multiple V, D, and J regions as a source of diversity*

Chuchana P., Blancher A., Brockly F., Alexandre D., Lefranc G., and Lefranc M.P. 1990. Definition of the human immunoglobulin variable lambda (IGLV) gene subgroups. *Eur. J. Immunol.* **20:** 1317–1325.

Max E.E., Seidman J.G., and Leder P. 1979. Sequences of five potential recombination sites encoded close to an immunoglobulin κ constant region gene. *Proc. Natl. Acad. Sci.* **76:** 3450–3454.

Miller J., Ogden S., McMullen M. Andres H., and Storb U. 1988. The order and orientation of mouse λ-genes explains λ-rearrangement patterns. *J. Immunol.* **141:** 2497–2502.

Seidman J.G., Leder A., Edgell M.H., Polsky F., Tilghman S.M., Tiemeier D.C., and Leder P. 1978. Multiple related immunoglobulin variable-region genes identified by cloning and sequence analysis. *Proc. Natl. Acad. Sci.* **75:** 3881–3885.

Shimizu A., Takahashi N., Yaoita Y., and Honjo T. 1982. Organization of the constant-region gene family of the mouse immunoglobulin heavy chain. *Cell* **28:** 499–506.

Storb U., Haasch D., Arp B., Sanchez P., Cazenave P.A., and Miller J. 1989. Physical linkage of mouse λ genes by pulsed-field gel electrophoresis suggests that the rearrangement process favors proximate target sequences. *Mol. Cell. Biol.* **9:** 711–718.

Weigert M., Gatmaitan L., Loh E., Schilling J., and Hood L. 1978. Rearrangement of genetic information may produce immunoglobulin diversity. *Nature* **276:** 785–790.

Vasicek T.J. and Leder P. 1990. Structure and expression of the human immunoglobulin λ genes. *J. Exp. Med.* **172:** 609–620.

## *Junctional diversity*

Early P., Huang H., Davis M., Calame K., and Hood L. 1980. An immunoglobulin heavy chain variable region gene is generated from three segments of DNA: VH, D and JH. *Cell* **19:** 981–992.

Gerstein R.M. and Lieber M.R. 1993. Extent to which homology can constrain coding exon junctional diversity in V(D)J recombination. *Nature* **363:** 625–627.

Sakano H., Hüppi K., Heinrich G., and Tonegawa S. 1979. Sequences at the somatic recombination sites of immunoglobulin light-chain genes. *Nature* **280:** 288–294.

Weigert M., Perry R., Kelley D., Hunkapiller T., Schilling J., and Hood L. 1980. The joining of V and J gene segments creates antibody diversity. *Nature* **283:** 497–499.

## *Somatic mutation*

Becker R.S. and Knight K.L. 1990. Somatic diversification of immunoglobulin heavy chain VDJ genes: Evidence for somatic gene conversion in rabbits. *Cell* **63:** 987–997.

Bernard O., Hozumi N., and Tonegawa S. 1978. Sequences of mouse immunoglobulin light chain genes before and after somatic changes. *Cell* **15:** 1133–1144.

Both G.W., Taylor L., Pollard J.W., and Steele E.J. 1990. Distribution of mutation around rearranged heavy-chain antibody variable-region genes. *Mol. Cell. Biol.* **10:** 5187–5196.

Bothwell A.L.M., Paskind M., Reth M., Imanishi-Kari T., Rajewsky K., and Baltimore D. 1981. Heavy chain variable region contribution to the $NP^b$ family of antibodies: Somatic mutation evident in a γ2a variable region. *Cell* **24:** 625–637.

Crews S., Griffin J., Huang H., Calame K., and Hood L. 1981. A single VH gene segment encodes the immune response to phospho-

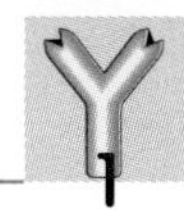

rylcholine: Somatic mutation is correlated with the class of the antibody. *Cell* **25:** 59–66.

Dildrop R., Bruggemann M., Radbruch A., Rajewsky K., and Beyreuther K. 1982. Immunoglobulin V region variants in hybridoma cells. II. Recombination between V genes. *EMBO J.* **1:** 635–640.

Gearhart P.J. 1993. Somatic mutation and affinity maturation. In *Fundamental immunology* (ed. W.E. Paul), pp. 865–885. Raven Press, New York.

Gearhart P.J., Johnson N.D., Douglas R., and Hood L. 1981. IgG antibodies to phosphorylcholine exhibit more diversity than their IgM counterparts. *Nature* **291:** 29–34.

Gershenfeld H.K., Tsukamoto A., Weissman I.L., and Joho R. 1981. Somatic diversification is required to generate the Vk genes of MOPC 511 and MOPC 167 myeloma proteins. *Proc. Natl. Acad. Sci.* **78:** 7674–7678.

Golding G.B., Gearhart P.J., and Glickman B.W. 1987. Patterns of somatic mutations in immunoglobulin variable genes. *Genetics* **115:** 169–176.

Insel R.A. and Varade W.S. 1998. Characteristics of somatic hypermutation of human immunoglobulin genes. *Curr. Top. Microbiol. Immunol.* **229:** 33–44.

Kallberg E., Jainandunsing S., Gray D., and Leanderson T. 1996. Somatic mutation of immunoglobulin V genes in vitro. *Science* **271:** 1285–1289.

Kim S., Davis M., Sinn E., Patten P., and Hood L. 1981. Antibody diversity: Somatic hypermutation of rearranged VH genes. *Cell* **27:** 573–581.

Lebecque S.G. and Gearhart P.J. 1990. Boundaries of somatic mutation in rearranged immunoglobulin genes: 5′ boundary is near the promoter, and 3′ boundary is about 1 kb from V(D)J gene. *J. Exp. Med.* **172:** 1717–1727.

Maizels N. 1995. Somatic hypermutation: How many mechanisms diversify V region sequences? *Cell* **83:** 9–12.

O'Brien R.L., Brinster R.L., and Storb U. 1987. Somatic hypermutation of an immunoglobulin transgene in κ transgenic mice. *Nature* **326:** 405–409.

Pech M., Hochtl J., Schnell H. and Zachau H.G. 1981. Differences between germ-line and rearranged immunoglobulin Vk coding sequences suggest a localized mutation mechanism. *Nature* **291:** 668–670.

Rada C., Yelamos J., Dean W., and Milstein C. 1997. The 5′ hypermutation boundary of κ chains is independent of local and neighboring sequences and related to the distance from the initiation of transcription. *Eur. J. Immunol.* **27:** 3115–3120.

Reynaud C.-A., Dahan A., Anquez V., and Weill J.-C. 1989. Somatic hyperconversion diversifies the single VH gene of the chicken with a high incidence in the D region. *Cell* **59:** 171–183.

Reynaud C.A., Garcia C., Hein W.R., and Weill J.C. 1995. Hypermutation generating the sheep immunoglobulin repertoire is an antigen-independent process. *Cell* **80:** 115–125.

Rogerson B., Hackett J., Peters A., Haasch D., and Storb U. 1991. Mutation pattern of immunoglobulin transgenes is compatible with a model of somatic hypermutation in which targeting of the mutation is linked to the direction of DNA replication. *EMBO J.* **10:** 4331–4341.

Selsing E. and Storb U. 1981. Somatic mutation of immunoglobulin light-chain variable-region genes. *Cell* **25:** 47–58.

Siekevitz M., Huang S.Y., and Gefter M.L. 1983. The genetic basis of antibody production: A single heavy chain variable region gene encodes all molecules bearing the dominant anti-arsonate idiotype in the strain A mouse. *Eur. J. Immunol.* **13:** 123–132.

Storb U. 1996. The molecular basis of somatic hypermutation of immunoglobulin genes. *Curr. Opin. Immunol.* **8:** 206–214.

Storb U., Peters A., Klotz E., Kim N., Shen H.M., Kage K., and Martin T.E. 1998. Somatic hypermutation of immunoglobulin genes is linked to transcription. *Curr. Top. Microbiol. Immunol.* **229:** 11–19.

Valbuena O., Marcu K.B., Weigert M., and Perry R.P. 1978. Multiplicity of germline genes specifying a group of related mouse κ chains with implications for the generation of immunoglobulin diversity. *Nature* **276:** 780–784.

Weigert M.G., Cesari I.M., Yonkovich S.J., and Cohn M. 1970. Variability in the λ light chain sequences of mouse antibody. *Nature* **228:** 1045–1047.

## Mechanism of VJ/VDJ joining

Agrawal A. and Schatz D.G. 1997. RAG1 and RAG2 form a stable postcleavage synaptic complex with DNA containing signal ends in V(D)J recombination. *Cell* **89:** 43–53.

Aguilera R.J., Akira S., Okazaki K., and Sakano H. 1987. A pre-B cell nuclear protein that specifically interacts with the immunoglobulin V-J recombination sequences. *Cell* **51:** 909–917.

Alt F.W. and Baltimore D. 1982. Joining of immunoglobulin heavy chain gene segments: Implications from a chromosome with evidence of three D-JH fusions. *Proc. Natl. Acad. Sci.* **79:** 4118–4122.

Difilippantonio M.J., McMahan C.J., Eastman Q.M., Spanopoulou E., and Schatz D.G. 1996. RAG1 mediates signal sequence recognition and recruitment of RAG2 in V(D)J recombination. *Cell* **87:** 253–262.

Early P., Huang H., Davis M., Calame K., and Hood L. 1980. An immunoglobulin heavy chain variable region gene is generated from three segments of DNA: VH, D and JH. *Cell* **19:** 981–992.

Eastman Q.M., Leu T.M., and Schatz D.G. 1996. Initiation of V(D)J recombination in vitro obeying the 12/23 rule. *Nature* **380:** 85–88.

Hiom K. and Gellert M. 1997. A stable RAG1-RAG2-DNA complex that is active in V(D)J cleavage. *Cell* **88:** 65–72.

Kurosawa Y., von Boehmer H., Haas W., Sakano H., Trauneker A., and Tonegawa S. 1981. Identification of D segments of immunoglobulin heavy-chain genes and their rearrangement in T lymphocytes. *Nature* **290:** 565–570.

Lafaille J.J., DeCloux A., Bonneville M., Takagaki Y., and Tonegawa S. 1989. Junctional sequences of T cell receptor γδ genes: Implications for γδ T cell lineages and for a novel intermediate of V-(D)-J joining. *Cell* **59:** 859–870.

Max E.E., Seidman J.G., and Leder P. 1979. Sequences of five potential recombination sites encoded close to an immunoglobulin κ constant region gene. *Proc. Natl. Acad. Sci.* **76:** 3450–3454.

McCormack W.T., Tjoelker L.W., Carlson L.M., Petryniak B., Barth C.F., Humphries E.H., and Thompson C.B. 1989. Chicken IgL gene rearrangement involves deletion of a circular episome and addition of single nonrandom nucleotides to both coding segments. *Cell* **56:** 785–791.

Oettinger M.A., Schatz D.G., Gorka C., and Baltimore D. 1990. RAG-1 and RAG-2, adjacent genes that synergistically activate V(D)J recombination. *Science* **248:** 1517–1523.

Ramsden D.A., Paull T.T., and Gellert M. 1997. Cell-free V(D)J recombination. *Cell* **388:** 488–491.

Reth M., Gehrmann P., Petrac E., and Wiese P. 1986. A novel VH to VHDJH joining mechanism in heavy-chain-negative (null) pre-B cells results in heavy-chain production. *Nature* **322:** 840–842.

Sakano H., Hüppi K., Heinrich G., and Tonegawa S. 1979. Sequences at the somatic recombination sites of immunoglobulin light-chain genes. *Nature* **280:** 288–294.

Sakano H., Kurosawa Y., Weigert M., and Tonegawa S. 1981. Identification and nucleotide sequence of a diversity DNA segment (D) of immunoglobulin heavy-chain genes. *Nature* **290:** 562–565.

Sakano H., Maki R., Kurosawa Y., Roeder W., and Tonegawa S. 1980. Two types of somatic recombination are necessary for the generation of complete immunoglobulin heavy-chain genes. *Nature* **286:** 676–683.

Schatz D.G. and Baltimore D. 1988. Stable expression of immunoglobulin gene V(D)J recombinase activity by gene transfer into 3T3 fibroblasts. *Cell* **53:** 107–115.

Spanopoulou E., Zaitseva F., Wang F.H., Santagata S., Baltimore D., and Panayotou G. 1996. The homeodomain region of Rag-1 reveals the parallel mechanisms of bacterial and V(D)J recombination. *Cell* **87:** 263–276.

van Gent D.C., Mizuuchi K., and Gellert M. 1996. Similarities between initiation of V(D)J recombination and retroviral integration. *Science* **271:** 1592–1594.

van Gent D.C., Ramsden D.A., and Gellert M. 1996. The RAG1 and RAG2 proteins establish the 12/23 rule in V(D)J recombination. *Cell* **85:** 107–113.

## Sequence of VJ/VDJ joining and allelic exclusion

Alt F.W., Enea V., Bothwell A.L.M., and Baltimore D. 1980. Activity of multiple light

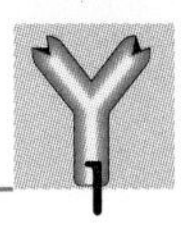

chain genes in murine myeloma cells producing a single, functional light chain. *Cell* **21:** 1–12.

Alt F., Rosenberg N., Lewis S., Thomas E., and Baltimore D. 1981. Organization and reorganization of immunoglobulin genes in A-MuLV-transformed cells: Rearrangement of heavy but not light chain genes. *Cell* **27:** 381–390.

Alt F.W., Yancopoulos G.D., Blackwell T.K., Wood C., Thomas E., Boss M., Coffman R., Rosenberg N., Tonegawa S., and Baltimore D. 1984. Ordered rearrangement of immunoglobulin heavy chain variable region segments. *EMBO J.* **3:** 1209–1219.

Cebra J.J., Colberg J.E., and Dray S. 1966. Rabbit lymphoid cells differentiated with respect to α-, γ- and μ-heavy polypeptide chains and to allotypic markers Aa1 and Aa2. *J. Exp. Med.* **123:** 547–558.

Coleclough C., Perry R.P., Karjalainen K., and Weigert M. 1981. Aberrant rearrangements contribute significantly to the allelic exclusion of immunoglobulin gene expression. *Nature* **290:** 372–378.

Costa T.E., Suh H., and Nussenzweig M.C. 1992. Chromosomal position of rearranging gene segments influences allelic exclusion in transgenic mice. *Proc. Natl. Acad. Sci.* **89:** 2205–2208.

Early P. and Hood L. 1981. Allelic exclusion and nonproductive immunoglobulin gene rearrangements. *Cell* **24:** 1–3.

Hieter P.A., Korsmeyer S.J., Waldmann T.A., and Leder P. 1981. Human immunoglobulin κ light-chain genes are deleted or rearranged in λ-producing B cells. *Nature* **290:** 368–372.

Kitamura D. and Rajewsky K. 1992. Targeted disruption of μ chain membrane causes loss of heavy-chain allelic exclusion. *Nature* **356:** 154–156.

Maki R., Kearney J., Paige C., and Tonegawa S. 1980. Immunoglobulin gene rearrangement in immature B cells. *Science* **209:** 1366–1369.

Neuberger M.S., Caskey H.M., Pattersson S., Williams G.T., and Surani M.A. 1989. Isotype exclusion and transgene down-regulation in immunoglobulin-λ transgenic mice. *Nature* **338:** 350–352.

Nussenzweig M.C., Shaw A.C., Sinn E., Danner D.B., Holmes K.L., Morse H., and Leder P. 1987. Allelic exclusion in transgenic mice that express the membrane form of immunoglobulin μ. *Science* **236:** 816–819.

Pernis B., Chiappino G., Kelus A.S., and Gell P.G.H. 1965. Cellular localization of immunoglobulins with different allotypic specificities in rabbit lymphoid tissues. *J. Exp. Med.* **122:** 853–875.

Perry R.P., Kelley D.E., Coleclough C., and Kearney J.F. 1981. Organization and expression of immunoglobulin genes in fetal liver hybridomas. *Proc. Natl. Acad. Sci.* **78:** 247–251.

Picarella D., Serunian L.A., and Rosenberg N. 1991. Allelic exclusion of membrane but not secreted immunoglobulin in a mature B cell line. *Eur. J. Immunol.* **21:** 55–62.

Ritchie K.A., Brinster R.L., and Storb U. 1984. Allelic exclusion and control of endogenous immunoglobulin gene rearrangement in κ transgenic mice. *Nature* **312:** 517–520.

Rusconi S. and Köhler G. 1985. Transmission and expression of a specific pair of rearranged immunoglobulin μ and κ genes in a transgenic mouse line. *Nature* **314:** 330–334.

Weaver D., Costantini F., Imanishi-Kari T., and Baltimore D. 1985. A transgenic immunoglobulin μ gene prevents rearrangement of endogenous genes. *Cell* **42:** 117–127.

### *Class switch*

Cogne M., Lansford R., Bottaro A., Zhang J., Gorman J., Young F., Cheng H.L., and Alt F.W. 1994. A class switch control region at the 3′ end of the immunoglobulin heavy chain locus. *Cell* **77:** 737–747.

Coleclough C., Cooper D., and Perry R.P. 1980. Rearrangement of immunoglobulin heavy chain genes during B-lymphocyte development as revealed by studies of mouse plasmacytoma cells. *Proc. Natl. Acad. Sci.* **77:** 1422–1426.

Cory S. and Adams J.M. 1980. Deletions are associated with somatic rearrangements of immunoglobulin heavy chain genes. *Cell* **19:** 37–51.

Davis M.M., Kim S.K., and Hood L.E. 1980. DNA sequences mediating class switching in α-immunoglobulins. *Science* **209:** 1360–1365.

Davis M.M., Calame K., Early P.W., Livant

D.L., Joho R., Weissman I.L., and Hood L. 1980. An immunoglobulin heavy-chain gene is formed by at least two recombinational events. *Nature* **283:** 733–739.

Dunnick W., Rabbits T.H., and Milstein C. 1980. An immunoglobulin deletion mutant with implications for the heavy-chain switch and RNA splicing. *Nature* **286:** 669–675.

Gerstein R.M., Frankel W.N., Hsieh C.L., Durdik J.M., Rath S., Coffin J.M., Nisonoff A., and Selsing E. 1990. Isotype switching of an immunoglobulin heavy chain transgene occurs by DNA recombination between different chromosomes. *Cell* **63:** 537–548.

Honjo T. and Kataoka T. 1978. Organization of immunoglobulin heavy chain genes and allelic deletion model. *Proc. Natl. Acad. Sci.* **75:** 2140–2144.

Hurwitz J.L., Coleclough C., and Cebra J.J. 1980. CH gene rearrangements in IgM-bearing B cells and in the normal splenic DNA component of hybridomas making different isotypes of antibody. *Cell* **22:** 349–359.

Iwasato T., Shimizu A., Honjo T., and Yamagishi H. 1990. Circular DNA is excised by immunoglobulin class switch recombination. *Cell* **62:** 143–149.

Jung S., Rajewsky K., and Radbruch A. 1993. Shutdown of class switch recombination by deletion of a switch region control element. *Science* **259:** 984–987.

Kataoka T., Miyata T., Honjo Y. 1981. Repetitive sequences in class-switch recombination regions of immunoglobulin heavy chain genes. *Cell* **23:** 357–368.

Kataoka T., Kawakami T., Takahashi N., and Honjo T. 1980. Rearrangement of immunoglobulin $\gamma$ 1-chain gene and mechanism for heavy-chain class switch. *Proc. Natl. Acad. Sci.* **77:** 919–923.

Lawton A.R., Kincade P.W., and Cooper M.D. 1975. Sequential expression of germ line genes in development of immunoglobulin class diversity. *Fed. Proc.* **34:** 33–39.

Lorenz M., Jung S., and Radbruch A. 1995. Switch transcripts in immunoglobulin class switching. *Science* **267:** 1825–1828.

Marcu K.B., Lang R.B., Stanton L.W., and Harris L.J. 1982. A model for the molecular requirements of immunoglobulin heavy chain class switching. *Nature* **298:** 87–89.

Matsuoka M., Yoshida K., Maeda T., Usuda S., and Sakano H. 1990. Switch circular DNA formed in cytokine-treated mouse splenocytes: Evidence for intramolecular DNA deletion in immunoglobulin class switching. *Cell* **62:** 135–142.

Nossal G.J.V., Warner N., and Lewis H. 1971. Incidence of cell simultaneously secreting IgM and IgG antibody to sheep erythrocytes. *Cell. Immunol.* **2:** 41–53.

Rabbitts T.H., Forster A., Dunnick W., and Bentley D.L. 1980. The role of gene deletion in the immunoglobulin heavy chain switch. *Nature* **283:** 351–356.

Reaban M.E. and Griffin J.A. 1990. Induction of RNA-stabilized DNA conformers by transcription of an immunoglobulin switch region. *Nature* **348:** 342–344.

Sakano H., Maki R., Kurosawa Y., Roeder W., and Tonegawa S. 1980. Two types of somatic recombination are necessary for the generation of complete immunoglobulin heavy-chain genes. *Nature* **286:** 676–683.

Snapper C.M. and Finkelman F.D. 1993. Immunoglobulin class switching. In *Fundamental immunology* (ed. W.E. Paul), pp. 837–863. Raven Press, New York.

Stavnezer J. 1996. Immunoglobulin class switching. *Curr. Opin. Immunol.* **8:** 199–205.

von Schwedler U., Jack H.M., and Wabl M. 1990. Circular DNA is a product of the immunoglobulin class switch rearrangement. *Nature* **345:** 452–456.

# Antibody–Antigen Interactions

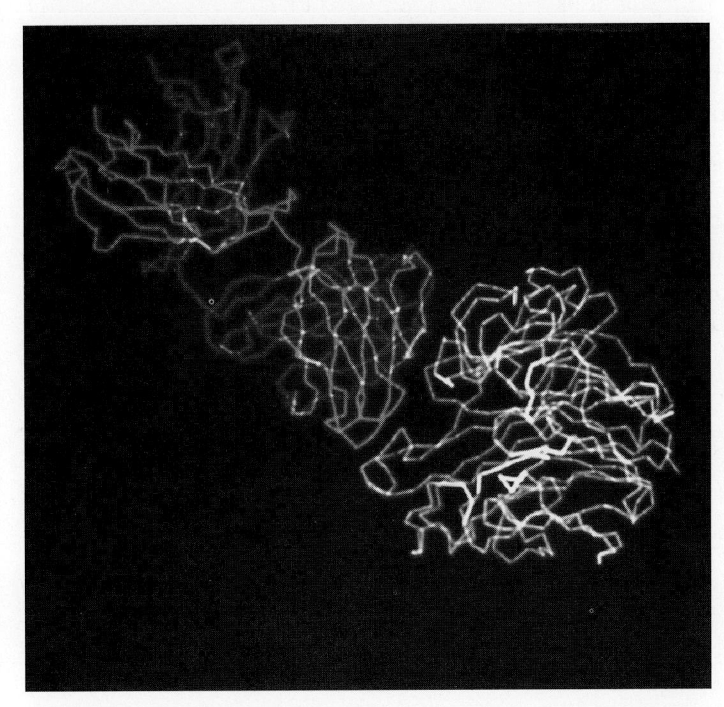

From Colman P.M., Laver W.G., Varghese J.N., Baker A.T., Tulloch P.A., Air G.M., and Webster R.G. 1987. Three-dimensional structure of a complex of antibody with influenza virus neuraminidase. *Nature* **326:** 358–363. (Reprinted with permission [copyright Macmillan].)

Fig. 5. Stereo image of one quarter of the promoter, showing the Fab bound to the side of the active site cavity on the enzyme. The enzyme active centre is facing the viewer, below and to the left [now right] of the antibody binding site.

To understand how to use antibodies as an effective research tool, it is essential to learn how they bind to their cognate antigens. There is a large and important literature using protein-chemistry approaches to define the binding sites that allow antibodies and antigens to interact. This earlier work has been expanded dramatically by the molecular detail provided by the determination of the structure of protein cocrystals formed between antibodies and antigens. X-ray studies such as the one shown here have shown us that the interaction face between antibodies and antigens can be quite large and that the interactions can be extensive. These structural studies have been complemented by extensive biophysical work that has determined the kinetics of interaction, the affinity of an antigen-binding site on an antibody for its epitope on the antigen, and the avidity of the complete antibody–antigen interaction. These studies allow researchers to establish and modify experimental designs to use antibodies effectively.

The interaction of an antibody with an antigen forms the basis of all immunochemical techniques. This chapter discusses the properties of the antibody–antigen interaction and is divided into three sections. The first summarizes the structure of the antibody–antigen bonds, the second covers the strength of these interactions, a characteristic known as affinity, and the third presents the factors that contribute to the overall stability of immune complexes, a property called avidity.

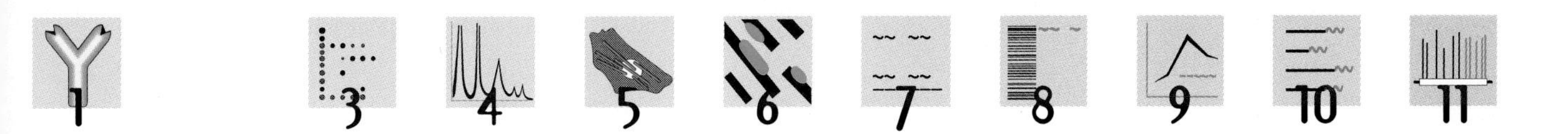


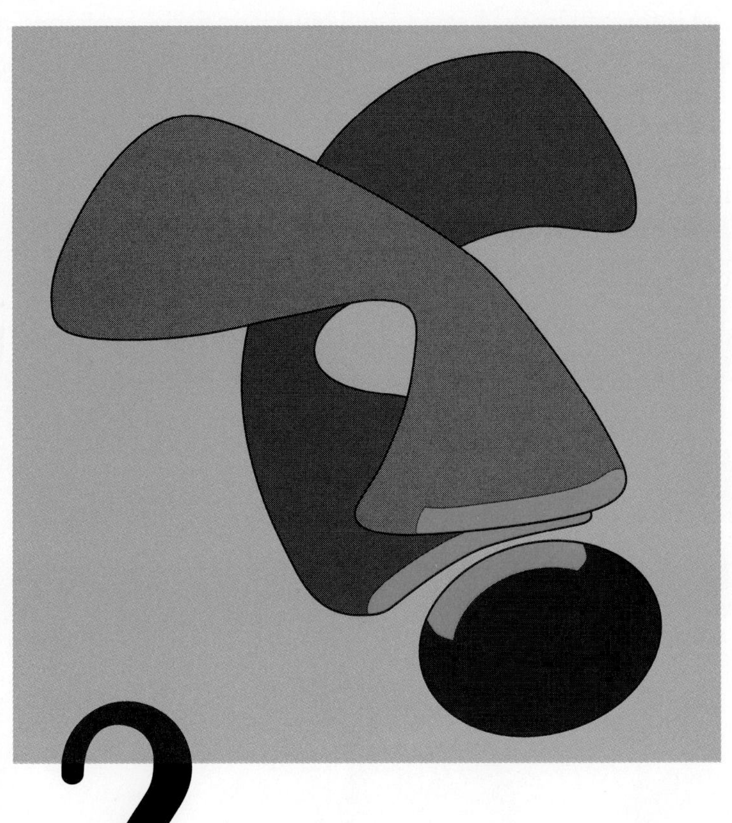

# 2 Antibody–Antigen Interactions

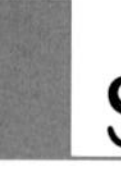

# Structure of the antibody-antigen complex

*The different binding specificities of antibodies for their antigens are established by an elegant series of mechanisms that generate sequence diversity in the combining site of the antibody. These mechanisms include (1) different heavy and light chains combine to form the final antibody; (2) during lymphocyte differentiation genetic recombination brings portions of the CDRs together to form the final transcription unit and produces a large array of different coding regions; (3) imprecise joining during these recombination steps produces new sequence variations; and (4) high rates of somatic mutation allow introduction and selection of new sequences in these regions. The outcome of these variations is a vast array of potential interaction surfaces that can be used to bind to foreign immunogens. The mechanisms that promote this diversity are described in more detail in Chapter 1.*

The structure of the antibody–antigen complex has been studied by measuring the affinity of binding between an antibody and a series of related antigens, by using affinity labeling reagents, by site-directed mutagenesis of the antibody combining site, by molecular modeling, and, most compellingly, by X-ray diffraction studies of antibody–-antigen cocrystals. Together, these techniques have delineated the region of the antibody molecule that is involved in antigen binding, the region of the antigen molecule that interacts with the antibody, and the molecular basis for antibody specificity.

## The antigen-binding site of an antibody is formed by the variable regions of the heavy and light chains

Affinity labeling and X-ray crystallography of immune complexes have established that the antigen-binding site is formed by the heavy- and light-chain variable regions. The two variable regions are tightly associated and are bound to each other by noncovalent interactions (Fig. 2.1). The remainder of the heavy and light chains provide other domains that are not involved in antigen binding but do contribute to how the antibody participates in an immune response (see Chapter 1). The amino acids forming the antigen-binding site are derived from both the heavy and light chains and correspond to the amino acids of the hypervariable regions determined from protein sequencing. The hypervariable regions are known as the complementarity determining regions (CDRs). There are six CDRs, three on the heavy and three on the light chain, and they form discrete loops anchored and oriented by the framework residues of the variable domains (Fig. 2.1).

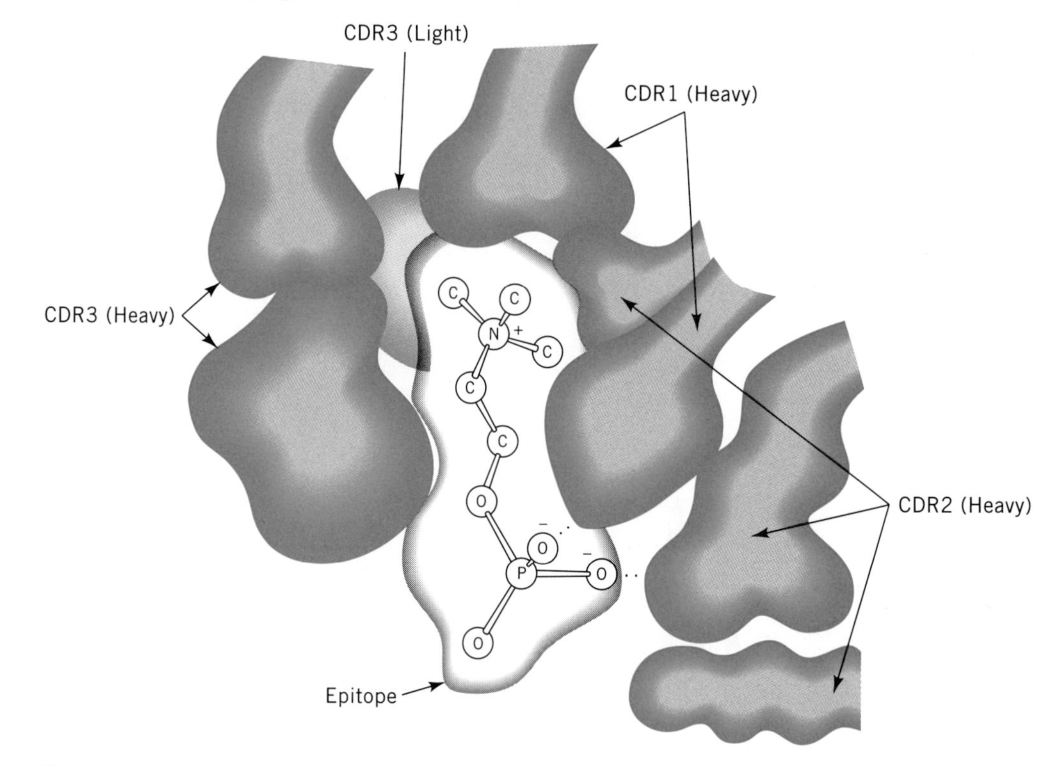


**Figure 2.1**
The six CDRs form the binding sites for antigen–antibody association. (Adapted from Capra and Edmundson 1977.)

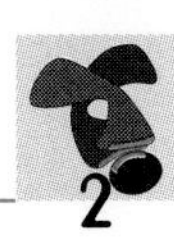


## The region of an antigen that binds to an antibody is called an epitope

The region of an antigen that interacts with an antibody is defined as an epitope. An epitope is not an intrinsic property of any particular structure, as it is defined only by reference to the binding site of an antibody. The size of an epitope is governed by the size of the combining site. From X-ray studies of the structures of cocrystals between small antigens bound to antibodies, the size of the combining site was thought to be relatively small. The site was visualized as a cleft or pocket into which the epitope docked. Relatively few of the amino acid side chains of the CDR were in close contact with the antigen. Later work using larger antigens showed that the area of these antigens in close apposition to the antibody can be quite large, occupying as much as 500–750 $Å^2$ and often involving contacts with multiple CDRs, and many times establishing contact with all six. Although these studies have shown that epitopes can be much larger than originally thought, it is still clear that high-affinity antibodies can be raised to small epitopes.

Because antibodies recognize relatively small regions of an entire antigen, occasionally they can find related structures on other molecules. This forms the molecular basis for cross-reaction. Cross-reactions can be helpful in finding related protein family members or distracting when they recognize unrelated proteins with a shared structural feature. For example, cross-reactions can detect highly related structures in common structural regions of protein family members. In this way, an antibody can be a useful tool to identify and study related proteins. However, cross-reactions may also detect similar spatial features in other antigens that do not represent shared structural domains. In these cases, the interactions may still be quite strong but the resulting interactions distracting rather than helpful. Therefore, it is always important to interpret cross-reactions in a conservative manner. Keep in mind that the presence of similar epitopes does not necessarily imply a functional relationship.

## Epitopes on protein antigens are local surface structures that can be formed by contiguous or noncontiguous amino acid sequences

Epitopes on an antigen can be formed either by a linear string of amino acid residues or by noncontinguous sequences that are folded into close proximity in the three-dimensional shape on the face of the antigen (Fig. 2.2). A good example of this is seen with one of the lysozyme–antibody cocrystals. Here, the amino acids of lysozyme that form the epitope come from two distant stretches of the primary sequence (residues 18–27 and residues 116–129). Although separated from each other in the primary sequence, these stretches of amino acids are adjacent on the protein surface. At the interface between the antigen and the antibody, a total of 16 amino acids of the antigen make close contacts with 17 amino acids of the antibody, the latter involving all six CDRs. The whole interface is tightly packed and excludes solvent. Strikingly, 748 $Å^2$ or 11% of the surface of lysozyme is covered by the antibody. Similar conclusions come from the study of the second lysozyme–antibody cocrystals and the neuraminidase–antibody cocrystals. Here, either three (lysozyme) or four (neuraminidase) stretches of distant primary sequence form portions of the epitope structure.

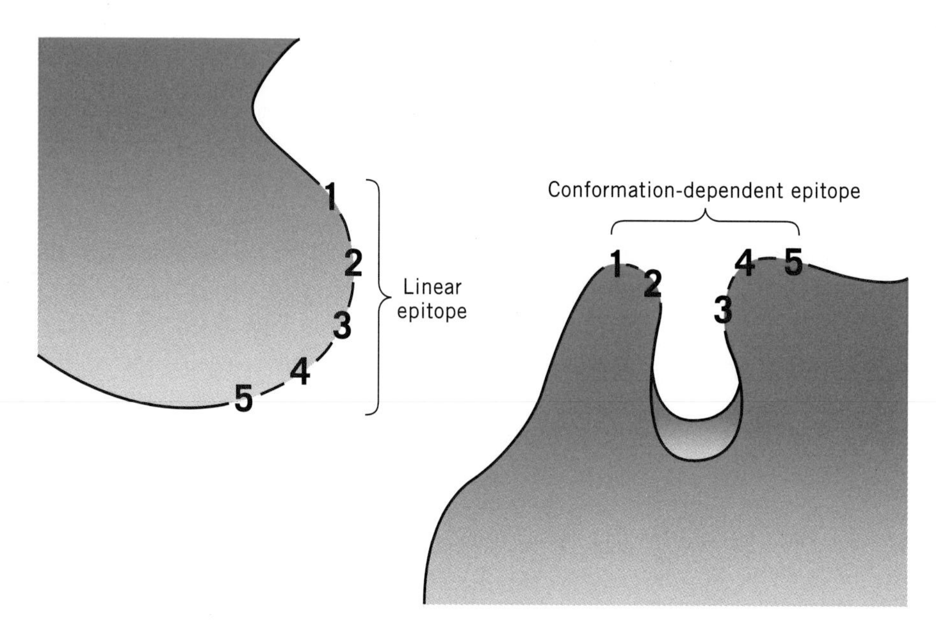


Figure 2.2
Epitopes on an antigen can be formed either by a linear string of amino acid residues or by non-continguous sequences that are folded into close proximity in the three-dimensional shape on the face of the antigen.

Work with antibodies raised against synthetic peptides or other small antigens provides a set of excellent examples for interactions between antibodies and small, well-defined epitopes. One set of commonly used antibodies that display this property are the anti-phosphotyrosine antibodies, which specifically recognize the phosphorylated side chain of this amino acid in different local regions of many proteins. The ability of antibodies to recognize small epitopes in various structural environments shows the versatility of antibodies to recognize small discrete regions.

## Some immune complexes show no alterations in the structure of the antibody or antigen, whereas others show large conformational changes

Antibody–antigen interactions can occur either with large structural changes in the antibody or the antigen or with no detectable changes. From the structures of the first antibody–protein antigen cocrystals, it was clear that both flexible and rigid structures can form good epitopes. In the crystal structure of one of the lysozyme–antibody complexes, no distortion of either the antigen or antibody could be detected, even at high resolution. In sharp contrast, the crystal structure of a neuraminidase–antibody complex revealed substantial structural alterations of both the antigen and antibody. Because the crystallization process itself can induce structural alterations, it is difficult to

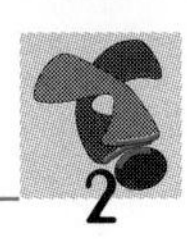


prove that these changes are due to antibody binding. However, many other studies have shown that antibodies can induce structural changes in antigens. Good examples of this are the removal of heme from myoglobin and the activation of enzymes by antibody binding.

## The antibody–antigen complex is held together by multiple, noncovalent bonds

The binding of the antibody to the antigen is entirely dependent on noncovalent interactions, and the antibody–antigen complex is in equilibrium with the free components. The immune complex is stabilized by the combination of weak interactions that depend on the precise alignment of the antigen and antibody. These noncovalent interactions include hydrogen bonds, van der Waals forces, coulombic interactions, and hydrophobic interactions. These interactions can occur between side chains or the polypeptide backbones.

Small changes in antigen structure can affect profoundly the strength of the antibody–antigen interaction. The loss of a single hydrogen bond at the interface can reduce the strength of interaction 1000-fold. The overall interaction is a balance of many attractive and repulsive interactions at the interface. This can be demonstrated in vitro by site-directed mutagenesis. Changing the amino acid residues that form the binding site can alter the strength of an antibody–antigen interaction. This is performed elegantly in vivo by the selection of cells secreting higher-affinity antibodies. By a still poorly understood process, the CDR residues from differentiating clones of B cells undergo extensive mutation, yielding antibodies that differ widely in the microstructure of their antigen-binding sites. Cells that express antibodies with higher affinity are stimulated preferentially to divide. This process continues during the exposure and reexposure to antigen and results in a stronger and more specific antibody response.

## Antibodies can bind to a wide range of chemical structures and can discriminate among related compounds

The microenvironment of the combining site can accommodate highly charged as well as hydrophobic molecules. Epitopes composed of carbohydrates, lipids, nucleic acids, amino acids, and a wide range of synthetic organic chemicals have all been identified. The repertoire of possible binding sites is enormous, and antibodies that are specific to novel compounds can be derived readily.

The specificity of antibodies has been demonstrated by a large number of experiments showing that small changes in the epitope structure can prevent antigen recognition. For example, antibodies have been isolated that will differentiate between conformations of protein antigens, detect single amino acid substitutions, or act as weak enzymes by stabilizing transition forms.

# Affinity

Affinity is a measure of the strength of the binding of an epitope to an antibody.

## The binding of antibodies to antigens is reversible, and the strength of the interaction can be described in terms of an equilibrium reaction

Antibody binding to antigen is noncovalent and reversible. The binding of antibody to antigen follows the basic thermodynamic principles of any reversible bimolecular interaction. Thus, if [Ab] = molar concentration of the unoccupied antibody-binding sites, [Ag] = molar concentration of the unoccupied antigen-binding sites, and [Ab-Ag] is the molar concentration of the antibody–antigen complex, then the affinity constant $K_A = [Ab\text{-}Ag]/[Ab]\cdot[Ag]$. In practical terms, affinity describes the amount of antibody–antigen complex that will be found at equilibrium.

The time taken to reach equilibrium is dependent on the rate of diffusion and does not vary from one antibody to another. However, high-affinity antibodies will bind larger amounts of antigen in a shorter period of time than low-affinity antibodies. In practice, this means that high-affinity interactions are substantially complete well before low-affinity interactions. High-affinity antibodies perform better in all immunochemical techniques. This is due not only to their higher capacity, but also to the stability of the complex. For example, the half-time for dissociation of an antibody binding to a small protein antigen with high affinity is 30 minutes or more, whereas for a low-affinity antibody this time may be a few minutes or less.

## The affinity of the antibody-antigen interaction varies over a wide range

The range of measured values of affinity constants for antibody–antigen binding is enormous and extends from below $10^5$ liter mol$^{-1}$ to above $10^{12}$ liter mol$^{-1}$. For comparison, the affinity of trypsin for its substrate is approximately $1.25 \times 10^4$ liter mol$^{-1}$, the affinity of λ repressor converting from monomer to dimer is $5 \times 10^7$ liter mol$^{-1}$, and the affinity of λ repressor for DNA is $10^{10}$ liter mol$^{-1}$. Like all equilibrium reactions, the affinity constant for antibody–antigen interactions is affected by temperature, pH, and solvent. Changes in these may increase or decrease the number of antibody–antigen complexes found at equilibrium. These alterations will change the affinity constant, either driving the reaction toward complete binding or releasing bound antigen.

The affinity of monoclonal antibodies can be determined exactly, but the affinity of polyclonal antibodies cannot. Because monoclonal antibodies are homogeneous, the exact measurement of their affinity is possible using a range of techniques. Polyclonal sera contain complex mixtures of antibodies of different affinities; therefore, the affinity of such sera cannot be exactly determined, but averages can be established.

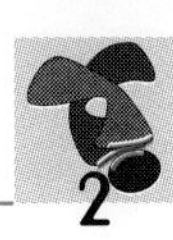


## Although the antibody-antigen affinity in a particular environment does not vary, the extent of complex formation can be manipulated

The easiest way to control the extent of complex formation is to vary the concentration of the antibody or antigen. Provided neither component is saturated, adding more antibody to a constant volume will increase the amount of antigen that is bound. Similarly, adding more antigen will increase the bound antibody. With suitably high affinities, the addition of excess antibody can be used to bind essentially all of the available antigen, but with low-affinity antibodies a significant fraction of the antigen will remain free. Increasing the reaction volume, thus lowering the concentration of both antibody and antigen, will decrease the amount of complex. The amount of complex decreases approximately with the square of the volume, when neither component is saturated. For low-affinity antibodies, reaction volume will greatly influence the amount of complex formed.

Table 2.1 lists typical affinity values for antibodies and compares these values with the required affinities for several of the common immunochemical techniques.

Table 2.1 *Factors affecting the strength of antibody binding*

| | |
|---|---|
| **Cell staining** | 1. Affinity, $10^6$ liter mol$^{-1}$ (weak signal) to $10^8$ liter mol$^{-1}$ (strong signal)<br>2. Possible bivalent binding<br>3. Possible multivalent binding to secondary reagent<br>4. Possible local concentration effects |
| **Immunoprecipitation** | 1. Affinity, $10^7$ liter mol$^{-1}$ (weak signal) to $10^9$ liter mol$^{-1}$ (strong signal)<br>2. Possible polyclonal binding<br>3. Possible multivalent binding to secondary reagents |
| **Immunoblotting** | 1. Affinity, $10^6$ liter mol$^{-1}$ (weak signal) to $10^8$ liter mol$^{-1}$ (strong signal)<br>2. Possible bivalent binding<br>3. Possible multivalent binding to secondary reagents<br>4. Possible local concentration effects |

# Avidity

Avidity is a measure of the overall stability of the complex between antibodies and antigens. The overall strength of an antibody–antigen interaction is governed by three major factors: the intrinsic affinity of the antibody for the epitope, the valency of the antibody and antigen, and the geometric arrangement of the interacting components. Since the avidity describes the complete reaction, this value ultimately determines the success of all immunochemical techniques.

## When the antibody and antigen can form multivalent complexes, the strength of the interaction is greatly increased

Most immunochemical procedures involve multivalent interactions. All antibodies are multivalent; IgGs and most IgAs are bivalent, and IgMs are decavalent (see Table 1.2). Antigens can be multivalent either because they contain multiple copies of the same epitope, as in the case of homopolymers, or because they contain multiple epitopes recognized by different antibodies. Multivalent interactions can greatly stabilize immune complexes, rendering the reactions practically irreversible.

Multimeric interactions allow even low-affinity antibodies to bind tightly. Because some techniques are more likely to allow multivalent interactions, low-affinity antibodies may work well in one technique, but not in another. When antibodies show this variation among different techniques, it is often due to differences in multivalent binding. Similarly, a cross-reaction that is undetectable in one technique may dominate the results of another assay.

It is not always easy to predict the effects of multivalency, as the reactions involve geometric arrangements that impose steric constraints. However, the effects of multivalency can be illustrated by considering several simple cases as described below: (1) where a monoclonal antibody interacts with a homopolymeric antigen (Fig. 2.3); (2) where polyclonal antibodies bind to an antigen that has multiple epitopes creating large multimeric complexes (Fig. 2.4); (3) where polyclonal antibodies bind to an antigen that has multiple epitopes creating a good target for multimeric binding by secondary reagents (Fig. 2.5); and (4) where an antibody binds to an antigen immobilized on a solid support (Fig. 2.6). There are other variations on these patterns, but they share the basic features illustrated by these examples.

## Homopolymeric antigens present identical, repeating epitopes that encourage bivalent binding

When a monoclonal antibody binds to a multimeric antigen, the initial reaction is identical to the bimolecular interactions discussed above. The antibody finds the antigen by diffusion. However, the second step of the reaction links the unoccupied combining site of the antibody with an identical epitope on the same antigen molecule. This reaction is an intramolecular conversion and does not depend on diffusion. It is restrained only by conformation (Fig. 2.3). Once this molecular complex is assembled,

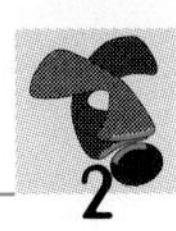

the rate of dissociation of the individual antibody–epitope interactions is similar to the normal bimolecular complex. However, since the antigen will still be held by the other interaction, the observed rate of dissociation will be much slower, thus forming a very stable antibody–antigen complex.

This type of multimeric interaction can occur in all immunochemical techniques.

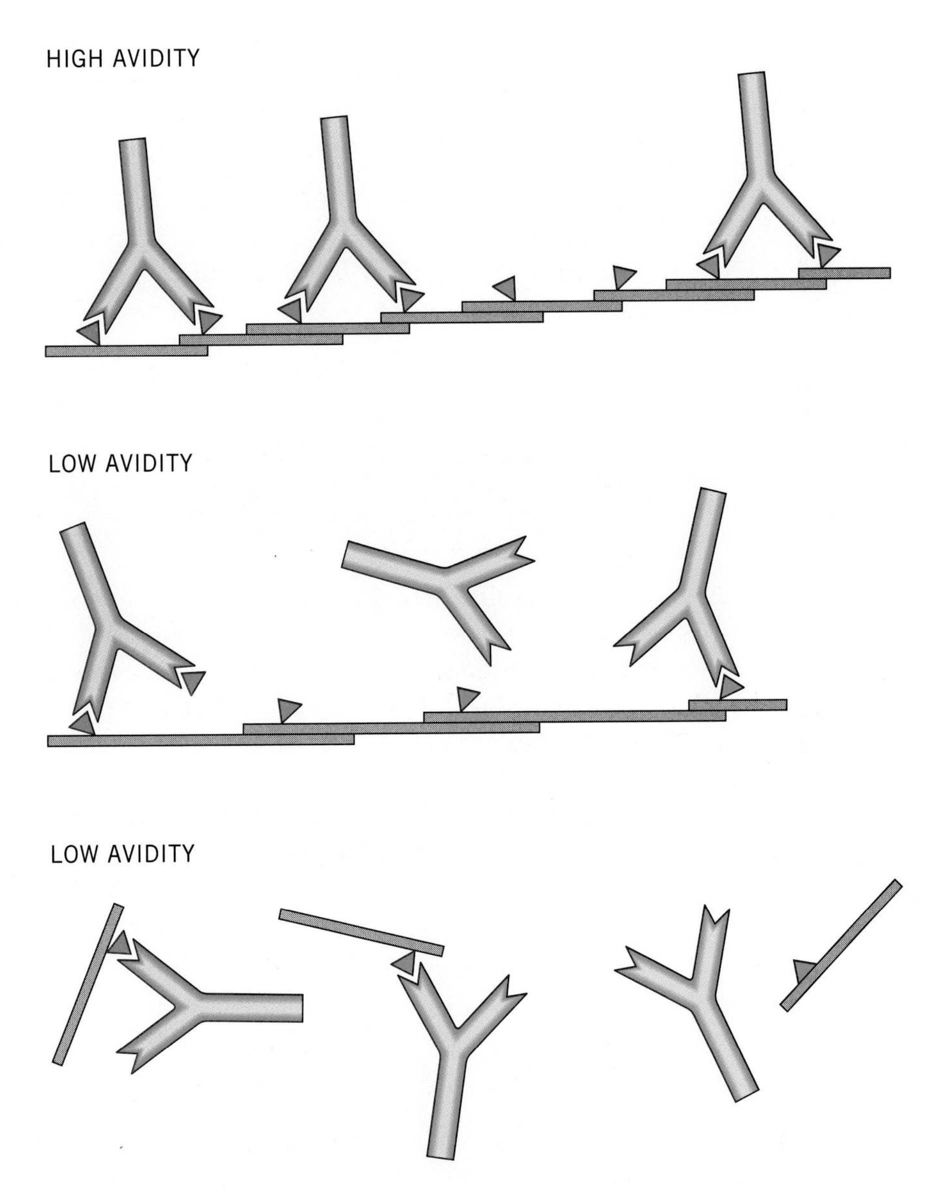


Figure 2.3
Bivalent binding of antibodies to polymeric antigens increases the avidity.

## Antibodies that bind to multiple sites on an antigen can form large, stable, multimeric complexes

When an antigen with more than one epitope is mixed with polyclonal antibodies, the complexes that form can be stabilized by intermolecular bridges (Fig. 2.4). During complex formation, one antibody binds more than one antigen molecule. If these antigen molecules are linked by the binding of a second antibody to other epitopes, a cyclic or lattice structure can be formed. The rate of dissociation of any one antibody–epitope binding is the same as for a simple interaction, but because the antigen is still held by other interactions, the overall rate of dissociation is very slow. These interactions form stable and often very large complexes. The formation of this type of complex is dependent on the relative molar ratios of the antigens and antibodies. Either used in excess will restrict the extent of cross-linking.

This type of multimeric interaction can occur in immunoprecipitation.

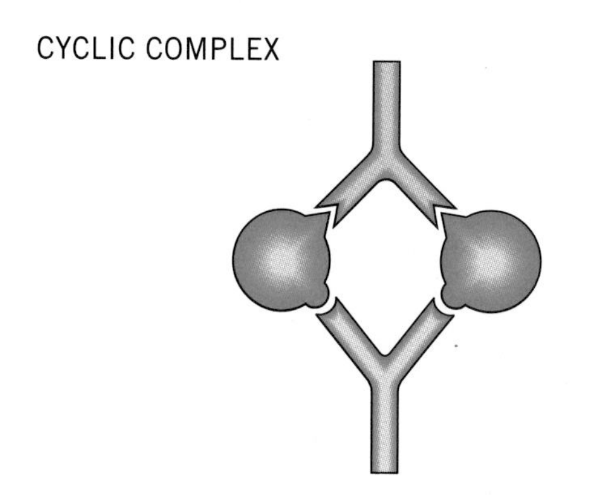


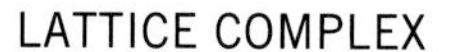


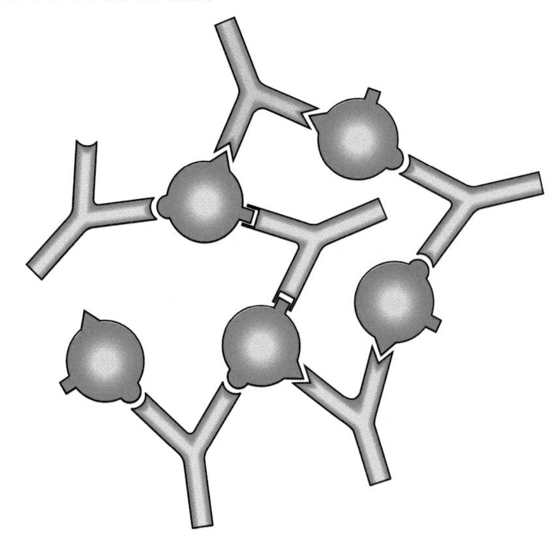

Figure 2.4
Polyclonal antibodies binding to multivalent antigens.

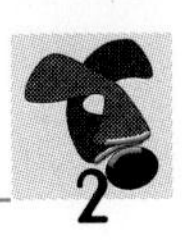


## Antibodies that bind to multiple sites on an antigen provide an excellent target for secondary reagents

When an antigen is coated by many antibodies, the complex provides multiple binding sites in a flexible geometric arrangement that allows many stable interactions with secondary reagents such as anti-immunoglobulin antibodies or protein A beads (Fig. 2.5). This provides a particularly useful target to interact with any secondary reagent.

This type of multimeric interaction can occur in most immunochemical techniques using secondary reagents.

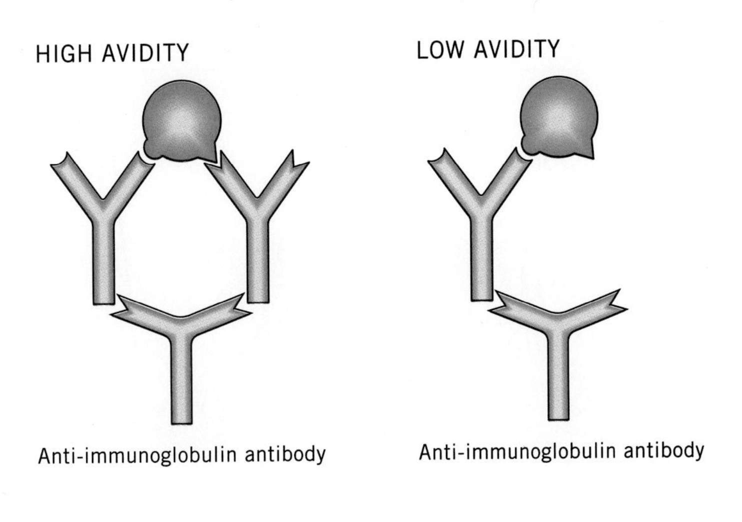


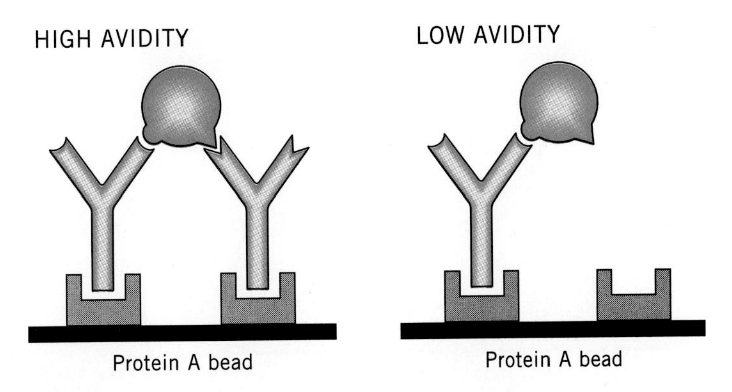


Figure 2.5
Polyclonal antibodies binding to multivalent antigens provide good targets for secondary reagents.

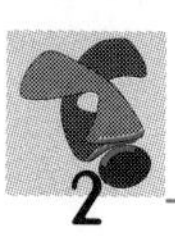



## Antigens immobilized on solid supports at high concentrations promote high-avidity, bivalent binding

When an antibody binds to an antigen on a solid phase, the interaction is biphasic, and two factors, in addition to the intrinsic affinity, control the strength of the interaction. These are the high local concentration of the antigen and the possibility of bivalent binding. The initial binding of the antibody to the immobilized antigen is limited by diffusion, but after the first antibody–epitope interaction occurs, the formation of the second bond may be an intramolecular conversion if sterically possible (Fig. 2.6). In addition, the high local concentration of antigen increases the chance that any dissociated antibodies will rebind to neighboring antigens. In essence, diffusion occurs, but the high concentration of antigen acts as a trap to hold the antibody to the solid phase. These factors combine to yield a high avidity.

This type of multimeric interaction can occur in cell staining, immunoblotting, and many types of immunoassays.

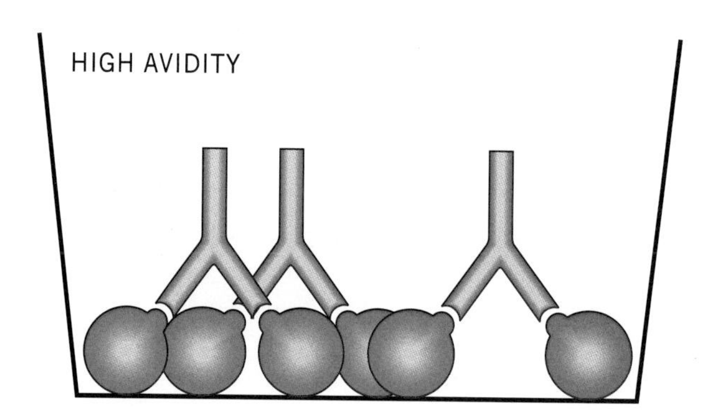


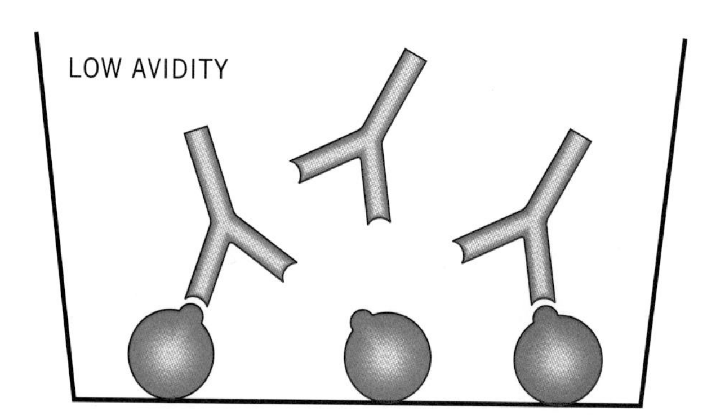


Figure 2.6
Bivalent binding to antigens immobilized on a solid phase increases the avidity.

## References

Capra J.D. and Edmundson A.B. 1977. The antibody combining site. *Sci. Am.* **236:** 50–59.

Colman P.M., Laver W.G., Varghese J.N., Baker A.T., Tulloch P.A., Air G.M., and Webster R.G. 1987. Three-dimensional structure of a complex of antibody with influenza virus neuraminidase. *Nature* **326:** 358–362.

## Further readings

### Antibody–antigen interactions

Berzofsky J.A. and Berkower I.J. 1993. Immunogenicity and antigen structure. In *Fundamental immunology*, 3rd edition (ed. W.E. Paul), pp. 235–282. Raven Press, New York.

Berzofsky J.A., Berkower I.J., and Epstein S.L. 1993. Antigen-antibody interactions and monoclonal antibodies. In *Fundamental immunology*, 3rd edition (ed. W.E. Paul), pp. 421–465. Raven Press, New York.

### Antigenic structure

Air G.M. and Layer W.G. 1989. The neuraminidase of influenza virus. *Proteins* **6:** 341–356.

Atassi M.Z. 1975. Antigenic structure of myoglobin: The complete immunochemical anatomy of a protein and conclusions relating to antigenic structures of proteins. *Immunochemistry* **12:** 423–438.

Barlow D.J., Edwards M.S., and Thornton J.M. 1986. Continuous and discontinuous protein antigenic determinants. *Nature* **322:** 747–748.

Benjamin D.C., Berzofsky J.A., East I.J., Gurd, F.R.N., Hannum C., Leach S.J., Margoliash E., Michael J.G., Miller A., Prager E.M., Reichlin M., Sercarz E.E., Smith-Gill S.J., Todd P.E., and Wilson A.C. 1984. The antigenic structure of proteins: A reappraisal. *Annu. Rev. Immunol.* **2:** 67–101.

Berzofsky J.A. 1985. Intrinsic and extrinsic factors in protein antigenic structure. *Science* **229:** 932–940.

Berzofsky J.A., Buckenmeyer G.K., Hicks G., Gurd F.R.N., Feldman R.J., and Minna J. 1982. Topographic antigenic determinants recognized by monoclonal antibodies to sperm whale myoglobin. *J. Biol. Chem.* **257:** 3189–3198.

Colman P.M. 1994. Influenza virus neuraminidase: Structure, antibodies and inhibitors. *Protein Sci.* **3:** 1687–1696.

Colman P.M., Varghese J.N., and Laver W.G. 1983. Structure of the catalytic and antigenic sites in influenza virus neuraminidase. *Nature* **303:** 41–44.

Colman P.M., Laver W.G., Varghese J.N., Baker A.T., Tulloch P.A., Air G.M., and Webster R.G. 1987. Three-dimensional structure of a complex of antibody with influenza virus neuraminidase. *Nature* **326:** 358–363.

Crumpton M.J. 1974. Protein antigens: The molecular basis of antigenicity and immunogenicity. In *The antigens* (ed. M. Sela), vol. 2, pp. 1–79. Academic Press, New York.

Crumpton M.J. and Wilkinson J.M. 1965. The immunological activity of some of the chymotryptic peptides of sperm-whale myoglobin. *Biochem. J.* **94:** 545–556.

Green N., Alexander H., Wilson A., Alexander S., Shinnick T.M., Sutcliffe J.G., and Lerner R.A. 1982. Immunogenic structure of the influenza virus hemagglutinin. *Cell* **28:** 477–487.

Landsteiner K. 1936. *The specificity of serological reactions.* C.C. Thomas, Springfield, Illinois.

Maron E., Shiozawa C., Arnon R., and Sela M. 1971. Chemical and immunological characterization of a unique antigenic region in lysozyme. *Biochemistry* **10:** 763–771.

### Structural studies of antibodies with haptens

Arevalo J.H., Taussig M.J., and Wilson I.A. 1993. Molecular basis of crossreactivity and the limits of antibody-antigen complementarity. *Nature* **365:** 859–863.

Garcia K.C., Ronco P.M., Verroust P.J., Brunger A.T., and Amzel L.M. 1992. Three-dimensional structure of an angiotensin II-Fab complex at 3 Å: Hormone

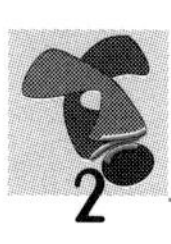



recognition by an anti-idiotypic antibody. *Science* **257:** 502–507.

Jeffrey P.D., Schildbach J.F., Chang C.Y., Kussie P.H., Margolies M.N., and Sheriff S. 1995. Structure and specificity of the anti-digoxin antibody 40–50. *J. Mol. Biol.* **248:** 344–360.

Keitel T., Kramer A., Wessner H., Scholz C., Schneider-Mergener J., and Hohne W. 1997. Crystallographic analysis of anti-p24 (HIV-1) monoclonal anitbody cross-reactivity and polyspecificity. *Cell* **91:** 811–820.

Lerner R.A., Benkovic S.J., and Schultz P.G. 1991. At the crossroads of chemistry and immunology: Catalytic antibodies. *Science* **252:** 659–667.

Marquart M., Deisenhofer J., Huber R., and Palm W. 1980. Crystallographic refinement and atomic models of the intact immunoglobulin molecule Kol and its antigen-binding fragment at 3Å and 1Å resolution. *J. Mol. Biol.* **141:** 369–391.

Patten P.A., Gray N.S., Yang P.L., Marks C.B., Wedemayer G.J., Boniface J.J., Stevens R.C., and Schultz P.G. 1996. The immunological evolution of catalysis. *Science* **271:** 1086–1091.

Satow Y., Cohen G.M., Padian E.A., and Davies D.R. 1986. Phosphocholine binding immunoglobulin Fab McPC603: An X-ray diffraction study of 2.7 Å. *J. Mol. Biol.* **190:** 593–604.

Saul F.A., Amzel L.M., and Poljak R.J. 1978. Preliminary refinement and structural analysis of the Fab fragment from human immunoglobulin new at 2.0 Å resolution. *J. Biol. Chem.* **253:** 585–597.

van den Alsen J.M., Herron J.N., Hoogerhout P., Poolman J.T., Boel E., Logtenberg T., Wilting J., Crommelin D.J., Kroon J., and Gros P. 1997. Bactericidal antibody recognition of a PorA epitope of *Neisseria meningitis:* Crystal structure of a Fab fragment in complex with a fluorescein-conjugated peptide. *Proteins* **29:** 113–125.

Wade H. and Scanlon T.S. 1997. The structural and functional basis of antibody catalysis. *Annu. Rev. Biophys. Biomol. Struct.* **26:** 461–493.

Wedemayer G.J., Patten P.A., Wang L.H., Schultz P.G., and Stevens R.C. 1997. Structural insights into the evolution of an antibody combining site. *Science* **276:** 1665–1669.

### *Structural studies of antibodies with antigens*

Amit A.G., Mariuzza R.A., Phillips S.E.V., and Poljak R.J. 1986. Three-dimensional structure of an antigen-antibody complex at 2.8 Å resolution. *Science* **233:** 747–753.

Amzel L.M., Poljak R.J., Saul F., Varga J.M., and Richards F.F. 1974. The three dimensional structure of a combining region-ligand complex of immunoglobulin NEW at 3.5-Å resolution. *Proc. Natl. Acad. Sci.* **71:** 1427–1430.

Bentley G.A. 1996. The crystal structures of complexes formed between lysozyme and antibody fragments. *EXS* **75:** 301–319.

Berzofsky J.A. and Schechter A.N. 1981. The concepts of cross-reactivity and specificity in immunology. *Mol. Immunol.* **18:** 751–763.

Bhat T.N., Bentley G.A., Fischmann T.O., Boulot G., and Poljak R.J. 1990. Small rearrangements in structures of Fv and Fab fragments of antibody D1.3 on antigen binding. *Nature* **347:** 483–485.

Braden B.C. and Poljak R.J. 1995. Structural features of the reactions between antibodies and protein antigens. *FASEB J.* **9:** 9–16.

Colman P.M., Laver W.G., Varghese J.N., Baker A.T., Tulloch P.A., Air G.M., and Webster R.G. 1987. Three-dimensional structure of a complex of antibody with influenza virus neuraminidase. *Nature* **326:** 358–363.

Colman P.M., Air G.M., Webster R.G., Varghese J.N., Baker A.T., Lentz M.R., Tulloch P.A., and Laver W.G. 1987. How antibodies recognize virus proteins. *Immunol. Today* **8:** 323–326.

Davies D.R. and Cohen G.H. 1996. Interactions of protein antigens with antibodies. *Proc. Natl. Acad. Sci.* **93:** 7–12.

Fields B.A., Goldbaum F.A., Ysern X., Poljak R.J., and Mariuzza R.A. 1995. Molecular basis of antigen mimicry by anti-idiotope. *Nature* **374:** 739–742.

Getzoff E.D., Geyson H.M., Rodda S.J., Alexander H., Tanner J.A., and Lerner R.A. 1987. Mechanisms of antibody binding to a protein. *Science* **235:** 1191–1196.

Herron J.N., He X.M., Ballard D.W., Blier P.R., Pace P.E., Bothwell A.L., Voss E.W., Jr., and Edmundson A.B. 1991. An autoantibody to single-stranded DNA: Compari-

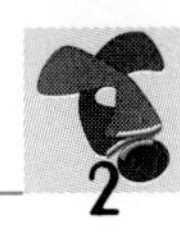

son of the three-dimensional structures of the unliganded Fab and a deoxy nucleotide-Fab complex. *Proteins* **11:** 159–175.

MacCallum R.M., Martin A.C., and Thornton J.M. 1996. Antibody–antigen interactions: Contact analysis and binding site topography. *J. Mol. Biol.* **262:** 732–745.

Rees A.R. 1987. The antibody combining site: Retrospect and prospect. *Immunol. Today* **8:** 44–45.

Rini J.M., Schulze-Gahment U., and Wilson I.A. 1992. Structural evidence for induced fit as a mechanism for antibody–antigen recognition. *Science* **255:** 959–965.

Sheriff S., Silverton E.W., Padlan E.A., Cohen G.H., Smith-Gill S.J., Finzel B.C., and Davies D.R. 1987. Three-dimensional structure of an antibody-antigen complex. *Proc. Natl. Acad. Sci.* **84:** 8075–8079.

Stanfield R.L., Fieser T.M., Lerner R.A., and Wilson I.A. 1990. Crystal structure of an antibody to a peptide and its complex with peptide antigen at 2.8 Å. *Science* **248:** 712–719.

Wade H. and Scanlan T.S. 1997. The structural and functional basis of antibody catalysis. *Annu. Rev. Biophys. Biomol. Struct.* **26:** 461–493.

Wedemayer G.J., Patten P.A., Wang L.H., Schultz P.G., and Stevens R.C. 1997. Structural insights into the evolution of an antibody combining site. *Science* **276:** 1665–1669.

Wilson I.A. and Stanfield R.L. 1994. Antibody-antigen interactions: New structures and new conformational changes. *Curr. Opin. Struct. Biol.* **4:** 857–867.

# Choosing Antibodies

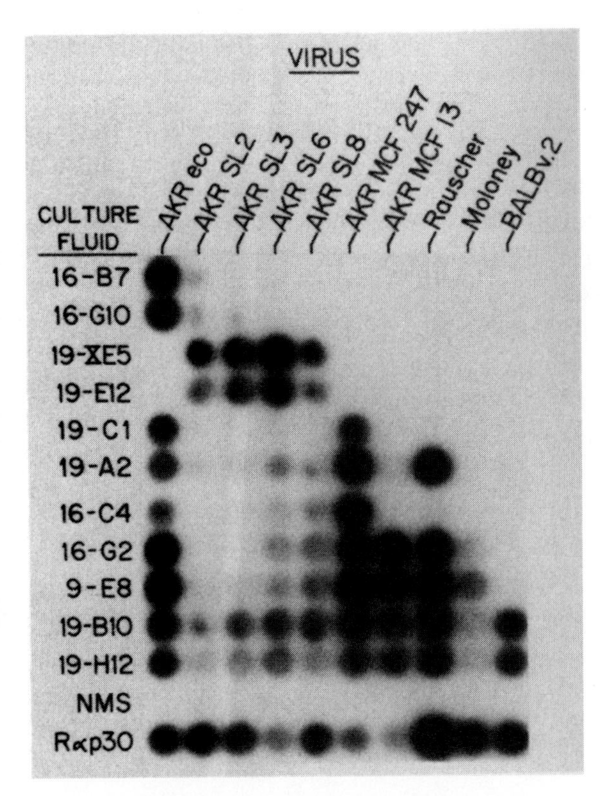


From Stone M.R., Lostrom M.E., Tam M.R., and Nowinski R.C. 1979. Monoclonal mouse antibodies as probes for antigenic polymorphism in murine leukemia viruses. *Virology* **96:** 286–290. (Reprinted with permission.)

Fig. 1. Antibody binding assays with culture fluids from hybrid cell lines. Nondiluted culture fluids from cloned hybrid cell lines were incubated in the wells of virus-adsorbed Microtest plates (see text for details). Immune reactions were detected by the addition of $^{125}$I-labeled proten A and subsequent autoradiography. Controls included tests with a 1/300 dilution of normal AKR mouse serum (NMS) and a 1/300 dilution of rabbit anti-Rauscher p30 antiserum (R α p30).

Choosing among the different antibodies that are available for a single antigen is one of the most critical steps in any immunochemical procedure. This figure is an early example of how different monoclonal antibodies all raised against a single viral immunogen compare in their binding properties for a series of closely related viruses. Even in this simple assay, the antibodies can be shown to fall into at least five classes of reactivity, emphasizing how seemingly idential antibodies can be shown to behave dramatically differently when tested in another assay. One of the most common problems encountered in immunochemistry today is the lack of appreciation of the widely different properties of antibodies in one assay compared to another. This problem has become more acute as panels of monoclonal antibodies and anti-peptide antibodies have become more widely used.

Every immunochemical technique presents the antigen in a different physical context. Immunostaining displays the antigen immobilized in its native, but complex, cellular context; immunoprecipitations present the antigen in solution surrounded by huge numbers of other contaminating molecules; immunoblotting leaves the antigen fully denatured and partially purified but bound to a solid support. Not surprisingly, given this diversity of antigen displays, each immunochemical technique requires antibodies with different properties. Even when used to study the same antigen, antibodies that work well for one method often are a poor choice for another. For example, antibodies that work exceptionally well in immunoblotting often fail completely when used for immunoprecipitations. In this chapter, the properties needed for each technique are compared, and we consider how to evaluate and choose a good antibody for your needs.

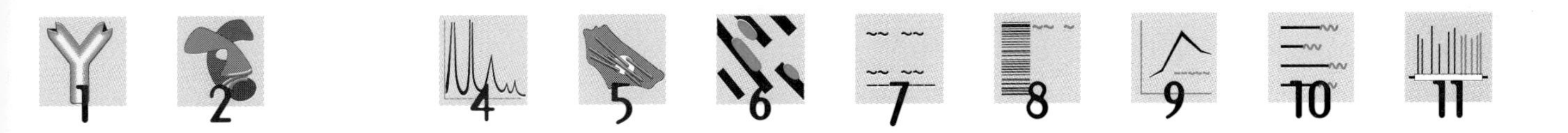




# 3 Choosing Antibodies

No single problem confounds the success of immunochemical techniques more than identifying the correct antibody to perform a desired task. No one source of antibodies will work for all methods described in this book. Multiple antibodies with different properties for an important antigen are essential to allow its study. One can dream of the time when every protein in all commonly studied organisms will have a set of well-characterized antibodies available for use. Short of this idealized time, we are stuck with carefully choosing and making antibodies to fit the requirements of a technique.

The particular requirements for a specific method are discussed in detail at the beginning of each technique chapter in this book. The information presented in this chapter is intended to be used in conjunction with the more specific information in each technique chapter.

This chapter is organized into three sections. The first section discusses the factors that determine the success of an immunochemical technique. The second section compares the requirements of the different techniques and suggests methods to compare antibodies and make selections. These first two sections are actually two views of the same problems. The first section is organized around the generalities of the problems themselves, whereas the second section discusses these issues as they pertain to each method. Consequently, many of the individual problems or their solutions appear in both sections. We have left this slightly redundant organization to allow each section to be complete on its own. The third and final section of this chapter discusses the choice of secondary reagents that are used in several methods in this book to locate the primary antibodies bound to your antigen.

## Success of an immunochemical technique

There are five main factors that influence how well an antibody will perform in an immunochemical technique. These factors are: (1) the avidity of antibodies for the antigen; (2) the specificity of the antibody for the antigen; (3) how the structures of the epitopes on the antigen are altered during the technique; (4) how easily the antibody can reach the antigen; and (5) in techniques that use them, the quality and type of secondary reagents.

### Antibody-antigen avidity

The most obvious factor that determines how well a particular antibody will perform in an immunochemical technique is its avidity for the antigen. Avidity is a measure of the total strength of the interaction between the antibody and its antigen in the context of a particular technique. The major component of avidity is the antibody–antigen affinity, a measure of how tightly the antigen-binding site of the antibody interacts with its cognate epitope on the antigen. However, the actual strength of the full interaction depends on many other factors, such as the number of interactions and the local concentration of epitopes. The structural explanations for the various factors that contribute to avidity are discussed in detail in Chapter 2.

### *Antibody–antigen affinity*

The primary component of the strength of the antibody–antigen interaction is affinity of the antibody for its epitope. These interactions are noncovalent bonds that can recognize many structural features of the antigen. When the antigen is a protein, the interactions frequently include bonds with amino acid side chains and the polypeptide chain backbone, and may even include interactions with sites of modification. Different immunochemical techniques require different degrees of affinity to achieve success. Generally, immunostaining requires the lowest-affinity interactions, whereas immunoprecipitation and immunoaffinity purification require the highest affinity. Immunoblotting requirements are intermediate between staining and immunoprecipitations.

### *Display architecture*

Another important factor in considering how well an antibody will succeed in an immunochemical method is the possibility of high-avidity interactions. Here, several factors of antigen display influence how strong the interaction will be. There are three general ways in which these interactions can be strengthened. Chapter 2 discusses these interactions in detail, so only a brief overview is included here. Table 3.1 lists which techniques are likely to generate high-avidity interactions.

If there is a high local concentration of the antigen, then every time an antibody and antigen interaction "breathes," the chances of the antibody rebinding with a nearby antigen are greatly increased. This occurs with many antigens in immunostaining and immunoblotting.

Table 3.1 *Antibody–antigen avidity requirements in the different immunochemical techniques*

| | | Avidity | | |
|---|---|---|---|---|
| **Technique** | **Affinity requirements** | **High local concentration of epitopes** | **Bridging through epitopes** | **Bridging through secondary reagents** |
| **Staining** | Lower-affinity antibodies often sufficient | With some antigens | Common | Common |
| **Immunoprecipitations** | Requires high-affinity antibodies | No, antigen in solution | Very rare | Only with polyclonal antibodies |
| **Immunoblots** | Lower-affinity antibodies often efficient | With some antigens | Occasionally | Common |
| **Immunoaffinity purification** | Requires high-affinity antibodies | No, antigen in solution | Try to avoid | Try to avoid |

A second situation in which the interaction is strengthened is when the antigen presents multiple epitopes that can be recognized simultaneously by the antibody. This can be as simple as a homodimer presenting two identical epitopes that allow interaction with both binding domains of an IgG (all techniques). Other situations that allow multiple interactions to be formed are when the antigen is bound to a solid substrate and the antibody can bridge two antigens that are held by the solid substrate (immunoblotting and immunostaining), when two or more antibodies can simultaneously link two antigens (any technique when polyclonal or pooled monoclonal antibodies are used), or when an antigen is a homopolymer and provides multiple identical binding sites (all techniques).

The third situation that drives high-avidity interactions is when secondary detection reagents can bind to multiple sites on the primary antibodies. If the secondary reagent can simultaneously bind to two sites on the primary antibody, the binding avidity is greatly enhanced. This can occur in both immunostaining and immunoblotting.

## Antibody specificity

Because antibodies recognize relatively small regions of their cognate antigens, it is not too surprising that they occasionally interact with molecules other than the immunogens used during their production. These cross-reactions either can recognize a related domain of the new antigen, suggesting some shared function or evolutionary relationship, or may detect an unexpected and generally unwanted interaction. You should be on the lookout for cross-reactions, both to make certain that you do not attribute properties of the cross-reacting molecule to your antigen and to take advantage of a potentially exciting lead on a related molecule (Table 3.2).

### *Structural similarities*

*It has been our experience that a cross-reaction seen with a denaturation-resistant epitope almost always is due to a spurious, and consequently uninformative, cross-reaction.*

How common are cross-reactions? This is best understood in the case of protein antigens. Here, cross-reactions are considerably more common for denaturation-resistant epitopes than for epitopes that are sensitive to changes in conformation. This is because denaturation-resistant epitopes are formed by linear stretches of amino acids, often as short as 5 amino acids, and therefore the frequency of random assortment suggests that finding another protein with a similar sequence is relatively common. Where large sets of antibodies to the same antigen are available, it has been shown that up to one in three or one in two of the antibodies specific for denaturation-resistant epitopes show some kind of spurious cross-reaction. This means that techniques such as immunoblotting, where denaturation is an important step in the procedure, and immunostaining, when denaturation occurs frequently, are highly susceptible to problems of cross-reactions.

Table 3.2 *Antibody specificity in the different immunochemical techniques*

| Technique | Cross-reactions | Cautions | Comments |
|---|---|---|---|
| **Staining** | Common | Difficult to recognize, because secondary method to confirm antigen identity is difficult | Controls such as two independent antibody important |
| **Immunoprecipitations** | Occasional | Important to distinguish between cross-reactions and association | Good controls needed |
| **Immunoblots** | Common | Easy to recognize, because antigen also identified by size | |
| **Immunoaffinity purification** | Occasional | Cross-reacting antibodies should be avoided | |

### *Architecture of epitope display*

*Researchers should be aware that finding more than one cross-reaction between two antigens is a good sign of a highly related structure.*

Because cross-reactions do not necessarily represent exact matches to the intended epitope, the affinity of the antibody for the epitope on the cross-reacting molecule is normally not as high as for the original immunogen. Therefore, settings that favor high-avidity interactions more commonly lead to the detection of cross-reactions. Because immunostaining and immunoblotting succeed well with lower-affinity antibodies, these techniques are especially prone to exposing cross-reactions. Researchers should be especially careful with their conclusions in these settings.

## Damaged epitopes

Each immunochemical technique described in this book uses different methods of preparing the antigen for detection. Each of these preparation methods alters the structure of the antigen to different degrees and influences how well a particular antibody will recognize the antigen (Table 3.3). The major factors that lead to changes in the epitope structure are denaturation of the native structure of the antigen and chemical modification of the amino acid that forms the epitope. Both of these features are inherent to the procedures of the technique itself, thus the problems that they impose cannot be avoided completely, but in some cases minor modifications can be used that may help the success of the method.

### *Denaturation of epitopes*

Denaturation of the antigen destroys epitopes that are formed by secondary, tertiary, or quaternary structural features found only in the fully native molecule. Denaturation of the antigen can be fully intended, as in the case of immunoblots where

Table 3.3 *Epitope quality in the different immunochemical techniques*

| Technique | Location of epitopes available for antibody binding | Types of epitopes displayed | Complicating issues |
|---|---|---|---|
| **Staining** | Surface epitopes | Some native; some denatured | Extensive loss of epitopes during fixation<br>Many epitopes masked by other cellular structures |
| **Immunoprecipitations** | Surface epitopes | Most native | Some loss of epitopes during extraction<br>Some epitopes blocked by associated molecules |
| **Immunoblots** | All linear epitopes | All denatured | Little or no renaturation of denatured epitopes |
| **Immunoaffinity purification** | Surface epitopes | Most native | Antibody–antigen interaction must be easily reversible |

the antigens are boiled in SDS, or unintentional where, for example, an extraction buffer reacts deleteriously with the antigen to destroy the native structure. Unintended denaturation can be minimized by using the mildest conditions for extraction and by minimizing the oxidation of protein antigens by physical damage or contact with oxygen.

### *Chemical modification of epitopes*

The second source of epitope damage comes from changes in the chemical groups that make up the epitope. These are most commonly the amino acid side chains of the antigen. Side chains are relatively more reactive and more accessible than other portions of the antigen and are therefore more susceptible to chemical modification. The major changes that occur are oxidation of the sulfur-containing side chains in methionine or cysteine residues, reduction of disulfide linkages, or attacks on the primary amines. In addition, the amino-terminal residue and the lysyl amino groups are frequently targets of fixation or coupling agents (for example, by paraformaldehyde fixation in cell staining, p. 123, or by coupling during the preparation of antigen affinity columns, p. 77). This destroys the epitopes that are composed of these residues. The best way to lessen problems of epitope loss by modification is primarily to keep exposure to the causative agents to a minimum. Fixation times can be reduced to the minimum needed to give a strong signal, and the fixative itself should be titrated to the lowest level that maintains antigen stability. For coupling reactions, the same guidelines apply: Allow the coupling reaction to incubate only long enough to achieve good antigen binding and use as little coupling agent as possible.

## Antibody access

Depending on the properties of the antigen under study and the method of preparing the antigen, some epitopes may not be accessible to an antibody. Steric blocks of antibodies to their cognate epitopes may be due to several different methods. The three most common reasons are (1) the presence of other molecules, particularly proteins or nucleic acids, that are already bound to the antigen and that compete for access to the epitope, (2) the modification of protein antigens, particularly protein phosphorylation, by cellular regulatory controls, and (3) problems in the orientation of the antigen in a complex setting such as found in cell or tissue staining.

### *Multimeric interactions*

One type of blockage is caused by the presence of other molecules that are bound to the antigen. This can easily be imagined by considering the case of protein–protein interactions. If the epitope for the antibody under study overlaps with the binding site for the interacting protein, no antibody–antigen interaction can be detected. This might be used as a method to determine whether a protein–protein interaction is present, but more often than not this competition is just a confusion to your studies. This competition for an epitope can be found with almost any molecular interaction but is most commonly seen with larger associated molecules such as protein or nucleic acid interactions. Multimeric interactions are problems in immunostaining, immunoprecipitations, and immunoaffinity purifications, but are not a problem for immunoblotting because here the antigens are fully denatured before the addition of the antibody (Table 3.4).

This problem can be overcome by one of several methods. Because this is a problem only for a specific antibody–antigen pair, it is often possible to change to an antibody that recognizes a different epitope. If there is no precise information about the binding sites for different antibodies, it is a simple matter to test several antibodies for the desired properties. Also, because polyclonal antibodies often recognize an antigen at multiple sites, these reagents seldom fail because of competition of the antigen with other molecules and therefore become an excellent choice to overcome this problem. A second solution to this problem is to disrupt the interaction before the addition of the antibody. Most protein–RNA, protein–DNA, and some protein–protein interactions can be disrupted by the addition of 400 mM or higher salt. This also is unlikely to damage the structure of the antigen dramatically, and most antibodies will still be able to target the antigen. For tighter interactions, harsher conditions can be used to break the antigen–competitor association. Chapter 9 discusses potential methods for breaking antibody–antigen interactions, and these are good starting points for testing dissociating conditions.

### *Posttranslational modification of protein antigens*

Another factor that may hinder the access of antibodies to their cognate protein antigen is posttranslational modifications. This has been most commonly reported with protein phosphorylation that may block the access of certain monoclonal antibodies to the antigen. This is normally just a problem that affects a subset of the proteins in

Table 3.4 *Antibody access in the different immunochemical techniques*

| | Multimeric interactions | | Protein modification | | Orientation of antigen | |
|---|---|---|---|---|---|---|
| **Technique** | **frequency?** | **common solution** | **frequency** | **common solution** | **common frequency?** | **solution** |
| **Immunoprecipitations** | Commonly seen | Change antibodies | Possible | Change antibodies, enzymatic removal | Never a problem | N/A |
| **Immunoblots** | Never a problem | N/A | Possible | Change antibodies, enzymatic removal | Never a problem | N/A |
| **Immunoaffinity purification** | Commonly seen | Change antibodies | Possible | Change antibodies, enzymatic removal | Never a problem | N/A |
| **Staining** | Possibly seen | Change antibodies, partial proteolysis, microwave | Possible | Change antibodies, enzymatic removal | Commonly seen | Change antibodies |

your cells or within your cell population, so often this type of steric change in the antigen structure only decreases the strength of the signal. In some cases, however, complete modification of the antigen is seen, and this fully blocks the access of the antibodies. This problem can be overcome by switching antibodies or by treating the protein antigens with enzymes that remove the modification; for example, with phosphatases in the case of phosphorylations of protein antigens.

### *Orientation*

A third type of problem of antibody access is caused by the orientation of an antigen in methods such as immunostaining. If the antigen is buried in a complex structure or is oriented behind an obstructing cellular structure, antibodies may not be able to reach the antigen physically. This is a problem encountered almost exclusively in cell or tissue staining.

Solving this problem is difficult. Each encounter with this problem needs a separate solution, because each setting in which antibodies are blocked from accessing an antigen is different. Therefore, each needs to be considered as a separate problem. All of the methods for solving these problems of antibody access involve some method of physically destroying the interfering structure. The two most common methods are partial proteolytic degradation and microwaving. The partial proteolysis is designed to clip off the inhibiting structures while leaving the targeted antigen mostly unaffected. For this to be effective, the amount of protease and timing of incubation need to be adjusted for each setting. Some help is provided by the fixation method, because many regions of the antigen are physically bound to adjacent structures through the cross-linker, and so even if some proteolytic clipping of the antigen takes place, at least portions of it will be still tethered to other local structures. Nonetheless, this is an effective method only if a suitable window of access can be achieved.

The second commonly used method to allow access is to microwave the specimen briefly. Here access is achieved by partially denaturing the cell structure. As with proteolytic access, the timing and intensity of the microwaving need to be adjusted carefully to allow access but not destroy the antigen or recognizable cell morphology.

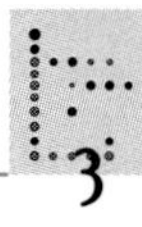

### Secondary reagents

The fifth factor that influences the success of an immunochemical method is specific to immunoblots and immunostaining. Both of these methods rely on primary antibodies to bind to and locate the antigen. In the case of immunoblots, antigens are displayed on a nitrocellulose filter and in immunostaining antigens are fixed in their normal position in the cell. To locate these antibodies, labeled secondary reagents are needed. These are most often purchased from a commercial source, and the qualities of these reagents greatly influence the success of your immunoblots or immunostaining assays. The major variables that are found with labeled secondary reagents are the background they produce in the assay, the sensitivity to detect antigen presence, their titer, and the specificity of their interactions. These issues are discussed below beginning on p. 57.

## Selecting the right antibody

Each immunochemical method described in this book relies on different properties of the antibody–antigen interaction to achieve success. Therefore, different antibodies perform to various degrees of success in each of these methods. In this section, we compare what the requirements are for each of the different immunochemical methods, suggest methods to test for the antibody that best fits these requirements, and discuss when to choose between polyclonal, monoclonal, and pooled monoclonal antibodies (Tables 3.5, 3.6, and 3.7).

### Comparing the different immunochemical methods

#### *Immunoblotting*

The three features of immunoblotting that influence the success of a particular antibody are the denaturation of the antigens during the procedure, the display of the antigen on the nitrocellulose membrane, and the specificity of the antibody. These features influence how well your antibodies will perform.

The most severe change in antigen structure in any immunochemical technique is found with immunoblotting. In immunoblotting, proteins from any source are denatured in harsh conditions (most often boiling in 2% SDS), separated by SDS-polyacrylamide gel electrophoresis, transferred to a nitrocellulose membrane, and then located by antibody binding. The three-dimensional structure of the antigen is destroyed by boiling in SDS, and renaturation is unlikely to be due to the physical attachment to the nitrocellulose membrane and the continued presence of residual SDS bound to the proteins on the membrane. Therefore, the antigens can be considered fully denatured by this method, and only epitopes that are formed by a linear stretch of amino acids will be available for antibody binding.

The second key feature of immunoblotting that affects the choice of antibody is that the antigen will be bound to a nitrocellulose membrane at a position corresponding to its molecular weight in the SDS-polyacrylamide gel. This creates a high local concentration of the antigen bound to the membrane. This provides a good setting for antibodies to bind through two binding sites of their Fab fragments. Having an antibody

Table 3.5 *Kinetics of antibody–antigen interaction in the various immunochemical techniques*

| Technique | Local epitope concentration | Antigen fixed? | Antibody fixed? | Binding kinetics | Comments |
|---|---|---|---|---|---|
| **Staining** | Concentrations mixed | Fixed | Free | Slow | Regular display allows lower affinity antibody to work<br>Possible higher local concentration allows lower affinity antibody to work |
| **Immunoprecipitations** | Generally very low | Free | Free | Fast | |
| **Immunoblots** | Mixed | Fixed | Free | Slow, incubation times greater than 1 hr are recommended | Possible higher local concentration promotes high avidity interactions |
| **Immunoaffinity purification** | Generally very low | Free | Fixed | Slow, but high local concentrations of the antibody drive the reaction | |

Table 3.6 *Methods for changing epitope display in the various immunochemical techniques*

| Technique | Method | Rationale | Comments |
|---|---|---|---|
| **Staining** | Protease treatment | Light protease treatment will remove sterically hindering proteins and may allow antibody access | Difficult to standardize<br>Many new epitopes displayed so excellent controls are required |
| | Microwave | Light irradiation distorts the local environment of the antigen and may allow antibody access | Many new epitopes displayed so excellent controls are required |
| **Immunoprecipitations** | Alter extraction conditions | Different lysis buffers will alter the presentation of the antigen | |
| | Boil samples in SDS prior to immunoprecipitation | Denaturation will expose epitopes | Need antibodies against denatured antigen<br>Will lose native interactions |
| **Immunoblots** | None | | |
| **Immunoaffinity purification** | Alter extraction conditions | Different lysis buffers will alter the presentation of the antigen | |
| | Boil samples in SDS prior to adding beads | Denaturation will expose epitopes | Need antibodies against denatured antigen<br>Will lose native interactions |

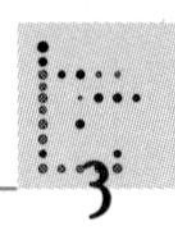

Table 3.7 *Factors that influence the success of immunochemical techniques*

| Technique | Antibody–antigen avidity a problem? | Specificity requirements | Epitope damage | Antigen accessibility |
|---|---|---|---|---|
| **Staining** | Normally no, but severe problems with architecture | Severe problems, and controls difficult | Medium | |
| **Immunoprecipitations** | Needs high-affinity antibody for antigen clearance | Examine antibody binders by SDS-PAGE | In most cases, antibody must see native structure | |
| **Immunoblots** | Generally no | Must see denatured structure | All antigen completely denatured | |
| **Immunoaffinity purification** | Must see native structure | Can examine antibody binders by SDS-PAGE | In most cases, antibody must see native structure | |

bound by two interactions greatly increases the avidity of the antibody for the antigen. This means that some antibodies that work poorly on soluble antigens may bind tightly in immunoblotting.

The features of immunoblotting put a severe pressure on the specificity of the antibodies. All antibodies that work in immunoblotting recognize short linear sequences of proteins, often six or fewer residues in length. Given that only a few of these residues are likely to contribute significant energy to the antibody–antigen interaction, it is not surprising to learn that antibodies in immunoblots frequently bind to other proteins in addition to the original immunogen. These may be formed by the random frequency with which several amino acids are found in the same order in a short peptide sequence. These denaturation-resistant cross-reactions are often exposed from the unfolding of the proteins during the immunoblotting procedures. Thus, a linear fragment that is well hidden in the three-dimensional structure of a protein may be uncovered during the display on the membrane. It is not uncommon to find that antibodies cross-react with unrelated proteins in immunoblots. These cross-reactions can often be identified by using other antibodies to your antigen. If cross-reacting proteins are well separated in size from your antigen, they are easy to ignore in your analysis, but if they are close in size, you may need to change antibodies.

Because immunoblots are rapid, it is simple to test various antibodies to ascertain their effectiveness. For most antigens, you should expect to find a good antibody source that will display interactions only with your antigen and with closely related family members. When needed, even closely related protein homologs can be distinguished by the careful choice of antibodies.

### *Immunoprecipitations and immunoaffinity purification*

These two methods rely on similar physical approaches to antibody–antigen interactions and therefore are discussed together here. Both methods are commonly used to collect native antigens in solution and can be complicated by problems of damaged epitopes, steric hindrance for antibody access, and antibody avidity for the antigen.

Because immunoprecipitations and immunoaffinity purifications are most often used to collect protein antigens in their native state, denaturation frequently destroys the antibody recognition sites. To keep the damage of the epitopes to a minimum, extraction conditions should be selected to find the mildest conditions that allow good release of the antigen.

These methods are often used to collect not only the antigen under study but also the associated molecules. For immunoprecipitations, this is done at an analytical stage, whereas immunoaffinity purifications are done for large-scale isolation. Antibodies should be evaluated based on the fraction of the total antigen that is removed from solution.

Both of these methods also are used to recognize antigens in solution, and thus high-affinity antibodies are required to bind the antigens quantitatively. Weaker-affinity interactions may allow the detection of the antigen, but will not allow its complete removal.

Choosing the best antibody for immunoprecipitations is easily done by running different antibody preparations side by side through a test protocol using a known source of antigen. This will indicate the relative titers and specificities of each antibody and give you a good measure of how these antibodies will perform with other samples. For immunoaffinity purification, it is easiest to prescreen potential antibodies by using immunoprecipitations to evaluate the possible antibody sources. Once antibodies are identified that give strong signals of the antigen, little or no background, and good selectivity, they will need to be tested further to determine which elution conditions are suitable. Methods for these tests are found in Chapter 9.

### *Cell staining and tissue staining*

Immunostaining of cells either in culture or in the organism poses the most difficult challenges in selecting useful antibodies. The literature presents many examples of inappropriate conclusions of subcellular localization or antigen presence due to inappropriate choices of antibodies. The methodology of immunostaining presents serious problems with establishing the specificity of the antibodies, with alteration of the epitope structure, and with steric hindrance of antibody access to the antigen.

One key factor that confounds the success of immunostaining is the inability to determine the specificity of a particular antibody. Methods such as immunoprecipitation or immunoblots separate the antigens by their relative molecular weights, and even immunoaffinity-purified proteins are commonly examined for purity by gel electrophoresis. This gives the researcher another method to distinguish the intended from the unintended interactions. No similar methods to determine which antigens

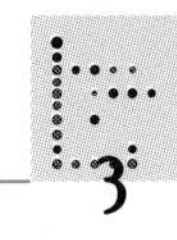

are recognized by the antibodies are possible with immunostaining. Positives are scored solely by the binding of the antibodies to the displayed cell structures. Unintended interactions are not readily distinguished from the desired binding. The problems of specificity in immunostaining are further amplified by the format of the antigen presentation. Because the antigens are physically bound to their respective subcellular compartments, it is quite common to find that multiple antigen-binding domains of the antibodies interact with the antigen. In addition, in cases where the antigen is present in a high local concentration, the chances of antibodies rebinding directly after "breathing" from their interaction with the antigen are more likely. These types of high-avidity interactions are discussed in detail in Chapter 2. Although these types of interactions increase the likelihood that lower-affinity antibodies will work successfully in immunostaining, they also raise the problem that undesired low-affinity interactions will score in your assays. The chapters that cover the immunostaining techniques discuss the use of potential controls to help in confirming that the staining pattern is due to the antigen under study. Briefly, these methods include showing that your antibodies are specific on immunoblots and immunoprecipitations, the use of multiple antibodies that bind to distinct regions of the antigen, comparing the staining pattern in antigen-negative cells, and comparing the staining pattern with GFP-fusion proteins (see Chapter 11).

The second factor that makes evaluating antibodies in immunostaining difficult is the problem encountered in fixation. The methods for fixing cells are harsh and are notorious both for distorting the epitopes and for chemically modifying the antigen. The preferred method of paraformaldehyde fixation covalently modifies the free amino groups of most antigens and therefore distorts the structure of many epitopes. Alternative methods for tissue-culture cells, such as use of organic solvents, acetone, or alcohols, dehydrate the samples and precipitate protein antigens. There are no surefire methods to reverse these effects, but several precautions can help. The most important factor is to keep these problems in mind and run sufficient controls to minimize them. The two most helpful approaches to overcome any difficulties encountered with fixation are to keep fixation times to a minimum and to use as low a concentration of fixative as retains your antigen. Because both of these variations can only be evaluated after a clear and reliable signal has been discovered, they are more helpful in troubleshooting than in evaluating the various antibodies sources.

The last major problem posed by immunostaining is the frequent steric hindrance of antibody access. This includes the interaction of target antigens with other molecules that block the access to key epitopes as well as the presence of cellular structures that often do not allow full access of the antibodies to the site of antigen. Again, these problems are inherent in the method and need to be remembered in designing the experiment and in planning controls. There are several methods that may lessen the problems of steric hindrance, including limited protease treatment and microwaving (see above). However, like the problems of fixation, these approaches cannot be successfully used before confirming the correct location and signal from your antigen.

*Using appropriate controls*

| Technique | Positive controls | Negative controls | Other needed controls |
|---|---|---|---|
| **Staining** | Stain known source of antigen for pattern | Nonimmune antibody | Omit primary antibody |
| **Immunoprecipitations** | Immunoprecipitate known source of antigen for size comparison | Nonimmune antibody | |
| **Immunoblots** | Immunoblot known source of Ag for size comparison | Nonimmune antibody | |
| **Immunoaffinity purification** | Run pure antigen on gel for size control[1] | Nonimmune antibody[1] | Resin alone[1] |

[1] All three controls for immunoaffinity purification should be used for each new antigen source or when changing epitope.

## Comparisons to help select the best antibodies

One key problem in choosing the best antibody to use in an immunochemical method is to learn which methods to use for evaluating the antibodies. Some of these decisions are straightforward, such as for immunoprecipitations and immunoblots. Potential antibodies sources for other techniques, such as immunostaining, are more difficult to assess. Table 3.8 summarizes the potential methods to assess antibodies for the various immunochemical techniques.

### *Immunoblots and immunoprecipitations*

For immunoblots and immunoprecipitations, it is simple to use the method itself to test the specificity and relative strengths of the response because the antigens that are bound are separated by SDS-polyacrylamide gel electrophoresis. This gives a reliable display of the group of antigens that are recognized by the antibodies, and it is easy to compare the antibodies to each other. Therefore, immunoblots and immunoprecipitations are the easiest assays for comparing and choosing the best antibodies.

### *Immunoaffinity purification*

For antibodies that might be used in immunoaffinity purification, there are several key steps that should be used to assess the various potential sources. In general, immunoaffinity purifications rely on monoclonal antibodies. This is because the single site for interaction provided by the monoclonal antibody is simpler to break during elution of the antigen than with polyclonal antibodies. The exception to this recommendation is the use of anti-peptide antibodies (see Chapter 9).

Table 3.8 *Techniques to compare antibody specificity*

| Method | Test by immunoblot | Test by immunoprecipitation | Test by immunostaining | Test by immunoaffinity purification | Comments |
|---|---|---|---|---|---|
| **Immunoblots** | Best test of success | Poor predictor | Not recommended | Not recommended | Immunoblots themselves give good test of signal strength and specificity |
| **Immunoprecipitations** | Poor predictor | Best test of success | Not recommended | Not recommended | Immunoprecipitations themselves give good test of signal strength and specificity |
| **Immunostaining** | Helpful, but not sufficient | Helpful, but not sufficient | Helpful, but not sufficient | Not recommended | Need multiple controls; immunoprecipitation, immunoblotting, and immunostaining all required but should include other controls; genetic nulls for the antigen are especially helpful |
| **Immunoaffinity purification** | Not recommended | Best test of success | Not recommended | Not recommended | Immunoprecipitations give good test of signal strength and specificity |

To test various sources of antibodies for immunoaffinity purifications, the easiest and best first step is to use immunoprecipitations. This will simulate the use of antibodies binding to native sources of antigens in solution. Antibodies that are efficient at binding most of the antigens in solution and that show few or no background bands on SDS-polyacrylamide gels of the immunoprecipitated proteins should be considered for the next steps of evaluation. These steps should include the determination of appropriate elution conditions (Chapter 9).

### *Immunostaining*

Staining of cells in culture or tissues provides the most difficult settings for assessing antibodies. As discussed above, immunostaining provides few of the opportunities for checking for specific detection of antigens that other methods do. For comparisons, it is best to test antibodies that might be used in immunostaining both by immunoprecipitation and immunoblots prior to use in immunostaining. No background bands here suggest that background problems may be minimal. This needs to be followed by careful use of controls for antigen presence (Chapters 5 and 6).

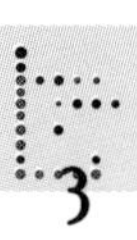



## Comparing commercial antibodies

Not all antibodies sold by companies are useful for all methods. An increasingly annoying problem has been the rapid production and sale of poorly characterized antibodies by some commercial houses. All buyers should be aware that claims made by companies need to be evaluated in your lab. Just because a company claims good use of antibody in a particular technique does not mean that you can assume that this claim is correct. We strongly urge all researchers to check the references for each commercial source prior to purchase. And if antibodies do not perform as advertised, complain! Let the supplier know that their products are not performing as expected. A reputable supplier will help you reach their predicted results, supply antibodies that will fulfill your needs, or provide restitution in some other way.

A good caution in purchasing antibodies is always to calculate the amount of antibodies needed to perform your experiments. For some approaches, such as immunoaffinity purification, it may not be possible to afford the amount of antibody needed and you will need to seek other sources.

Researchers should also remember that many hybridoma cell lines are available from the American Type Culture Collection and European Collection of Animal Cell Cultures. These may provide a useful source for reagents or controls.

## Using polyclonal, monoclonal, or pooled monoclonal antibodies

Each of these sources does not perform equally in the various immunochemical techniques. Table 3.9 lists the various techniques discussed in this book and suggests appropriate choices. In addition, in each technique chapter we compare the various sources of antibodies and make recommendations on their use.

Table 3.9 *Choice of polyclonal, monoclonal, or pooled monoclonal antibodies*

| Method | Polyclonal antibodies | Monoclonal antibodies | Pooled monoclonal antibodies |
|---|---|---|---|
| Immunoblots | Good choice, if correct antibodies are available | Good choice, if correct antibody is available | Best choice, if multiple specific monoclonal antibodies are available |
| Immunoprecipitations | Good choice, if correct antibodies are available | Good choice, if correct antibody is available | Best choice, if multiple specific monoclonal antibodies are available |
| Immunostaining | Good choice, if correct antibodies are available | Better choice, because of specificity | Not recommended, unless signal strength a problem |
| Immunoaffinity purification | Not recommended, unless using antipeptide antibodies | Best choice | Not recommended; dissociating the antigen is very difficult |

# Selecting the best secondary reagents

Often the success of an immunochemical technique rests on the selection of a good labeled secondary reagent. These reagents are used to identify the position of unlabeled primary antibodies in immunoblots and immunostaining methods (Chapters 5, 6, and 8). There are four main issues to consider in selecting the best secondary reagent. These factors are (1) the background that arises from the secondary reagent, (2) the sensitivity of the detection reagent, (3) the titer of commercial sources, and (4) the specificity of interaction with the primary antibodies.

## Background arising from the secondary reagent

Background problems in any assay that relies on a secondary reagent can be assessed by omitting the primary antibody and running the assay as per normal. The best secondary reagents will give no detectable signal without the presence of the primary antibody. In practice this ideal is seldom achieved, but a useful source should give very low backgrounds on its own.

This test is an important one to include not only in assessing potential commercial sources of secondary reagents, but also routinely in your assays. Long-term storage of secondary reagents often leads to aggregation or denaturation, so continued monitoring of the background levels is important. This is particularly true with cell and tissue immunostaining, where omitting the primary antibody should be included as a control in every assay.

## Sensitivity of commercial sources

The sensitivity of a secondary detection reagent is due to two factors. These are the choice of the appropriate tag and the care with which the coupling reaction has been done. The choice of appropriate tags is discussed in each technique chapter, but the efficiency of the coupling of the labeled tag to the secondary reagent should be tested by comparing different commercial sources.

You should purchase several lots of potential secondary reagents from different companies and compare these in side-by-side tests run in conditions identical to those that will be used in your lab. The assay used for these comparisons should be robust and easily repeated. Try to select batches or lots that are in reasonable supply at the different companies. After you have identified a good lot and purchased a suitable supply, set aside a small sample to use as a standard for your next round of testing, once this lot is exhausted. Be sure to save the lot number for reordering. After a few rounds of testing, you will begin to develop confidence in a small subset of suppliers.

## Titer of commercial sources

An important variable to consider in analyzing different sources of products from various suppliers is the effective titer at which to use the reagent. For example, the cost of 1 mg of labeled antibody may vary widely between various commercial houses. How-

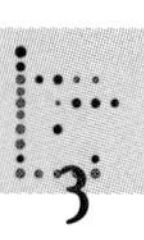



ever, a reagent that can be used at a 10-fold higher dilution may be a significantly better value even though the cost per weight is higher.

In addition, using higher dilutions of secondary reagents produces much cleaner backgrounds. Therefore, any opportunity to select secondary reagents that can be used at a lower titer is advantageous. Be sure to do all your dilutions in protein-containing buffers such as 3% BSA/PBS. Low concentrations of proteins have a tendency to denature, raising the possibilities of nonspecific interactions and lessening the advantages of using higher dilutions.

## Specificity

The final factor that may influence your choice of secondary reagent is the specificity of recognizing the primary antibody. This will not always be a problem, but if you need to be able to recognize your species of primary antibody in a setting of other potentially competing proteins, it will be important to test for these cross-reactions. This is most frequently seen when immunostaining samples contain antibodies from the host organism or in double-label immunofluorescence experiments.

### Conventions for discussing antibodies

Over the years, several standard conventions for describing the species of origin, the immunogen, and the antibody type have evolved. This shorthand makes some order from a confusing set of information, but to the uninitiated, some explanation may be needed. The immunogen is commonly identified by the species of origin and is always preceded by the prefix *anti-*. So if you were discussing antibodies specific for the vertebrate morphogen *sonic hedgehog*, which had been isolated from the mouse, you would describe your reagents as *anti-mouse sonic hedgehog antibodies* or *anti-mouse sonic hedgehog immunoglobulins.* The species in which the antibody was raised is always given before the antibody name. Therefore, if you were raising your antibodies in the ibex, the resulting reagents would be called *ibex anti-mouse sonic hedgehog antibodies.* The next level of complication comes if the antibodies have been further modified. All modifications to the antibodies are given before the immunized animal. So, *FITC-conjugated ibex anti-mouse sonic hedgehog antibodies* gives you a labeled primary antibody to look for sonic hedgehog in immunostaining.

In this book, we have followed an additional convention to discuss antibodies that have been raised against antibodies isolated from other species. These are always discussed as *anti-immunoglobulin antibodies*, using the more formal name *immunoglobulin* to describe the immunogen and the more conversational *antibodies* to identify the product. If the antibodies have been raised to only a subset of the immunoglobulins, this is indicated in the immunogen descriptor. Thus, *goat anti-mouse immunoglobulin* $IgG_{2a}$ *antibodies* are antibodies raised in the goat against purified mouse $IgG_{2a}$.

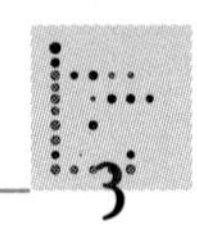


## The etiquette of antibody requests

All antibodies that are described in the published literature should be available following a polite request to the authors. The only reasonable denial from authors will be when a polyclonal antibody has run out or is in very short supply. All monoclonal antibodies should be provided without question, and just because only a polyclonal antibody was made is not sufficient argument for not supplying a sample to a qualified researcher. If the makers of the antibody have arranged for supply from a commercial source, a requester should be prepared to pay the standard rate for this antibody. The only case that is somewhat confusing is when large amounts of the antibody are needed; for example, for an antibody affinity column. Somewhere between an expectation to receive sufficient antibody to run several experiments and obtaining multiple milligrams of purified antibody, the etiquette of reagent exchange breaks down. In these more difficult cases, both the requester and the antibody provider need to search for an acceptable solution.

To ensure a respectful response to a request for an antibody, the inquiry should contain a careful description of the desired antibody, an offer to cover the costs for shipping using a simple method for payment (normally including your account number for a commercial shipper is sufficient, but a pre-addressed shipping form is best), and an indication of how much antibody is required. The amount of antibody requested should be modest. If you need large amounts you should either consider making the antibody yourself or offer to establish a collaboration. Please also remember that many labs who specialize in antibody production receive several requests per day. Even if your request will be honored, you should be prepared to wait several weeks before expecting a reply.

After receiving the antibody, two follow-up steps will show your gratitude. A simple note to the supplying lab that indicates the antibody arrived safely and an acknowledgment in any publication that comes from the experiments are sufficient thanks for antibody producers.

### Making the right antibody

If no source of antibodies correctly fulfills their needs for a particular immunochemical technique, researchers should be prepared to make the correct antibodies. The production of good reagents not only solves the researchers' immediate needs, but also can provide needed reagents for the field as a whole. Researchers should also be aware that all companies that sell antibodies are constantly on the lookout for good sources of important new reagents. When contacting these companies, be sure to rely on companies who provide good reagents for you. Companies that you do not respect for delivery of good antibodies do not deserve the access to your new reagents.

# Handling Antibodies

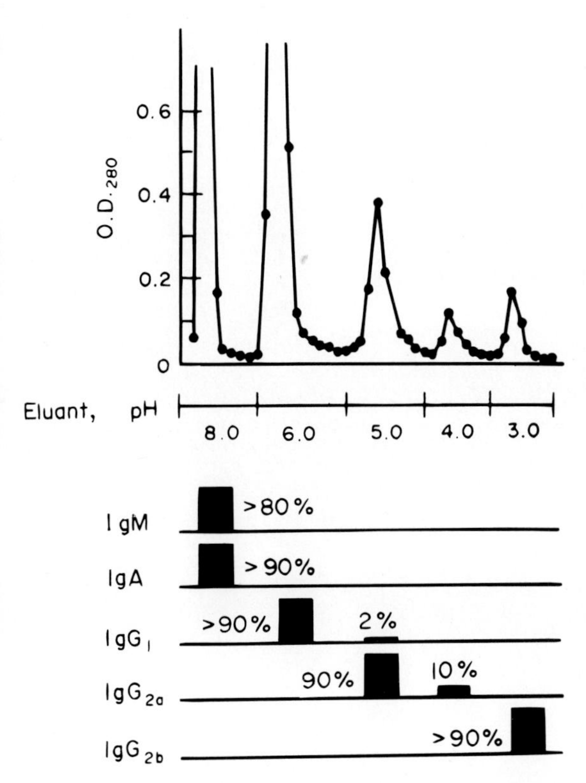


From Ey P.L., Prowse S.J., and Jenkin C.R. 1978. Isolation of pure $IgG_1$, $IgG_{2a}$, $IgG_{2b}$ immunoglobulins from mouse serum using protein A-Sepharose. *Immunochemistry* **15:** 429–436. (Reprinted with permission.)

Fig. 1. Elution of Igs from protein A-Sepharose. Serum (0.8 ml) from mice immunized with *N. dubius* larvae was mixed with 2 ml 0.14 *M* phosphate, pH 8.0 and applied to the protein A-Sepharose column. The column was washed with 0.14 *M* phosphate, pH 8.0 and then sequentially with buffers of pH 6.0, 5.0, 4.0, and 3.0. The flow rate was 0.46 ml/min and fractions of 3.9 ml were collected. Their optical density at 280 nm ($O.D._{280}$) was measured and they were then pooled as indicated. Each pool was analysed for Ig by radial immunodiffusion. The results are shown as block histograms depicting the proportion of Ig recovered as a percentage of that applied to the column.

Antibodies have been in use as common research tools for over a half century, and thus there is an extensive practical lore on their handling and storage. These empirical trial- and error-tests have led to a good understanding of how to handle antibodies—tasks that are not difficult and are helped greatly by the stability of antibodies. Antibodies are more resistant to denaturation than most other proteins, and this makes their storage, purification, and labeling easy. Such tasks have become even more accessible with the discovery of antibody-binding proteins such as protein A and protein G. As shown in this figure, protein A makes an excellent matrix for purifying antibodies in a simple one-step procedure. This procedure has made the isolation of all antibodies a straightforward task. The availability of high-quality commercial reagents that provide access to labeling immunochemical reagents of all types is another major advantage.

This chapter presents techniques that are recommended to store, purify, and label antibodies. In general, these techniques are sufficient for handling antibodies that are made in your or your colleagues' labs. Most commercial suppliers who provide antibodies, either labeled or unlabeled, provide suggestions on how to store, handle, and use their antibody products.

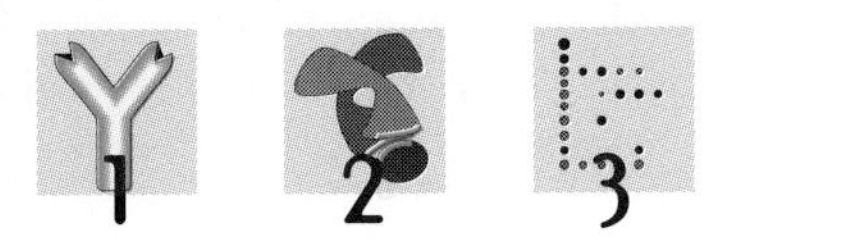


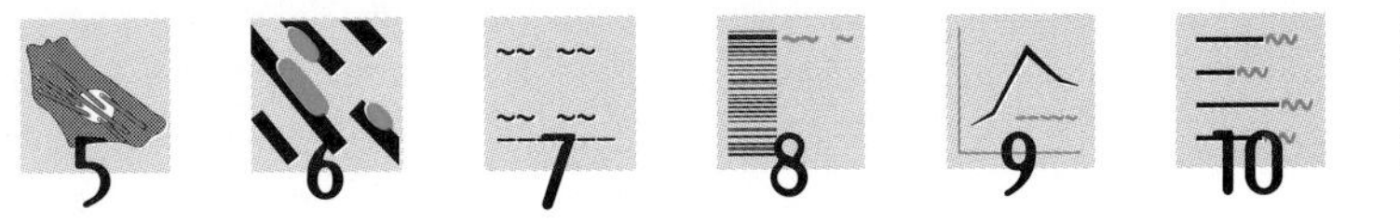


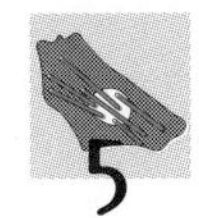
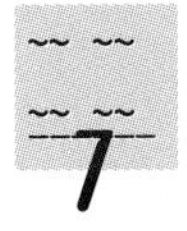
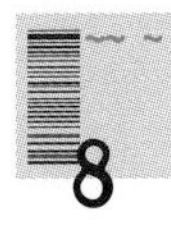
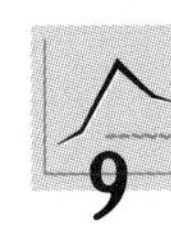
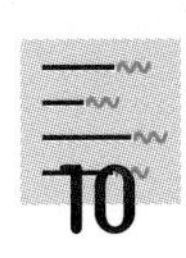
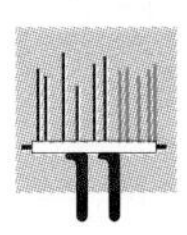

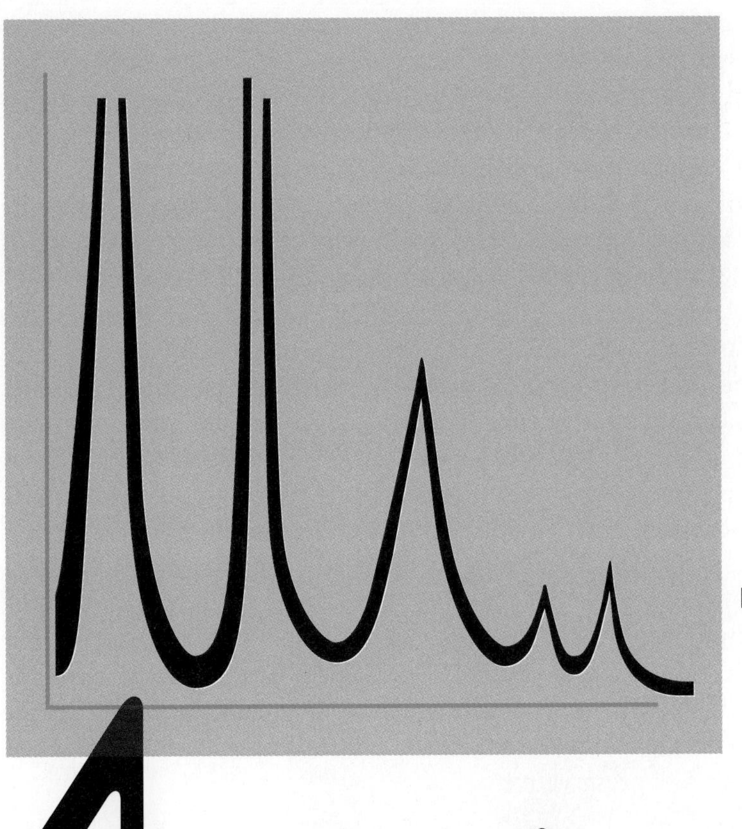



# 4 Handling Antibodies

# Storing antibodies



Antibodies have a compact three-domain structure that has evolved to retain activity in most biological settings, even at sites of major body trauma. One practical advantage of such compact and stable protein domains is that they are resistant to a broad range of mildly denaturing conditions, making long-term storage of antibodies relatively easy. Storage buffers seldom need to be supplemented with glycerol or other stabilizing compounds that are commonly added to help maintain the activity of proteins purified in the lab.

## Contamination

The only problem commonly encountered in storing antibodies is contamination of these solutions with bacteria or fungi. This can be prevented by the addition of antimicrobial agents; for example, by adding sodium azide to 0.02% or, as an alternative, Merthiolate to 0.01%. Although useful and effective for most settings, sodium azide is not appropriate in some assays, because it blocks the cytochrome electron transport system and therefore is toxic to most organisms. In addition, the primary amine on the azide interferes with many coupling methods. For coupling reactions in which the amino group interferes with the chemical reactions, sodium azide should not be added until after purification. If sodium azide is already present in a solution, it can be removed by dialysis or gel filtration.

If antibodies will be used in biological assays (for example, microinjection of antibodies), we recommend that no preserving agents be used. Instead, the antibodies should be purified and stored frozen in small aliquots for these tests. For in vivo tests (for example, antibody imaging), it is extremely important not to add any preservative. However, sterility is important, and in these cases, the antibody solution should be purified and filter-sterilized. Filters made with materials that do not bind appreciable amounts of proteins are best. The sterile antibody solution then should be handled aseptically.

In several of the techniques in this book, we have suggested that antibody conjugates or antibody matrices should be stored in 0.01% Merthiolate. This is an alternate preservative that does not have a primary amine which would attack the stability of the antibody's interaction with the conjugate or matrix. For most purposes, however, we recommend sodium azide as a preservative.

## Caution

Sodium azide, see Appendix IV.

## Temperature for storage

For long-term storage, antibodies can be kept conveniently at –20°C in the serum, tissue culture supernatant, or ascitic fluid in which they are collected. Lower temperatures will not hurt the antibody activities, but there is no significant advantage in lower-temperature storage.

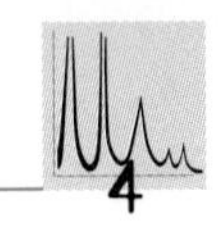


*Many workers prefer to store ascites fluid at −70°C. This helps with long-term storage and ensures that no proteolytic activity can continue.*

Working solutions of antibodies are conveniently stored at 4°C. At this temperature they are stable for months to years without loss of activity.

Antibody solutions should not be frozen and thawed repeatedly, because this can lead to partial denaturation of the antibodies that may lead to unwanted protein–protein aggregation. Aggregation of antibodies can cause the loss of activity due to steric interference of the antigen combining site or by generating insoluble material that is lost during centrifugation or filtration.

The only group of antibodies that should not be stored at 4°C are the so-called cryoproteins, which are sensitive to low-temperature storage, where they precipitate. Some mouse antibodies of the $IgG_3$ subclass may fit these characteristics. If antibodies precipitate at 4°C over time, they should be kept at room temperature with the addition of sodium azide.

## Time of storage

Antibodies are remarkably stable. If tightly sealed to avoid evaporation, they can be stored at 4°C for months with no loss of activity. Antibodies stored at –20°C have been shown to keep their activity for decades.

## Storing sera

● STORING
○ PURIFYING, 70
○ LABELING, 81

*Serum is prepared by incubating a freshly drawn sample of blood at 37°C for 30 minutes to 1 hour to allow the clot to form. The clot is loosened from the tube by ringing the side of the tube with a pasteur pipet, straightened paper clip, or similar instrument. Transfer to 4°C overnight, allowing the clot to contract. The serum is separated by centrifugation at 10,000g for 10 minutes at 4°C.*

*Many sera generate an insoluble lipid component with prolonged storage at 4°C. This may look like microbial contamination, but this is unlikely if sodium azide has been included. The precipitate can be removed by centrifugation at 10,000g. In some cases, the lipids will form a layer above the aqueous phase. Remove the aqueous phase and store as described above.*

Serum is the fluid phase of blood that remains after it has been allowed to clot.

### Thinking ahead

It is important to consider how you plan to use the serum in your various applications, because this will dictate the size of the samples that you will prepare and whether or not a preservative will be used. Also, it is always important to try to collect as much serum as possible. Many researchers stop serum collection, even from animals that are producing excellent antibodies, too early. Polyclonal antibodies are not a renewable resource, and most investigators who have prepared good antibodies find that they run out much too soon. Be forewarned; collect as many samples as possible from animals that are producing useful antibodies.

### Caution

Sodium azide, see Appendix IV.

1. Serum is already well buffered, so no addition of any buffer is needed.

2. If there is no reason to avoid the use of sodium azide, add to 0.02%.

3. Aliquot antibodies into smaller samples and freeze multiple tubes. For serum, suitable sizes would be 100–500 μl per tube. Most antibodies are stable for years when stored at –20°C.

4. Thaw individual tubes at room temperature or below and store at 4°C. Working solutions can be stored conveniently at 4°C for months. Cap tightly to avoid evaporation.

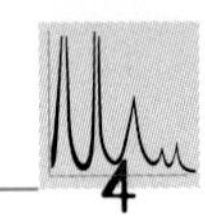


## Storing tissue culture supernatants



Hybridoma cells secrete their antibodies into the tissue culture supernatants just as plasma cells do in the body. These supernatants can be collected and used for most standard immunochemical tests.

### Caution

Sodium azide, see Appendix IV.

*Hybridoma tissue culture supernatants are prepared simply by removing the hybridoma cells by centrifugation at 1000g for 5 minutes at 4°C. Remove the supernatant and respin at 10,000g for 10 minutes at 4°C and carefully collect the supernatant.*

1. Hybridoma tissue culture supernatants should be buffered by the addition of 1/20 volume of 1 M Tris (pH 8.0).

2. If there is no reason to avoid the use of sodium azide, add to 0.02%.

3. Dispense the antibodies in convenient volumes and store at –20°C. For tissue culture supernatants, tubes of 2–5 ml are convenient. Most antibodies are stable for years when stored at –20°C.

4. Thaw individual tubes for use and store them at 4°C. Working solutions stored at 4°C are stable for months.

## Storing ascitic fluid



Acsites are tumors that normally form in the peritoneal cavity due to the growth of a leukemic cell. The acsites contain both the large number of tumor cells that are proliferating and the fluids that are secreting into the peritoneum in response to the tumor cells. If the tumor derives from a B cell, these fluids will contain most of the antibodies that are secreted by this cell. This ascitic fluid is an extremely concentrated solution of specific antibodies.

### Caution

Sodium azide, see Appendix IV.

*Ascitic fluid is prepared by injecting into the peritoneal cavity an oil, most often pristane, that acts as an irritant and then a selected hybridoma cell line. The cell line proliferates and the cells and fluid are removed. The fluid is separated from the hybridoma cells by centrifugation at 10,000g at 4°C and any remaining oil is removed.*

1. Ascitic fluids are well buffered without any further addition.

2. If there is no reason to avoid the use of sodium azide, add to 0.02%.

3. Dispense the antibodies in convenient volumes and store at –20°C or –70°C. For ascites, suitable sizes would be 100–500 μl per tube. Most ascites fluids are stable for years when stored at –70°C.

4. We do not recommend storing working samples of ascites at 4°C, because these preparations are often heavily contaminated with proteases. For long-term storage or repeated use, the antibodies present in ascites should be purified and used in this form.

## Storing purified antibodies



Purified antibodies can come from many different sources. For most purposes described in this book, these antibodies will be prepared as described in the next section or purchased from a commercial source. Antibodies from commercial sources are normally supplied with proper storage conditions.

### Caution

Sodium azide, see Appendix IV.

1. Purified preparations of antibodies are stable in most commonly used buffers. The pH should be kept near neutral; pHs between 7 and 8 show no deleterious effects, even over many years of storage. Salt concentrations between 0 and 150 mM are suitable for most applications, but little harm is caused with long-term storage in salt concentrations up to 500 mM. If no other indications are known, we recommend long-term storage in PBS or 50 mM Tris, pH 8.0.

2. If there is no reason to avoid the use of sodium azide, add it to 0.02%. Aliquot samples of the purified antibodies into convenient volumes and store frozen at –20°C.

3. Solutions of purified antibodies should be stored at relatively high concentrations (i.e., ≥ 1 mg/ml) at neutral pH. Concentrations up to 10 mg/ml are commonly used. Antibodies at lower concentrations should be concentrated prior to freezing. Any of the standard methods for concentration, such as ultrafiltration, can be used. Another simple method is to use protein A or protein G affinity column purification as a method of concentration (p. 74). If purified antibodies will not be labeled, they can be stored at lower concentrations with the addition of 1% BSA.

4. Working solutions can be thawed and stored conveniently at 4°C, where they are stable for months.

# Purifying antibodies

STORING, 64
PURIFYING
LABELING, 81

For most immunochemical techniques, crude preparations of monoclonal or polyclonal antibodies are perfectly useful and reliable. However, purified antibodies are required for a number of techniques. Table 4.1 lists the commonly used immunochemical techniques and the types of antibodies needed for each. Several techniques rely on purified antibodies, at least in some variations. There are several instances where purification of antibodies is needed.

Table 4.1 *Antibody requirements for commonly used techniques*

| Technique | Antibody use | Required antibodies | Preparatory action | Comments |
|---|---|---|---|---|
| **Immunostaining** | Direct localization of antigen | Labeled primary antibody | Purify and label yourself | Use only when needed |
| | Indirect localization of antigen | Unlabeled primary antibody and labeled secondary antibody | Buy commercial labeled secondary antibody | Recommended approach when possible |
| **Immunoassays** | Direct detection of antigen | Labeled primary antibody | Purify and label antibody | Use when needed |
| | Indirect detection of antigen | Unlabeled primary antibody and labeled secondary antibody | Buy commercial labeled secondary antibody | Use when needed |
| **Immunoblots** | Direct detection of antigen | Labeled primary antibody | Purify and label antibody | Use only when needed |
| | Indirect detection of antigen | Unlabeled primary antibody and labeled secondary antibody | Buy commercial labeled secondary antibody | Recommended approach |
| **Immunoaffinity** | Purification of antigen | Purified antibody | Purify yourself | |
| **Immuno-precipitation** | Small-scale purification of antigen | Unlabeled primary antibody and protein A/G beads | Buy commercial protein A/G beads | |

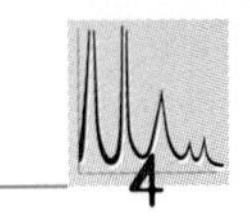


One common use for purified antibodies is in the direct detection method. Here an antibody is labeled with an easily identifiable "tag" and then used to bind and detect the antigen under study. In the indirect detection method, a primary antibody is not labeled but is detected by a labeled secondary antibody (an anti-immunoglobulin antibody). In general, the indirect method is recommended whenever possible, because reliable labeled secondary antibodies can be purchased cheaply from many commercial suppliers, and the indirect method demands less work but provides similar results.

Several methods do require labeled primary antibodies, however. For example, in immunostaining when the relative location of more than one antigen needs to be determined, it is often necessary to purify and label each antibody with a different tag. This allows the location of more than one antigen to be compared. In these cases, using an indirect detection method, in which a secondary reagent is used to locate an unlabeled primary antibody, is inappropriate. Another example, where tagging of a primary antibody is required, occurs when the sample has large amounts of irrelevant antibodies that would interfere with the detection of the primary antibody. This might occur when a mouse monoclonal antibody is used to locate an antigen in a mouse tissue section. In cases such as these, the primary antibody will need to be purified and then labeled directly as discussed below (p. 81).

A second technique that may require purified antibodies is immunoaffinity purification. In this technique, antibodies are covalently linked to a solid-phase matrix such as a cross-linked agarose or polyacrylamide bead. In one of the commonly used approaches, the antibodies are purified first and then added to beads that have been chemically activated to contain a combining site. Here a good preparation of purified antibodies is essential to allow the procedure to succeed.

A third instance that requires antibody purification is isolation of antigen-specific antibodies from a polyclonal serum. A polyclonal serum contains a complicated assortment of antibodies including those raised against the immunogen as well as the entire collection of antibodies that were present when the serum was collected. For some purposes, it is necessary to isolate the antibodies that are specific for the antigen under study. The most common example of this need is when using antipeptide antibodies. It is often important to isolate only those antibodies that recognize the peptide sequences. These types of purification allow the selection of antibodies with very specific activities.

Another use for purified antibodies is to lower background. Using purified antibodies in almost any technique will lower the nonspecific background. This effect is due primarily to the removal of contaminating proteins that are scoring inappropriately in the assay as well as to the ability to control precisely the amount of antibody needed to generate a positive signal. In no case does using purified antibodies cause an increase in the background, so this can be a potential troubleshooting step in any immunochemical assay.

Finally, purification of antibodies is often the easiest method to concentrate a preparation of antibodies. Any source of antibodies can be concentrated by using the protein A or protein G purification methods discussed below.

## Recommended methods for purification

Although there are a wide variety of methods to purify antibodies, we recommend purification on either protein A or protein G beads as the most useful technique. This

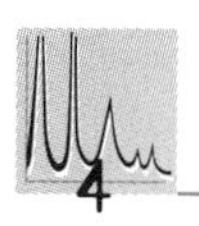



## Quantity and quality of purified antibodies

During the purification of antibodies, several variables need to be monitored. These include the purity, the amount, and the antigen-binding activity of the antibody. The individual methods to assess these variables are found in other sections, as noted below.

**Purity.** At any stage, the simplest method to determine the purity of an antibody solution is to run a portion of the sample on an SDS-polyacrylamide gel. The gel can be stained either with Coomassie blue (sensitivity 0.1–0.5 μg/band) or silver (sensitivity 1–10 ng/band) (see pp. 420–428).

**Quantitation.** If the antibody is not yet pure, a convenient method for quantitation will be to separate the heavy and light chains by SDS-polyacrylamide gel electrophoresis and compare the staining to known standard controls. If many samples need to be analyzed, it is easier to quantitate the amount of antibody in a immunoassay.

If the antibody is pure, either of these methods can be substituted by techniques that measure the total amount of protein. These include the methods described on pp. 448–453. A convenient method is UV absorbance. The amount of antibody can be determined by an absorbance measurement at 280 nm (1 OD = approximately 0.75 mg/ml of purified antibody).

**Antigen-binding activity.** In general, we recommend using the purified antibodies without worrying about changes in antigen-binding capacity. Purification using protein A or protein G resin seldom causes loss of activity. However, if the final antibody product is not functioning as you expect, it will be important to check loss of activity through the purification process. Compare the purified antibody to the starting material in a series of titrations, normalizing to the total amount of antibody in each preparation. This should give a good estimate of the loss of activity through purification.

technique is robust, offers sufficient purification for commonly used applications, and, with the commercial availability of both protein A and protein G matrices, allows all antibody sources to be purified. There are any number of methods that rely on conventional chromatography methods, and these are potentially useful in some settings. These methods include DEAE ion-exchange chromatography, ammonium sulfate precipitation, and many others. However, purification on either protein A or protein G affinity columns is as easy or easier than other methods and provides a fold purification that cannot be reached with other methods. Therefore, for all common applications, we recommend this approach.

One application where protein A or protein G affinity purification is not appropriate is when polyclonal antibodies need to be further separated and the fraction that is specific for the antigen under study needs to be isolated. Here an antigen-affinity column is used to bind and purify the antigen-specific antibodies. A simple method for this purification is included below for this specific need.

Table 4.2 summarizes the possible sources of antibodies for purification. Also included in this table are the possible sources of antibody contamination and the expected level of purity.

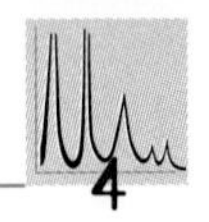

Table 4.2 *Sources for purifying antibodies*

| Source | Antibody type | Concentration, total antibody (in mg/ml) | Concentration, specific antibody (in mg/ml) | Contaminating antibodies | Possible purity of specific antibodies |
|---|---|---|---|---|---|
| **Serum** | Polyclonal | 10 | 1 at best (10% max) | Other serum antibodies | 10% at best[a] |
| **Tissue culture supernatant with 10% FBS** | Monoclonal | 1 | 0.05 (5% max) | Calf antibodies | >95%[b] |
| **Tissue culture supernatant with serum-free media** | Monoclonal | 0.05 | 0.05 (100%) | None | 95% |
| **Ascites** | Monoclonal | 1–10 | 0.9–9 (90%) | Mouse antibodies | 90% |

[a]Except for antigen affinity purification, where purity = 100%.
[b]On protein A affinity columns, bovine antibodies present in fetal serum will not bind efficiently.

## Antibody purification of protein A or protein G columns*

STORING, 64
PURIFYING
LABELING, 81

Protein A and protein G are bacterial cell wall proteins that bind to a domain in the Fc region of antibodies. This interaction is quite strong, but the affinity is sensitive to changes in pH. At neutral or slightly basic pH values, antibodies bind tightly to protein A or protein G. The antibody/protein A or antibody/protein G affinity is dramatically decreased by lowering the pH. The purification of antibodies on protein A or protein G affinity columns is based on these pH-sensitive changes in affinity.

Many commercial sources provide protein A or protein G covalently coupled to a variety of resins. For most purification strategies, a cross-linked agarose or polyacrylamide bead is the best choice, because these matrices have good chemical resistance, stand up well to the physical pressures of column chromatography, and are relatively inexpensive. In this procedure, these protein A or protein G beads are loaded into a column and a crude source of antibodies is passed down the column at a slightly basic pH. The antibodies bind to the protein A or protein G in the column. The column is then washed, and the antibodies are eluted with an acidic buffer. The pH of the eluate is adjusted to neutral, and the antibodies are now ready for further use. The method is rapid and nearly foolproof.

The only major variable that needs to be considered is the choice of protein A or protein G (Table 4.3). Each of these proteins binds a different spectrum of antibodies. In general, we recommend protein A for mouse monoclonal antibodies from the $IgG_{2a}$, $IgG_{2b}$, and $IgG_3$ subclasses and protein G for $IgG_1$. For monoclonal antibodies from other species, protein G is recommended. For polyclonal antibodies, protein A should be used for samples from rabbit, human, horse, donkey, pig, guinea pig, dog, or cow, whereas protein G is recommended for mouse, rat, and goat polyclonal antibodies.

Table 4.3 *Choice of protein A or protein G*

| Antibody source | Protein A | Protein G |
|---|---|---|
| **Monoclonal antibodies** | | |
| mouse $IgG_1$ | | ✓ |
| mouse $IgG_{2a}$, $IgG_{2b}$, $IgG_3$ | ✓ | |
| rat | | ✓ |
| **Polyclonal antibodies** | | |
| human | ✓ | |
| rabbit | ✓ | |
| mouse | | ✓ |
| rat | | ✓ |
| horse | | ✓ |
| goat | | ✓ |
| donkey | | ✓ |
| pig | ✓ | |
| guinea pig | ✓ | |
| dog | ✓ | |
| cow | | ✓ |

*Adapted from Ey et al. (1978).

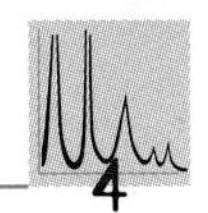


### Needed solutions

1.0 M Tris (pH 8.0)
100 mM Tris (pH 8.0)
10 mM Tris (pH 8.0)
50 mM glycine (pH 3.0)

### Special equipment

Simple column chromatography setup

### Cautions

Lithium chloride, SDS, see Appendix IV.

*Serum contains approximately 10 mg/ml of total IgG, tissue culture supernatants contain 20–50 μg/ml of monoclonal antibody, and ascites contains between 1 and 10 mg/ml.*

1. Adjust the pH of the crude antibody preparation (serum, tissue culture supernatant, or ascites) to 8.0 by adding 1/10 volume of 1.0 M Tris (pH 8.0).

2. Pass the antibody solution through a protein A or protein G bead column. These columns bind approximately 10–20 mg of antibody per milliliter of wet beads (each protein A or protein G molecule binds two molecules of antibody). Note the approximate volume of the column bed because the wash and elution buffers are measured in relative values compared to the volume of beads being used.

*As with all protein solutions, avoid excess mechanical action or contact with the air to minimalize protein denaturation.*

3. Wash the beads with 10 column volumes of 100 mM Tris (pH 8.0).

4. Wash the beads with 10 column volumes of 10 mM Tris (pH 8.0).

5. Elute the column with 50 mM glycine (pH 3.0). Add this buffer stepwise at approximately 1/2 column volume per step (see Fig. 9.2 for example). Collect the eluate from each step in tubes containing 1/10 column volume of 1 M Tris (pH 8.0). Mix each tube gently to bring the pH back to neutral.

6. Identify the immunoglobulin-containing fractions by absorbance at 280 nm (1 OD = approximately 0.75 mg/ml) or by Bradford dye binding spot test (pp. 451 and 459). Combine the antibody-containing fractions and measure purity by running 2 μg of total protein in a SDS-polyacrylamide gel and staining with Coomassie blue. Good purification should yield essentially pure heavy- and light-chain bands (Fig. 4.1).

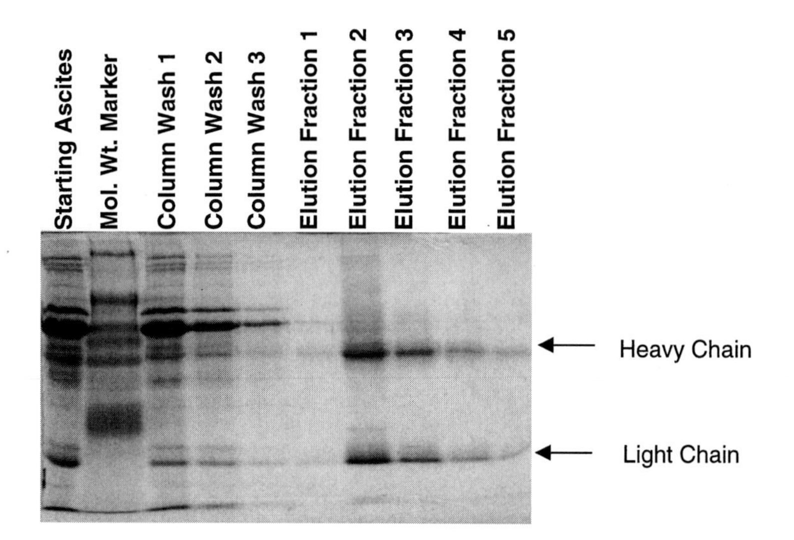


Figure 4.1
Purification of antibodies from a protein A/G column.

## Common problems

The only common problem encountered in using protein A or protein G columns is the rare antibody source that does not bind well to these resins. In this case, we recommend raising the salt concentration in the binding and wash buffers. The interactions between the protein A or protein G with the Fc of the antibody are primarily hydrophobic. Adding high salt will favor these interactions and increase the binding capacity. Sodium chloride concentrations to 3.3 M are appropriate.

In some cases, the antibodies that are being collected may be damaged by the low pH elution. Different species of antibodies or different subclasses will elute at different acidic pHs. The method above uses one pH for elution, and this should be appropriate in all but the rarest of cases. However, less acidic pH values can often be used to elute. Use a gradient of increasingly lower pH values to determine the mildest conditions for the elution of the desired antibodies.

For analytical work in which more than one antibody will be purified on the same column, extreme care must be taken. Because different antibodies have varied affinities for protein A or protein G, it is easy to contaminate one batch with the residual from a previous run. For bulk purification we recommend dedicating one column to the particular antibody source. The column can be stored in the presence of Merthiolate at 4°C and reused when needed. If the same column must be used for multiple antibody sources, washing columns sequentially with 2 M urea, 1 M lithium chloride, and 100 mM glycine (pH 2.5) will be sufficient for most needs.

# Purification of antibodies on an antigen column*

STORING, 64
PURIFYING
LABELING, 81

Immunoaffinity purification is the only method commonly used to purify antigen-specific antibodies from a preparation of polyclonal antibodies. In this procedure, pure antigen is bound covalently to a solid support. The antibodies within the polyclonal pool that are specific for the antigen are allowed to bind. The unbound antibodies are removed by washing, and the specific antibodies are eluted. This method is not appropriate for monoclonal antibodies, which are already homogeneous in their antigen-binding activity.

There are two situations in which immunoaffinity purifications of antibodies are commonly needed. The first is in the preparation of antipeptide antibodies. For these approaches, synthetic peptides representing a sequence for which antibodies are needed are coupled to a carrier protein to produce an effective immunogen. After polyclonal antibodies are raised against the peptide–conjugate complex, they frequently are not ready for use until the antibodies that specifically recognize the peptide are separated from the bulk of the antibodies in the sera. Thus, immunoaffinity purification serves two needs here. It separates the desired antibodies from those that have been raised against the carrier protein, and it concentrates the specific antipeptide antibodies, changing their relative concentration from being dilute in the sera to being the prominent species.

The second major use of immunoaffinity purification of antibodies is the more general need to remove an unwanted activity in a polyclonal antibody preparation. Both specific and nonspecific background problems are normally much worse when using polyclonal antibodies. One useful method to remove an unwanted nonspecific activity is to purify the desired antibodies on an antigen column. This will greatly reduce the spurious antibodies that confuse an immunochemical result. The method is cumbersome, but the results can turn a poor antiserum into a valuable reagent.

## Needed solutions

100 mM glycine (pH 2.5)
0.5 M sodium phosphate (pH 7.5)
1 M NaCl, 0.05 sodium phosphate (pH 7.5)
10 mM Tris (pH 7.5)
500 mM sodium chloride, 10 mM Tris (pH 7.5)
10 mM Tris (pH 8.8)
1 M Tris (pH 8.0)
100 mM ethanolamine (pH 7.5)
PBS
100 mM triethylamine (pH 11.5, prepared fresh)

## Special equipment

Simple column chromatography setup

## Cautions

Ethanolamine, potassium thiocyanate, SDS, sodium azide, triethylamine, see Appendix IV.

*Adapted from Campbell et al. (1951).

*The antibody preparations must not contain extraneous compounds in the buffer that will combine with reactive groups on the activated beads. Most often the coupling reactions will target amino groups in the antibody (or thiol groups, if using tosyl chloride). If these compounds have been used during the purification, the antibody preparation should be extensively dialyzed against the binding buffer of 0.5 M sodium phosphate (pH 7.5).*

1. Covalently attach the antigen to a solid support. The easiest approach is to couple the antigen to an activated bead. A number of different supports are available commercially, and use of these activated matrices is discussed in Chapter 9. If there are no reasons to avoid their use, our first recommendation would be to use a matrix with a flexible spacer arm which will keep the active site for binding to the antigen a reasonable distance from the bead itself. Commercial sources of these activated beads are shown in Table 9.4.

   If using a polypeptide antigen, the antigen should be linked directly to the activated bead.

   If using a peptide antigen, it is preferable to link the peptide directly to the bead without first linking it to a carrier molecule. If your synthesis has left a single free amino or cystyl group at either end, it is best to bind the peptide directly to the bead through this group. In the unlikely event that these groups were not part of the synthesis, the peptide should first be coupled to a carrier molecule in the same manner that the antigen was prepared. The carrier must be distinct from that used for immunization (e.g., one could use BSA-peptides for purification of antibodies raised against KLH-peptides). If not, you will also be purifying the antibodies specific for the carrier. Although any type of molecule could theoretically be used as a carrier, we recommend using another large protein that will resemble how the peptide-conjugate was presented during the immunization.

2. Prepare a solution of antigen in 0.5 M sodium phosphate (pH 7.5). Save a small sample to determine the binding efficiency (to be checked in step 5). The amount of antigen to be coupled will vary depending on the individual experiment. For most purposes, 10 mg of antigen per milliliter of beads will yield a high-capacity column.

*As with all protein solutions, avoid excess mechanical action or contact with the air to minimalize protein denaturation.*

3. Add the activated beads prepared as described by the manufacturer.

4. Mix gently for 2 hours at room temperature or overnight at 4°C on a rocker.

5. Wash the beads twice with 0.5 M sodium phosphate (pH 7.5). Save the supernatant from the overnight binding. Compare the amount of protein from the "before" and "after" samples of the binding buffers. This is usually done by comparing the absorbance at 280 nm if the antigen contains tyrosine, tryptophan, or phenylalanine residues. Alternatively, SDS-polyacrylamide gels stained with Coomassie blue can be used.

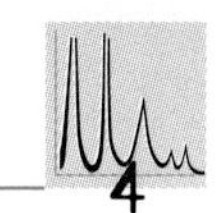

6. Wash the beads once with 1 M sodium chloride, 0.05 M sodium phosphate (pH 7.5).

7. Add 10 volumes of 100 mM ethanolamine (pH 7.5). Incubate at room temperature for 4 hours or overnight at 4°C with gentle mixing.

8. Wash twice with PBS.

9. Transfer the beads with the bound antigen to a column. In a preliminary wash, it is important to remove any antigen that might be removed by the conditions used to elute the antibodies. In this example, the antibodies are released by both low pH and high pH, so the column is washed first with these buffers.

   Wash the column with 10 bed-volumes of 10 mM Tris (pH 7.5). Then wash with 10 bed-volumes of 100 mM glycine (pH 2.5), followed by 10 volumes of 10 mM Tris (pH 8.8). Check the pH of the last drops of the Tris wash. If it is not 8.8, continue the wash. Then add 10 bed-volumes of 100 mM triethylamine (pH 11.5, prepared fresh). Wash with 10 mM Tris (pH 7.5) until the pH reaches 7.5.

*High-pH and low-pH cycles will elute only a portion of the antibodies that are bound to the column. Some high-affinity antibodies will not be eluted under these conditions, and so these columns eventually will lose antibody-binding capacity. If this becomes a serious practical problem and making a new column is prohibited, then elution in harsher reagents such as 1.5 M potassium thiocyanate, 4 M urea, or 3.5 M $MgCl_2$ may regenerate the column and may produce useful antibody preparations depending on the characteristics of the antibodies.*

10. Pass the polyclonal serum through the column to bind the antibody. The serum should be free of any debris prior to loading on the column. If there is any debris, remove it by centrifugation or purification of the antibodies by protein A or protein G chromatography (p. 74). If using whole serum, dilute the serum 1 in 10 in 10 mM Tris (pH 7.5) prior to loading. The antibody solution should be passed through the column at a slow flow rate using a peristaltic pump.

11. Wash the column with 20 bed-volumes of 10 mM Tris (pH 7.5), and then with 20 bed-volumes of 500 mM sodium chloride, 10 mM Tris (pH 7.5).

12. Elute the antibodies that are bound by acid-sensitive interactions by passing 10 bed-volumes of 100 mM glycine (pH 2.5) through the column. Collect the eluate in a tube containing 1 bed-volume of 1 M Tris (pH 8.0).

13. Wash the column with 10 mM Tris (pH 8.8) until the pH rises to 8.8.

14. Elute the antibodies that are bound by base-sensitive interactions by passing 10 bed-volumes of 100 mM triethylamine (pH 11.5, prepared fresh) through the column. Collect the eluate in a tube containing 1 bed-volume of 1 M Tris (pH 8.0).

15. Wash the column with 10 mM Tris (pH 7.5) until the pH is 7.5. The column may be reused by storing it in buffers with 0.01% Merthiolate.

16. Combine the antibody fractions and dialyze against PBS with 0.02% sodium azide. If necessary, concentrate the antibody solution by running on a protein A or protein G column (p. 74).

## Common problems

The major strength of this method is its unique ability to isolate specific antibodies from a mixed population. Its principal disadvantages are that it requires large amounts of antigen and that elution of the specific antibody requires conditions that can lead to some loss of activity.

If only minor amounts of antigen are available, there may not be a suitable method to immunoaffinity-purify the desired antibodies. One potential source that is often overlooked is the purification of antibodies from antigens transferred to nitrocellulose after immunoblotting. This will not yield large sources of antibodies but may provide sufficient quantities for analytical studies.

If the antibodies do not elute readily from the column or the eluted antibodies no longer will bind to the antigen, other elution conditions must be tried. Immunoaffinity purification is discussed in detail in Chapter 9, where it is used to isolate antigens. The principles for both types of affinity purifications are identical, and the elution conditions suggested there can be tried.

In some cases, small amounts of antigen will leach off the antigen columns. If the assays for which the affinity-purified antibodies are being prepared are sensitive to contamination with the antigen (e.g., enzyme assays), then the individual batches of eluted antibodies will need to be tested for the presence of the antigen.

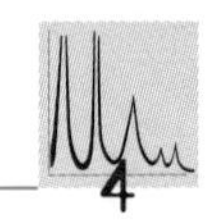


# Labeling antibodies

STORING, 64

PURIFYING, 70

LABELING

A wide range of immunological techniques depend on the use of labeled antibodies. The main reason for labeling an antibody is to locate and, in some cases, quantitate an antigen when it is displayed among a complicated array of other molecules. Because antibodies have high affinity for their antigen partners, having an easily detected label attached to the antibody allows the antigen to be localized, ideally in a rapid, cheap, and quantitative manner.

The three methods discussed in this manual that may need labeled antibodies are immunostaining, immunoblotting, and immunoassays. In all three of these cases, antigens in a complex setting can be located and, with appropriate controls, quantitated. For immunostaining, the goal is to locate the antigen while it is displayed in its normal cellular environment. In this setting, all antigens are exposed to the antibody, which then binds to its cognate antigen. When the antibody is labeled, the location of the antigen can be accurately determined. For immunoblotting, all the proteins in a complex mixture are denatured and separated by gel electrophoresis. All of the separated proteins are transferred to a membrane, and the antigen under study is then located by using a labeled antibody to find it among the array of displayed proteins. For immunoassays, a wide variety of formats are used to display or capture the antigen, which is then located and quantitated by using a labeled antibody. All of these techniques rely on labeled antibodies to locate the antigen.

The major decisions that need to be made when preparing for these methods are whether direct or indirect methods will be used to locate the antigen and what type of label will best fit the demands of the technique. These two issues are discussed below.

## Direct versus indirect detection

Detection techniques can be divided into two general classes—direct and indirect methods. In the direct method, an antibody is purified, labeled with an easily detected tag, and used to bind directly to the antigen. The antigen is then detected by whatever label has been added to the antibody. In the indirect method, the antibody is unlabeled and need not be purified. It binds to the antigen, unbound antibodies are removed by washing, and the antigen/antibody complex is detected by a secondary reagent, such as labeled anti-immunoglobulin antibodies or labeled protein A or protein G. In all of these settings, the antibody that binds to the antigen is referred to as the primary antibody, and it is labeled in the direct detection methods but unlabeled in the indirect methods. An antibody that binds to the primary antibody is known as a secondary antibody, and in these cases it will always be labeled (Fig. 4.2).

The choice of the direct or indirect method depends on the circumstances of the experiment (Table 4.4). The use of a labeled primary antibody in a direct detection method involves fewer steps and is less prone to background problems, but is less sensitive than indirect methods. It also requires a new labeling step for each antibody to be studied. In contrast, indirect methods offer the advantages of stronger signals and widely available labeled reagents. Also, the primary antibody is not modified so the loss of activity is avoided. Therefore, for the majority of applications the indirect methods are the most useful.

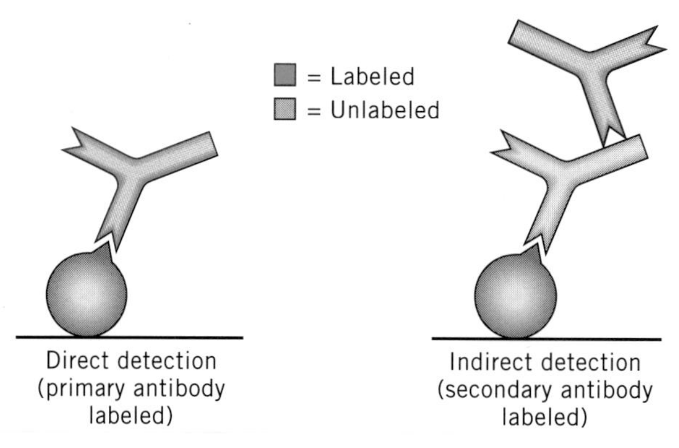


Figure 4.2
Direct versus indirect detection.

When labeled secondary antibodies are used, it is seldom worthwhile to prepare and label these reagents yourself. They can be purchased from a number of commercial sources, where they are prepared and tested in large, economic batches. Therefore, whenever possible, we recommend using indirect methods of detection and commercial reagents.

There are several cases in which directly labeled antibodies are essential. The most common use is for colocalization studies in which two or more antigens need to be localized in the same cell or tissue sample. Here, each antibody must be purified and labeled with a different tag to allow comparison of the location of each antigen. In addition, there are times when the background of an assay interferes with the readout, and labeled primary antibodies may be a useful approach. Finally, for immunoassays where good quantification is needed, labeled primary antibodies may be essential.

Table 4.4 *Choice of direct or indirect method*

| Detection method | Direct detection | Indirect detection |
|---|---|---|
| **Location of label** | Labeled primary antibodies | Labeled secondary antibodies |
| **Advantages** | Fewer steps<br>Less prone to background | Stronger signals<br>Widely available labeled reagents<br>Primary antibody is not modified<br>Easier |
| **Disadvantages** | Less sensitive<br>New labeling step required for each antibody to be studied<br>More difficult | More prone to bad backgrounds |

## Choice of label

Regardless of whether the direct or indirect method will be used, the most crucial decision is the choice of label. Table 4.5 lists the most commonly used labels, their advantages and disadvantages, and their preferred use. The choice of label for some techniques is very straightforward. For example, fluorescent labels are essential for cell sorting or high-resolution immunostaining. Routine immunohistology is most satisfactory with enzyme-labeled antibodies. With the widespread use of chemiluminescence, enzyme-labeled reagents have become the agent of choice for immunoblots. For other techniques the choice is less clear, as, for example, both enzyme-labeled and iodinated antibodies perform well in immunoassays. As a very broad generalization, enzyme labels offer the advantage of an instant visual result and great sensitivity but are more difficult to use in quantitative assay. This is because of the need to measure the rate of the enzyme reaction to get a true measure of the amount of bound enzyme and because the enzyme-labeled reagents are not homogeneous. Fluorescence is an excellent method to determine the precise subcellular localization. Iodine-labeled reagents, in particular directly iodinated monoclonal antibodies, can give strikingly accurate quantitative results in immunoassays.

### Biotinylation

Biotinylation of the primary antibody is an underexploited solution to many labeling difficulties. The biotinylation reaction is simple and mild, and rarely inactivates the antibody. Biotinylated antibodies can be stored for years without loss of specific activity. The secondary reagents avidin and streptavidin, which bind to the biotin groups, are available commercially in essentially all labeled forms. In addition, avidin and streptavidin show very low levels of background binding and bind so tightly and with such speed that the disadvantages of a multistep procedure are greatly reduced. A major advantage of biotinylation is that after the primary antibody is labeled, a choice can be made later to determine which avidin or streptavidin-labeled secondary reagent will be used.

## Caution

Biotin, see Appendix IV.

Table 4.5 *Choice of label*

| Label | Recommended applications | Direct or indirect | Detection methods | Advantages | Disadvantages |
|---|---|---|---|---|---|
| **Fluorochromes** | Immunostaining | Direct or indirect | Fluorescence microscopy | Long shelf life<br>Good resolution | Autofluorescence |
| **Biotin** | Immunostaining<br>Immunoassays<br>Immunoblots | Direct or indirect | Avidin or streptavidin coupled to various labels | Long shelf life<br>High sensitivity<br>Universal detection<br>Many detection methods | Multiple steps<br>Endogenous biotin |
| **Enzyme** | Immunoblots<br>Immunostaining | Indirect | Chromogenic substrates | Long shelf life<br>High sensitivity<br>Can visualize by eye | Multiple steps<br>Endogenous enzymes<br>Low resolution |
| **Iodine** | Immunoassays | Direct or indirect | Gamma-counter<br>X-ray film | Easy to quantitate<br>High sensitivity | Short half-life<br>Potential health hazard |
| **Biosynthesis** | Immunoassays<br>Immunoblots | Direct | Beta-counter<br>X-ray film | No damage to antibody<br>Easy | Requires hybridomas<br>Low sensitivity<br>Short half life |

# Labeling antibodies with fluorochromes*

STORING, 64
PURIFYING, 70
LABELING

One of the most useful types of labels that are attached to antibodies are fluorochromes. Under the appropriate illumination, these labels fluoresce, allowing the localization of the antibodies and, through them, the distribution of the antigen under study. These methods for detection are described in Chapter 5 (p. 136). Most often these methods use indirect detection and rely on a labeled secondary antibody that is specific for unlabeled primary antibody. For indirect work, suitable secondary reagents labeled with a number of fluorochromes are available commercially. However, in some cases direct labeling of the primary antibody is needed. Direct labeling of purified antibodies is the method of choice when simultaneously visualizing two antibodies of the same species, class, or subclass. This allows the localization of two antigens to be compared in the same cell, tissue, or sample.

Four fluorochromes are in common use: fluorescein, rhodamine, Texas Red, and phycoerythrin. The properties of these fluorochromes are summarized in Table 5.3 (p. 129). A method for labeling of antibodies with the isothiocyanate derivatives of fluorescein and rhodamine is given below. Methods for labeling antibodies or other proteins with Texas Red or the phycoerythrins are not commonly used except for commercial applications.

## Thinking ahead

Before beginning this labeling method, you will need a source of purified antibodies (see p. 70). The antibody solution will need to be adjusted to pH 9.0 and should not contain any extraneous molecules with free amino groups. Dialysis against 0.1 M sodium borate or sodium carbonate at pH 9 is sufficient. The column for purification can be prepared days in advance and stored by equilibration with buffer containing 1% BSA and 0.02% sodium azide.

## Needed solutions

PBS
1 mg/ml FITC or TRITC in DMSO (made fresh)
1 M Ammonium chloride
1% Xylene cyanol
Glycerol
10% Sodium azide

## Special equipment

Simple gel filtration column

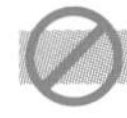

## Cautions

Ammonium chloride, DMSO, FITC, sodium azide, sodium borate, TRITC, xylene cyanol, see Appendix IV.

Prepare the gel filtration column that will be used to separate the labeled antibody from the free fluorochrome after the completion of the reaction. Use a gel matrix with an exclusion limit of 20,000–50,000 for globular proteins. Use fine-sized beads (approximately 50 μm in diameter). To

*Riggs et al. (1958); The and Feltkamp (1970a,b); Goding (1976).

determine the size of the column that is needed, multiply the total volume of the coupling reaction (see below) by 20. Prepare a column of this size according to the manufacturer's instructions (swelling, etc.). Pass 20 column volumes of PBS through the column. Allow the column to run until the buffer level drops just below the top of the bed resin. Stop the flow of the column either by using a valve at the bottom of the column or by plugging the end with modeling clay or Parafilm.

2. Prepare an antibody solution of at least 2 mg/ml in 0.1 M sodium borate or carbonate (pH 9.0). Be sure to avoid the presence of extraneous molecules with primary amines.

3. Dissolve the fluorescein isothiocyanate (FITC) or tetramethylrhodamine isothiocyanate (TRITC) in anhydrous dimethyl sulfoxide (DMSO) (best grade available) at 1 mg/ml. Prepare fresh for each labeling reaction.

4. For each 1 ml of protein solution, add 50 μl of the dye solution. The dye should be added very slowly in 5-μl aliquots, and the protein solution should be gently but continuously mixed during the addition.

5. Leave the reaction in the dark for 1 hour at 4°C.

6. Add ammonium chloride to 50 mM. Incubate for 2 hours at room temperature. Add xylene cyanol to 0.1% and glycerol to 5%.

7. Separate the unbound dye from the conjugate by gel filtration. Carefully layer the coupling reaction on the top of the column. Open the block to the column and allow the antibody solution to flow into the column until it just enters the column bed. Carefully add PBS to the top of the column and connect to a buffer supply. The conjugated antibody elutes first and can usually be seen under room light.

*The conjugated antibody can be seen more easily when viewed on a white background.*

8. Store the conjugate at 4°C in the column buffer in a lightproof container. If appropriate, add sodium azide to 0.02%.

9. For fluorescein coupling, the ratio of fluorescein to protein can be estimated by measuring the absorbance at 495 nm and 280 nm. For rhodamine, measure at 550 nm and 280 nm. The ratio of absorbance for fluorescein (495 nm/280 nm) should be between 0.3 and 1.0; for rhodamine (550 nm/280 nm), between 0.3 and 0.7. Ratios below these yield low signals, and higher ratios show high backgrounds. If the ratios are too low, repeat the conjugation using lower levels of antibody and higher levels of dye. If higher levels are found, either repeat the labeling with appropriate changes or purify

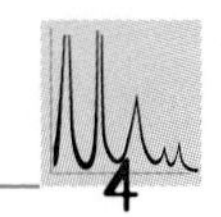


the labeled antibodies further on a DEAE ion-exchange column. Equilibrate and load the column with 10 mM potassium phosphate (pH 8.0). Elute with increasing salt concentrations. Measure the ratios (495/280 or 550/280) of each fraction and select and pool the appropriate fractions.

## Common problems

The major problem encountered is either over- or undercoupling. Overcoupling may block the antigen recognition site or may give high numbers of fluorochromes on the surface of the antibody molecule that will be sites for nonspecific binding. This will lead to more background. Undercoupling will reduce the signal strength and make detection more difficult. Therefore, for each antibody preparation, there will be an optimal ratio of fluorochromes to antibody that will balance these problems. Thankfully, there are simple methods to measure the coupling efficiency of these reactions using simple ratio of absorbance, so the amount of coupling can be adjusted accordingly.

# Labeling antibodies with biotin*

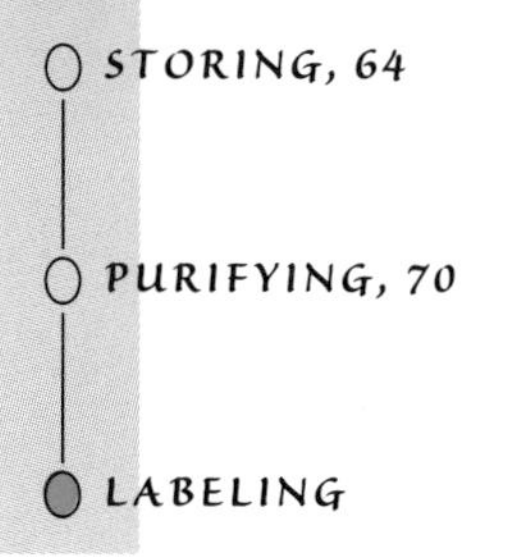


Antibodies can be easily modified to contain biotin. In turn, the biotin groups can act as binding groups for streptavidin or avidin, either of which is available commercially coupled with enzymes, fluorescent dyes, or iodine. This allows a single purified antibody, once coupled to biotin, to be detected with any of a wide variety of different labels. The affinity of streptavidin and avidin for biotin is exceptionally high ($K_a$ $10^{15}$ liter $mol^{-1}$), and therefore the interaction is essentially irreversible. Streptavidin is preferred for most applications because it has a more favorable pI, and therefore the backgrounds will be lower.

Labeling antibodies by covalent coupling of biotinyl groups is a very simple and straightforward technique. Biotinylation normally does not have any adverse affect on the antibody, and the coupling conditions are mild. The sensitivity of detection with the avidin- or streptavidin-labeled reagents is similar to those found when using equivalently labeled anti-immunoglobulin reagents. Becker and Wilchek (1972), Heitzmann and Richards (1974), and Heggeness and Ash (1977) all provide examples of the first uses of biotin and avidin complexes; Green (1963, 1990) has detailed reviews of biotin and avidin interactions.

Most biotinylations are performed using an *N*-hydroxysuccinimide ester of biotin. The succinimide group binds to free amino groups on the antibody, normally lysyl side

Table 4.6 *Available spacer arms and their characteristics*

| Coupling target | Compound type | Reactive group | Side chain | Comments | Sources |
|---|---|---|---|---|---|
| $-NH_2$ | NHS-biotin | Hydroxysuccinimide | 5 atoms | DMSO or DMF soluble | Pierce Chemical, Boehringer Mannheim, Bio-Rad, Zymed, Sigma, Calbiochem-Novabiochem, ICN Biomedicals, Molecular Probes |
| | Sulfo-NHS-biotin | Hydroxysuccinimide | 5 atoms | Water soluble | Pierce Chemical, Calbiochem-Novabiochem, Molecular Probes |
| | NHS-X-biotin | Hydroxysuccinimide | 12 atoms | DMSO or DMF soluble | Pierce Chemical, Boehringer Mannheim, LT Industries, Zymed, Sigma, Calbiochem-Novabiochem, Molecular Probes |
| | Sulfo-NHS-X-biotin | Hydroxysuccinimide | 12 atoms | Water soluble | Pierce Chemical, Calbiochem-Novabiochem, Molecular Probes |
| | NHS-X-X-biotin | Hydroxysuccinimide | 19 atoms | DMSO or DMF soluble | Pierce Chemical, CLONTECH, Calbiochem-Novabiochem, Molecular Probes |
| | Sulfo-NHS-X-X-biotin | Hydroxysuccinimide | 19 atoms | Water soluble | Pierce Chemical, Molecular Probes |
| –SH | Biotin-maleimide | Maleimide | 13 atoms | DMSO or DMF soluble | Molecular Probes |
| | Biotin-BMCC | Maleimide | 16 atoms | DMSO or DMF soluble | Pierce Chemical |
| | Iodoacetyl-X-biotin | Iodoacetyl | 14 atoms | DMSO or DMF soluble | Pierce Chemical, Molecular Probes |
| Any | Photobiotin | 35 nm visible light | 14 atoms | Water soluble | Pierce Chemical |

*Bayer et al. (1976); Guesdon et al. (1979); Bayer and Wilchek (1980).

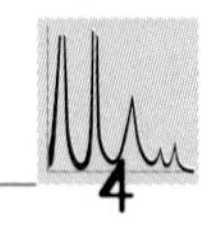

chains. Many biotinylated esters are now available. Most of these variations alter the size and characteristics of the spacer arm between the coupling group and the biotin. For some applications, the spacer arms may be critical. For example, a longer spacer arm will provide easier access to the biotin group and more flexibility, although longer arms will also provide more sites for nonspecific binding. Some spacer arms will be cleavable and, therefore, allow release of the antibody under controlled conditions. Table 4.6 lists many of the available spacer arms and their characteristics. All the esters are handled in a similar manner to the technique listed below. Unless there are reasons to the contrary, we recommend *N*-hydroxysuccinimide biotin as a starting reagent.

## Thinking ahead

Before beginning this labeling procedure you will need a source of purified antibodies (see p. 70). As discussed below, the antibodies will need to be adjusted to pH 8.8 with the addition of borate buffer. Any extraneous molecules with primary amines must be avoided. Before beginning, it is important to calculate the number of biotin ester molecules per antibody molecules that you wish to achieve. For most applications we recommend beginning at approximately 4:1.

## Needed solutions and compounds

PBS
1 M Ammonium chloride
10% Sodium azide
Your chosen biotin ester (see Table 4.6 and the discussion above)

## Caution

Ammonium chloride, biotin, DMF, DMSO, sodium azide, see Appendix IV.

1. Prepare a solution of *N*-hydroxysuccinimide biotin at 10 mg/ml in anhydrous DMSO.

2. Prepare an antibody solution of at least 1–3 mg/ml in sodium borate buffer (0.1 M, pH 8.8). If antibodies have been stored in sodium azide, the azide must be removed prior to coupling. Dialyze the solution extensively against the borate buffer to remove the azide.

*Using multiple reactions with different ester/antibody molar ratios (3:1, 10:1, 30:1) allows different levels of coupling to be tested side by side.*

3. Add the biotin ester to the antibody at a ratio of 25–100 μg of ester per mg of antibody. Mix well and incubate at room temperature for 4 hours. The DMSO concentration should not drop below a final concentration of 5% before the reaction is complete; otherwise the biotin ester precipitates.

   High concentrations of the biotin ester will lead to multiple biotin groups binding to the antibody and will increase the probability that all of the antibodies will be labeled. Lower ratios will keep biotinylation to a minimum (25 μg of ester per mg of antibody gives an initial molar ratio of ~10:1).

4. Add 20 μl of 1 M ammonium chloride per 250 μg of ester. Incubate for 10 minutes at room temperature.

5. Dialyze the antibody solution against PBS or other desired buffer to remove uncoupled biotin. The biotin dialyzes more slowly than would be expected for its size, so extensive dialysis is needed. Alternatively, repurify the antibody on a protein A or protein G column (p. 74).

6. Store as for pure antibody (p. 69).

## Common problems

After coupling, the activity of the antibody may have been decreased. This normally occurs when a free amino group forms a portion of the antibody that is essential for activity, normally in the antigen-combining site. In these cases, biotinylation lowers or destroys the antigen-binding capacity of the protein. This can be determined by comparing the activity of coupled antibodies in a titration with similar amounts of purified antibodies in assays commonly used in your lab.

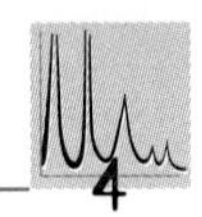


# Labeling antibodies with iodine*

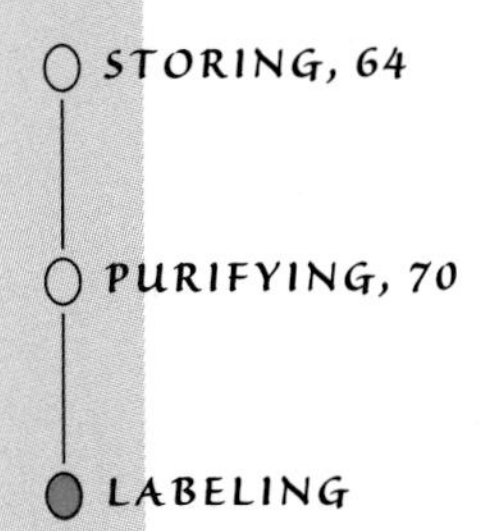


Iodination of antibodies or other proteins is a straightforward and effective method of labeling. Radioactive iodine is readily detectable using gamma counters or film. Although some forms of iodine are volatile and care must be used when handling this radionuclide, iodinated antibodies do not pose any unreasonable hazard if handled correctly. The ease of detection and quantitation makes them an ideal choice in some settings. The major use is in immunoassays, although other techniques can be adopted conveniently to iodine detection method.

The most commonly used radioisotope of iodine is $^{125}I$. The decay of $^{125}I$ yields low-energy gamma and X-ray radiation and, therefore, is easy to detect. The 60-day half-life of $^{125}I$ is a convenient compromise between effective shelf life and waste disposal.

When sodium iodide is exposed to a strong oxidant, the iodide is converted to iodine ($I_2$), which is then free to attack available moieties by a halogenation reaction. For proteins, the most frequent target is tyrosine, but some histidine residues will also be iodinated. These reactions are simple to manipulate, and high specific activities can be achieved routinely.

A number of approaches can be used to label proteins with iodine. Because this method of labeling antibodies is commonly used just for immunoassay work, we have given only a simple chemical oxidation method here. In the chemical iodination procedure, the iodide-125 (normally supplied as NaI) is oxidized to form iodine-125 ($I_2$), which attacks tyrosyl and histidyl side chains. The oxidation is initiated by a chemical oxidant. Chemical oxidants are normally harsher but are less troublesome to manipulate than enzymatic methods. In this method, the oxidant IODO-GEN (1,3,4,6-tetrachloro-3a,6α-diphenyl-glycoluril) is dissolved in a volatile organic solvent such as chloroform or methylene chloride. The solution is added to a test tube, and the solvent is allowed to evaporate. IODO-GEN is not soluble in water, so aqueous solutions will not remove it from the tube. Next, the reaction mixture of $Na^{125}I$ and protein is added. The oxidation is terminated by removing the mixture from the tube, and the iodinated proteins are separated from unincorporated label by gel filtration chromatography.

## Thinking ahead

Before beginning this procedure, it is extremely valuable to make sure the area in which the iodination will be done is completely set up for this procedure. In addition to meeting all of your institute's safety standards, make sure that you are completely familiar with potential problems and their solutions. It is a good idea to have all of your material laid out in a convenient manner. Have a suitable counter going to constantly monitor for any contaminated area and have extra gloves available to change into if any iodine should contaminate your outer glove.

Prior to the iodination, prepare the IODO-GEN tubes (step 1) and the gel filtration column (step 2). These can be prepared well in advance of the labeling. You will need a preparation of purified antibodies (0.2 to 1.0 mg/ml) in 0.5 M phosphate buffer at pH 7.5 (p. 465). Immediately before use, prepare the IODO-GEN stop tube (step 3).

*Fraker and Speck (1978)

## Special equipment

You will need a fume hood with appropriate ventilation for $^{125}I$, a handheld monitor to detect $^{125}I$, sufficient shielding to protect you and the area from radiation, and bins for proper storage and eventual disposal of $^{125}I$. In addition, you will need a simple disposable column that can be used for gel filtration.

## Needed solutions

PBS with 0.02% sodium azide
Carrier-free $Na^{125}$ iodide.

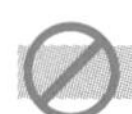

## Caution

Chloroform, $^{125}I$, sodium azide, xylene cyanol, see Appendix IV.

1. At any time prior to the iodination, prepare IODO-GEN-coated tubes (two 6-mm soda glass or 1.5-ml conical tubes are convenient). Dissolve the IODO-GEN (Pierce Chemical, 28600) at 0.5 μg/ml in chloroform. Dispense into appropriate tubes at 100 μl and at 20 μl per tube. Allow the chloroform to evaporate overnight in a fume hood. Store the tubes in a desiccator at room temperature; they are stable for several years. The tubes coated with 20 μl of IODO-GEN will give a slower rate of iodination, so they can be used if the normal reaction seems to cause damage to the antibody.

*A convenient column for one-time use can be prepared either in a 1-ml or 2-ml syringe barrel with a glass fiber filter cut to fit the bottom of the barrel, or in a disposable pipet with a portion of the cotton plug or some glass wool pushed to the bottom of the pipet.*

2. Immediately prior to the iodination, prepare a gel filtration column to separate the labeled antibody from the iodotyrosine generated during the addition of the stop buffer. Use a gel matrix with an exclusion limit of 20,000–50,000 for globular proteins. Use medium-sized beads (approximately 100 μm in diameter). Prepare the column with 1 ml of bead volume according to the manufacturer's instructions (swelling, etc.). This column will be discarded at the end of the labeling, so choose a suitable column. To keep the nonspecific binding of the iodinated proteins to a minimum, the column should be prerun with a minimum of 10 column volumes of 1% BSA/PBS with 0.02% sodium azide. Then wash the column with 10 volumes of PBS to remove the BSA. Alternatively, swell the beads in buffer containing BSA. Wash with PBS prior to use. Allow the column to run until the buffer level drops just below the top of the bed resin. Stop the flow of the column either by using a valve at the bottom of the column or by plugging the end with modeling clay.

3. Immediately prior to the iodination, prepare a "stop tube" that will be used to terminate the oxidation and capture all of the unincorporated iodine. To a 1.5-ml conical tube, add 50 μl of IODO-GEN-stop buffer (10 mg/ml of tyrosine [saturated], 10% glycerol, 0.1% xylene cyanol in PBS).

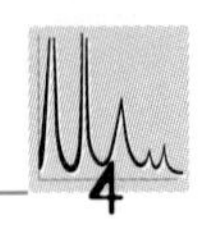

4. Behind appropriate shielding in a fume hood, add 50 μl of antibody to an IODO-GEN-coated tube at room temperature. The antibody should be at a concentration of 0.2–1 mg/ml in 0.5 M sodium phosphate buffer (pH 7.5).

*Other buffers can be used, but no reducing agents should be included.*

5. Add 500 μCi of $Na^{125}$ iodide to the IODO-GEN tube with the antibody. Dispose of the pipetting tip in a container for $^{125}I$ solid waste. Incubate the tube for 2 minutes. Longer times may be used, but may increase the chances of oxidative damage.

6. Using a pasteur pipet, transfer contents of the tube to the 50 μl of IODO-GEN stop buffer. Mix gently. Dispose of the pasteur pipet and the IODO-GEN-coated tube in a container for $^{125}I$ solid waste.

*Radioactive isotopes of iodine are available commercially in carrier-free solutions. Although other isotopes of iodine are available, $^{125}I$ is normally used for most immunochemical analyses. $^{125}I$ can be purchased from several commercial suppliers. Buy $Na^{125}I$ in alkaline solutions to keep oxidation to a minimum. $^{125}I$ can be stored for approximately 6 weeks at room temperature.*

7. Carefully apply the reaction mixture in the stop solution to the column. Dispose of the pipetting tip in a container for $^{125}I$ solid waste.

8. Release the flow of the column and begin collecting the eluate in a 1.5-ml conical tube. After the iodinated proteins have run into the beads, carefully add 0.3 ml of PBS with 0.02% sodium azide to the column. Continue to collect the eluate in the first tube. When the buffer reaches the top of the beads, change the collection tube to a second 1.5-ml conical tube, and then apply a second 0.3 ml of PBS with sodium azide to the column. Continue to collect the eluate in steps. Monitor the tubes using a minimonitor to identify the peaks of $^{125}I$-labeled antibody and unincorporated label. The antibody should come off in approximately the second to fourth fraction, well ahead of the blue xylene cyanol, which should run with the unincorporated label.

9. Pool the fractions containing the iodinated antibody. It is often convenient to dispose of the unincorporated label by leaving it on the column and putting the entire column into the $^{125}I$ solid waste.

10. The labeled antibody can be stored in the column buffer of 1% PBS/BSA at 4°C. Although the antibody is stable, the radioactive iodine is not; thus, the labeled antibody should be used within 6 weeks of preparation.

    Up to 90% of the input iodine can be incorporated. This labeling procedure will yield specific activities between 1 μCi/μg and 45 μCi/μg. These levels can be adjusted by varying the input iodine and protein concentrations.

## Common problems

The major problems stem from oxidative damage to the antibodies. Proteins can be damaged either by oxidation or by distortion due to the introduction of the bulky iodine atom on a critical tyrosine group. Oxidative damage can be minimized by using lower amounts of the oxidant IODO-GEN and by stopping the reaction sooner. Both of these remedies will also lower the specific activities of the iodinated product.

# Labeling monoclonal antibodies by biosynthesis*

STORING, 64
PURIFYING, 70
LABELING

If labeling monoclonal antibodies with any of the conventional techniques described above causes loss of activity, one convenient method for preparing tagged monoclonal antibodies is to label the polypeptide chain by growing the hybridomas in the presence of radioactive amino acids. This can only be done with antibodies for which the hybridoma cells are available, but the resultant antibodies have a number of potentially important properties, the most important of which is that the labeled antibodies will be essentially identical to the unlabeled antibodies. Therefore, these radioactively labeled antibodies will be useful for many of the techniques requiring labeled immunoglobulins.

Any amino acid can be used to label antibodies in this way. However, for most applications the use of $^{35}$S-containing amino acids is preferred. The half-life of $^{35}$S is sufficiently long (87 days) to allow a reasonable storage time, and the energy released by a $^{35}$S decay is high enough to allow relatively easy detection. Unless there is a reason to avoid its use, we recommend using [$^{35}$S]methionine over [$^{35}$S]cysteine because of the lower cost.

## Thinking ahead

This is a convenient method to label and compare a set of antibodies specific for the same antigen without resorting to purifying and labeling each individually. Since each antibody is labeled, a simple competition between a small amount of the labeled antibody and an excess of another unlabeled antibody on an immune blot (or similarly immobilized antigen) can be used to see if the two antibodies recognize overlapping epitopes. If these types of monoclonal antibodies are being prepared, it may be wise to label each antibody during the last stages of their initial single-cell cloning. Often the methionine and cysteine remaining in a used vial are sufficient to label these antibodies. Rinse the vial with the methionine-free medium to collect the remaining label.

## Special equipment

A standard tissue culture lab will have all of the equipment needed for this procedure.

## Caution

Radioactive substances, sodium azide, see Appendix IV.

---

1. The hybridoma cells should be healthy and rapidly growing at the time of labeling. Collect approximately $2 \times 10^6$ cells by centrifugation (300*g* for 10 minutes).

2. Wash the cells once by resuspending the cell pellet in medium without methionine (prewarmed to 37°C) and spinning at 300*g* for 10 minutes.

*Adapted from Cuello et al. (1982).

*The [$^{35}$S]methionine used to label these antibodies can be changed to other amino acids by using media lacking these precursors for the labeling.*

3. Resuspend the cells at approximately $10^6$ cells per milliliter of medium without methionine. Add [$^{35}$S]methionine (100 μCi per labeling will yield approximately $10^5$–$10^6$ cpm of antibody).

4. Incubate overnight at 37°C in a $CO_2$ incubator.

5. Centrifuge the cell suspension at 1000 *g* for 10 minutes to generate a tight cell pellet. Remove the supernatant and add 1/20 volume of 1 M Tris (pH 8.0) and sodium azide to 0.02%.

   The antibodies may be purified from the supernatants by standard techniques or used as crude preparations.

## Common problems

The only major problem encountered with metabolically labeled antibodies is that the specific activity will be relatively low. With other methods that use chemical labeling of purified antibodies, essentially every antibody in the preparation can be labeled. However, with metabolic labeling, only a fraction of the amino acids precursors are radioactive. For [$^{35}$S]methionine, even for the highest specific activity sources, only 1 in 10 molecules is radioactive. Also, the cells will continue to make methionine, so the pool of cold methionine in the cell will remain high. Therefore, the resulting population of antibodies will always show low specific activity compared to other methods.

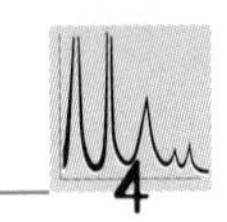


## References


Bayer E.A. and Wilchek M. 1980. The use of avidin-biotin complex as a tool in molecular biology. *Methods Biochem. Anal.* **26:** 1–45.

Bayer E.A., Wilchek M., and Skutelsky E. 1976. Affinity cytochemistry: The localization of lectin and antibody receptors on erythrocytes via the avidin-biotin complex. *FEBS Lett.* **68:** 240–244.

Becker J.M. and Wilchek M. 1972. Inactivation by avidin of biotin-modified bacteriophage. *Biochim. Biophys. Acta* **264:** 165–170.

Campbell D.H., Luescher E., and Lerman L.S. 1951. Immunologic adsorbents. I. Isolation of antibody by means of a cellulose-protein antigen. *Proc. Natl. Acad. Sci.* **37:** 575–578.

Cuello A.C., Priestley J.V., and Milstein C. 1982. Immunocytochemistry with internally labeled monoclonal antibodies. *Proc. Natl. Acad. Sci.* **79:** 665–669.

Ey P.L., Prowse S.J., and Jenkin C.R. 1978. Isolation of pure $IgG_1$, $IgG_{2a}$, and $IgG_{2b}$, immunoglobulins from mouse serum using protein A-sepharose. *Immunochemistry* **15:** 429–436.

Fraker P.J. and Speck J.C., Jr. 1978. Protein and cell membrane iodinations with a sparingly soluble chloroamide, 1,3,4,6-tetrachloro-3a,6a-diphenylglycoluril. *Biochem. Biophys. Res. Commun.* **80:** 849–857.

Goding J.W. 1976. Conjugation of antibodies with fluorochromes: Modifications to the standard methods. *J. Immunol. Methods* **13:** 215–226.

Green N.M. 1963. Avidin. I. The use of $^{14}C$ biotin for kinetic studies and for assay. *Biochem. J.* **89:** 585–591.

———. 1990. Avidin and streptavidin. *Methods Enzymol.* **184:** 51–67.

Guesdon J.-L., Ternynck T., and Avrameas S. 1979. The use of avidin-biotin interaction of immunoenzymatic techniques. *J. Histochem. Cytochem.* **27:** 1131–1139.

Heggeness M.H., and Ash J.F. 1977. Use of the avidin-biotin complex for the localization of actin and myosin with fluorescence microscopy. *J. Cell Biol.* **73:** 783–788.

Heitzmann H. and Richards F.M. 1974. Use of the avidin-biotin complex for specific staining of biological membranes in electron microscopy. *Proc. Natl. Acad. Sci.* **71:** 3537–3541.

Riggs J.L., Seiwald R.J., Burckhalter J.H., Downs C.M., and Metcalf T.G. 1958. Isothiocyanate compounds as fluorescent labeling agents for immune serum. *Am. J. Pathol.* **34:** 1081–1096.

The T.H. and Feltkamp T.E.W. 1970a. Conjugation of fluorescein isothiocyanate to antibodies. I. Experiments on the conditions of conjugation. *Immunology* **18:** 865–873.

———. 1970b. Conjugation of fluorescein isothiocyanate to antibodies. II. A reproducible method. *Immunology* **18:** 875–881.

# Antibody purification on protein A or protein G columns

| Antibody source | Protein A | Protein G |
|---|---|---|
| Monoclonal antibodies | | |
| mouse $IgG_1$ | | √ |
| Mouse $IgG_{2a}$, $IgG_{2b}$, $IgG_3$ | √ | |
| rat | | √ |
| Polyclonal antibodies | | |
| human | √ | |
| rabbit | √ | |
| mouse | | √ |
| rat | | √ |
| horse | √ | |
| goat | | √ |
| donkey | √ | |
| pig | √ | |
| guinea pig | √ | |
| dog | √ | |
| cow | √ | |

1. Adjust the pH of the crude antibody preparation by adding 1/10 volume of 1.0 M Tris (pH 8.0).

2. Pass the antibody solution through a protein A or protein G bead column. These columns bind approximately 10–20 mg of antibody per milliliter of wet beads. Serum contains approximately 10 mg/ml of total IgG, tissue culture supernatants contain 20–50 μg/ml of monoclonal antibody, and ascites between 1 and 10 mg/ml.

   Note the approximate volume of the column bed because the wash and elution buffers are measured in relative values compared to the volume of beads being used.

3. Wash the beads with 10 column volumes of 100 mM Tris (pH 8.0).

4. Wash the beads with 10 column volumes of 10 mM Tris (pH 8.0).

*Adapted from Ey et al. (1978).

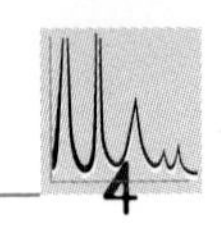

5 Elute the column with 50 mM glycine (pH 3.0). Add this buffer stepwise at approximately 1/2 column volume per step. Collect the eluate from each step in tubes containing 1/10 column volume of 1 M Tris (pH 8.0). Mix each tube gently to bring the pH back to neutral.

6 Identify the immunoglobulin-containing fractions by absorbance at 280 nm (1 OD = approximately 0.8 mg/ml).

Combine the antibody-containing fractions and measure purity by running 2 μg of total protein on a SDS-polyacrylamide gel and staining with Coomassie blue. Good purification should yield essentially pure heavy and light chain bands.

# Staining Cells

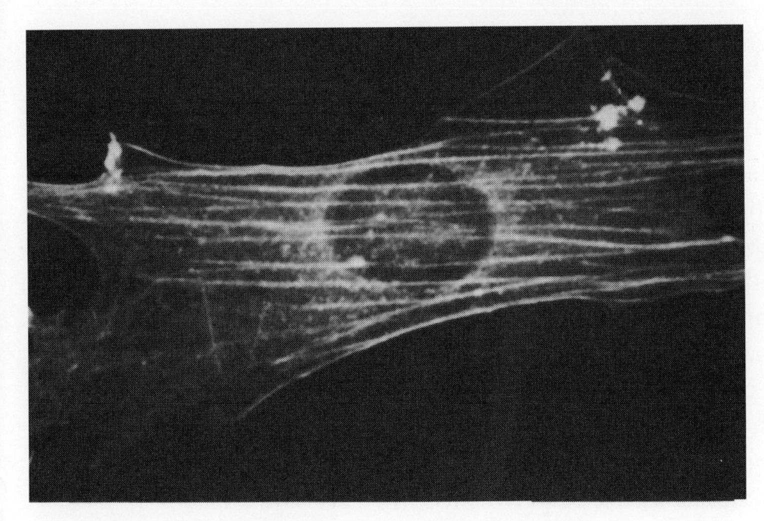

Lazarides E., and Weber K. 1974. Actin antibody: The specific visualization of actin filaments in non-muscle cells. *Proc. Natl. Acad. Sci.* **71:** 2268–2272. (Reprinted with permission.)

Fig. 3b. Indirect immunofluorescence using actin antibody....(*b*) A sparse hamster established hamster cell line (BHK). Cells were grown on coverslips in Dulbecco's modified Eagle's medium containing 10% calf serum.

Immunofluorescence became a widely used method for identifying the subcellular location of antigens when in the early 1950s the method was modified to include labeled secondary reagents to determine the site of antibody binding. Previous work had relied on the purification of the primary antibody and then labeling with a suitable fluorochrome. The wide availability of multiple fluorochromes, the impressive advances in microscopy, and creative use of fusion proteins have made immunofluorescence one of the key methods to characterize any antigen. In this early indirect immunofluorescence experiment, an antibody raised against actin purified from SDS-polyacrylamide gels is used to show the characteristic structure of actin filaments. To feel confident of the antibody's specificity, the authors carefully purified the actin to get a single polypeptide band for immunizations, and then tested the resulting antisera for cross-reactions in immunodiffusion assays. Careful experiments such as these provided wide support for immunofluorescence and quickly made these techniques the method of choice for localization studies, supplanting the more difficult methods of electron microscopy.

Immunostaining can be used to pinpoint the subcellular localization of a protein antigen, to follow its changing cellular address as cells respond to stimuli, or to compare its locale to other proteins in the same cell. With careful controls, you may also be able to get an idea of how much protein is present in the cell. In this book, the immunostaining procedures have been separated into two major variations based on the source of the cells to be examined. In this chapter, staining cells growing in tissue culture is discussed. In the next chapter, methods for staining tissues and whole organisms are presented. Immunostaining of tissue culture cells is simple and can be performed in less than half a day. However, immunostaining can be fraught with misinterpretations caused by inappropriate choice of antibodies or by sloppy use of controls, so particular care should be given to the experimental design and the characteristics of antibodies in use.

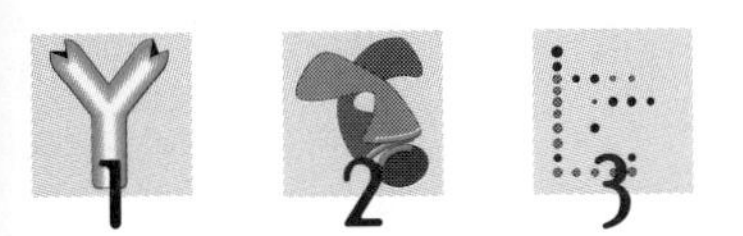
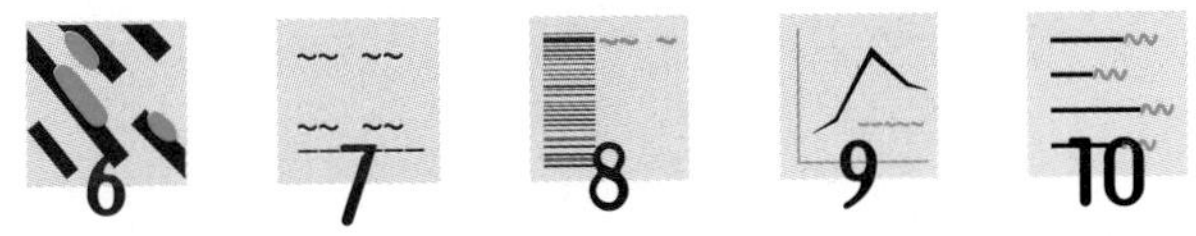
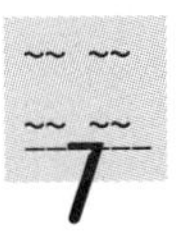

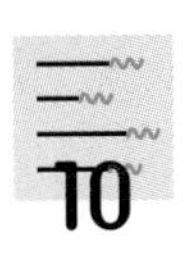
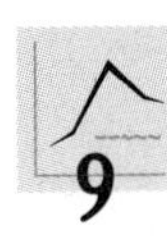
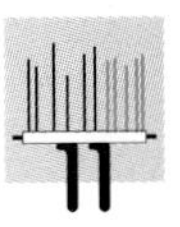

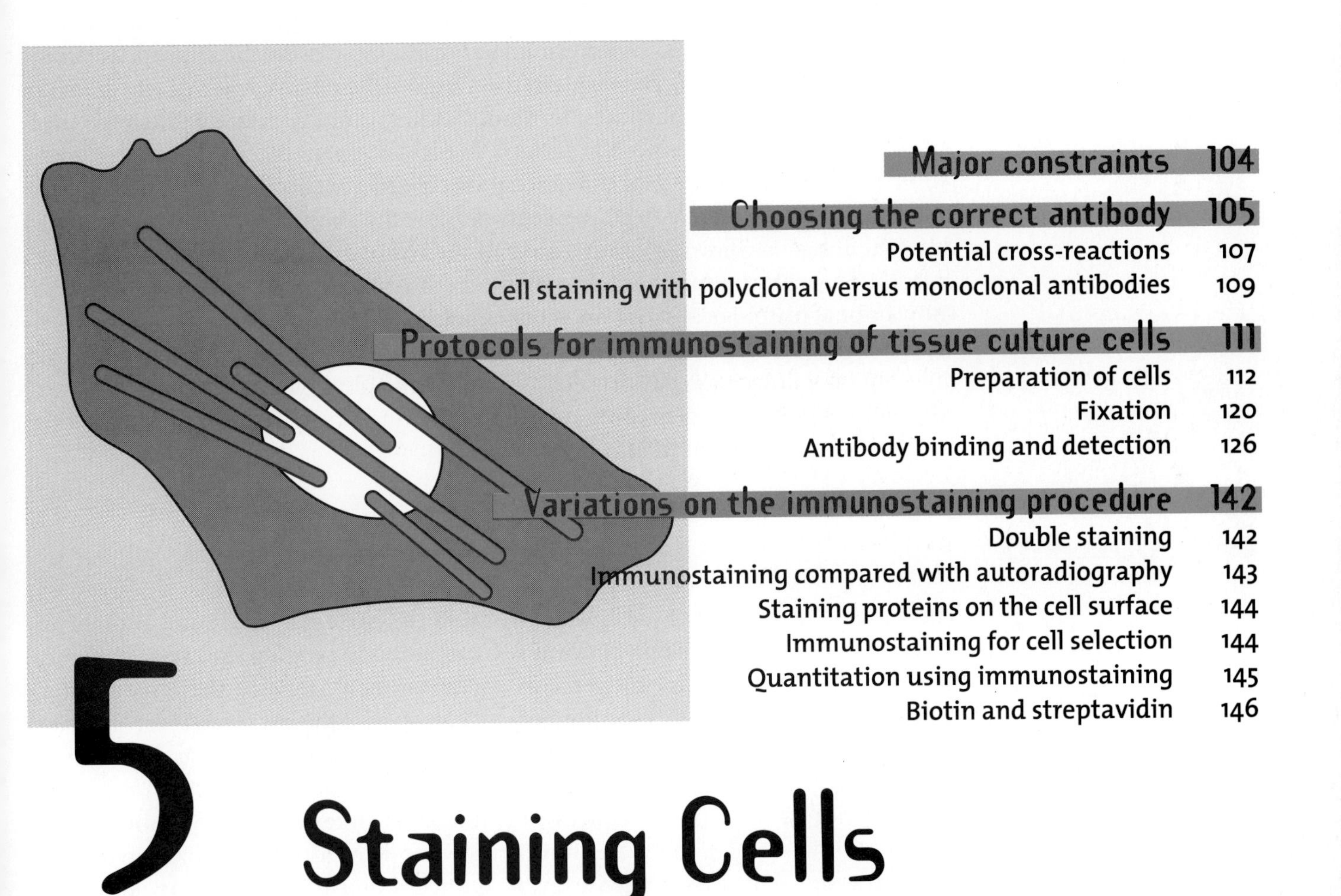



# 5 Staining Cells

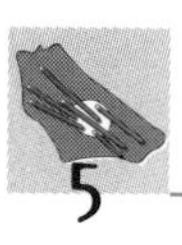



Antibodies can be used to detect the presence and localization of antigens in a wide variety of cells grown in culture. The overall strategy is to use a specific unlabeled primary antibody to locate the antigen in the cell, and then the position of the primary antibody, still bound to your antigen, is determined by using an easily detected secondary reagent that will interact with the primary antibody. To begin, cells are most often bound to a solid support so that the immunostaining techniques, which involve treating the samples with a series of antibody and wash solutions, can be performed easily and rapidly. Then the cells and their intracellular components are fixed in place with chemical cross-linkers, and the cells are permeabilized to ensure free access of the antibody. The cell preparations are then incubated with the primary antibody. Unbound primary antibody is removed by washing, and the bound antibody is detected using a labeled secondary reagent. Using a labeled secondary reagent allows a broad range of primary antibodies to be used without the need to label each one individually.

There are many variations of the immunostaining technique that allow other characteristics of the antigen to be determined. For example, with the appropriate comparisons, immunostaining can be used to determine the relative levels of an antigen in different sites. For most purposes, immunostaining is not accurate enough for measurements of absolute levels of the antigen, but it is useful to determine relative levels. Another use is to compare subcellular locations of different antigens. Here labeling the antibodies with different detection agents permits the simultaneous detection of two different antigens, allowing comparisons of the relative distribution of two antigens. In addition, many immunostaining methods can also be used in conjunction with conventional histological stains and autoradiographic methods to compare the localization of the antigen with other markers. Relocalization or loss of the antigen over time can be followed as cells proceed through some physiological change. With certain modifications, the procedure can also be used to purify cells on the basis of the antigenic composition of their cell surface.

## Major constraints

Three major factors determine how easily an antigen is detected using immunostaining. These are the local antigen concentration, the accessibility of the epitope(s) being studied, and the type of detection method employed.

The major factor that influences the strength of the signal is the local antigen concentration. Diffuse antigens, even when present at high concentrations, are difficult to detect or distinguish from background signals. The antigens that are easiest to detect have a characteristic structure and present a large number of identical antibody-binding sites in a small local environment. One of the most exciting changes over the last several years has been the dramatic improvements in sensitivity and image handling, particularly with confocal instruments. These new methods allow the detection and localization of lower concentrations of antigens and have greatly extended the quantitation and reliability of immunostaining methods.

The second factor that determines how easy an antigen is to detect is the ac-

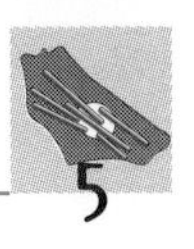


cessibility of the epitope(s) recognized by the primary antibody. This is determined by the type of fixative being used, the characteristics of the primary antibodies, and the presence of other physical structures around the epitope. Living cells are dynamic structures, and, with the exception of techniques that label live cells, most immunostaining methods require that the cells be fixed. Perfect fixation would immobilize the antigens, while retaining authentic cellular and subcellular architecture and permitting unhindered access of antibodies to all cells and subcellular compartments. No fixation method reaches this ideal. Many antigens are masked or altered by certain fixatives or require special methods to uncover their presence. In addition, many antibodies are specific for epitopes that are altered by the chemical properties of the fixation method itself. Fixatives work by bonding the antigen to other cellular structures. If the epitope recognized by your antibody is affected by the fixative, finding your antigen will be difficult or impossible. Finally, some epitopes are hidden by local subcellular structures or by interactions with other molecules that hinder the access of primary antibodies. All of these factors affect how accessible the epitope is to the primary antibody and create maddening situations where antibody recognition of the antigen fails, even when the antigen is highly expressed and nicely localized, or when seemingly excellent antibodies are available.

The resolution and sensitivity of immunostaining also depend on the method used for antibody detection. Enzyme-labeled antibodies are particularly useful for identifying small amounts of antigen and do not require any specialized microscopy, but they do not offer high resolution. On the other hand, high resolution can be obtained using fluorochrome-labeled antibodies, where images of subcellular structures can be studied at magnifications even beyond the limit of resolution of the transmitted light microscope. However, unless you have access to a confocal microscope, these methods are not as sensitive as enzyme-labeled methods.

Potential approaches to overcome the constraints of immunostaining methods and to achieve maximum specificity and signal strength are discussed in each section below.

## Choosing the correct antibody

Choosing the correct antibody to use in immunostaining is the most important decision in ensuring that an immunostaining protocol will succeed (Table 5.1). Two problems must be overcome by the correct choice of antibodies. The first is whether your antibody is capable of recognizing the antigen after fixation. The second problem is that both polyclonal and monoclonal antibodies often cross-react with other proteins on the partially denatured cell preparations that are used for staining, and you will need either to avoid antibodies that cross-react or to distinguish the cross-reactions from the correct signal. Both of these factors should be tested in choosing the correct antibodies for staining.

Table 5.1 *Antibody choice*

| | Polyclonal antibodies | Monoclonal antibodies | Pooled monoclonal antibodies |
|---|---|---|---|
| Signal strength | Excellent | Fair | Excellent |
| Specificity | Good, but some background | Excellent, but some cross-reactions | Excellent, by avoiding any antibodies with cross-reactions |
| Good features | Signal strength | Specificity | Signal strength<br>Specificity |
| Bad features | Background<br>Often need to titer | Lower signal strength | Availability |

## Fixation

To determine whether your antibodies will recognize the antigen after fixation, it is easiest just to test them in the standard immunostaining methods. Although there are potential methods to test whether your antibodies will recognize a purified sample of your antigen that has been treated by one of the fixation methods, this is seldom worth the effort. However, given that many antibodies will fail to recognize your antigen after fixation, it is helpful to consider why this occurs.

Fixation methods come in two varieties. Either they cause the protein components of the cells to be precipitated in their current local environment on existing components of the subcellular architecture, or they chemically cross-link the molecules of the cell to one another. Both methods maintain the antigens in their correct localization, but both approaches induce major structural changes to the shape of the antigens. The precipitation methods, which are all hydrophilic organic solvents, such as acetones or ethanols, rapidly solubilize lipids, thus allowing access, and dramatically change the hydration of the proteins. This results in the precipitation of the proteins on local structures, but will obviously alter many of the structural epitopes that are recognized by your antibodies. The cross-linking reagents are most frequently directed to free primary amino groups, and treatments make lattices of interconnected molecules to maintain localization. Free access in these cases is provided by detergent lysis of the cells after cross-linking. This approach will block any interacting antibody that relies on a primary amino group for binding.

If none of the antibodies that are available to your antigen perform well in immunostaining, there are three approaches you can use that may help. The first is the obvious advice to try both methods before panicking. Because the fixation methods are mechanistically so different, antibodies that fail in one may work well in the other. The second method to minimize the problems of fixation is to lower the concentration of the fixative in the reaction. Set up a series of test cases in which the fixative is tried at a wide range of lower concentrations. We have chosen methods below that are robust, but good fixation can be achieved with much lower concentrations. Third, it may be worthwhile to prepare antibodies that will take advantage of the fixation method. Preparations of your immunogen can be treated with a fixation method prior to injection. This will present the antigen in a form that most closely resembles the antigen as it will be presented in the immunostaining method.

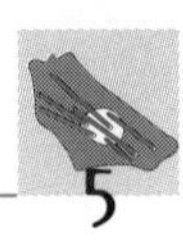


## Potential cross-reactions

Probably the biggest problem in immunostaining is the cross-reaction of your antibodies with antigens other than the protein you are studying. This poses a serious problem because of several issues. The complexity of the epitopes displayed in these preparations is vast, representing all of the proteins found in the cell, and each protein is likely to be displayed in a number of different states of denaturation. This type of fixed display of antigens is also ideally suited to capture low-affinity interactions. Many proteins will be seen in a very high local concentration and, because they are fixed to the substrate, the high local concentrations will promote binding of lower-affinity antibodies and therefore increase the probability of cross-reaction. In addition, this display is unlike any other similar method that might be used to test antibodies. All of these issues—a large number of epitopes displayed in many different states of denaturation, no easy method to test for the best antibody, and a binding exposure that enhances low-affinity interactions—make choosing the correct antibody for immunostaining an important task. There is no completely accurate method for determining which antibody to use to avoid cross-reactions, but there are several controls and tests that can help select the best antibody to use.

### *Negative antibody controls*

This is an essential control for all immunostaining tests, but it is an important comparison to begin the characterization of your antibody. Compare the staining pattern using your antibody with appropriate negative control antibodies, both at the same concentration. The negative control antibody should be as closely matched as possible to your immune antibody. Good negative control antibodies should be from the same species if you are using polyclonal antibodies and from the same species and isotype if you are using a monoclonal antibody. The staining pattern with the negative control should show none of the same pattern of immunolocalization given by the test antibody. Similar patterns, even at different intensities, indicate that this site of potential localization is not due to your antigen.

### *Antigen blocking*

This will test whether the staining pattern is due to antibodies that recognize your antigen. This is particularly important when using polyclonal antibodies, because these sources have a wide array of antibodies in the serum that are not specific for the immunogen. Add saturating amounts of the immunogen to a sample of the antibodies just before adding to the fixed cells. Blocking of the staining pattern means that the results are due to antigen-specific antibodies and allows you to conclude that the pattern is not due to any spurious antibodies that are found in your source of antibodies. Be cautious in interpreting these findings, because these tests help you ensure that the staining patterns are specific, but they do not allow the discrimination between the true localization of the antigen and a cross-reaction.

### *Immunoblot*

Of the commonly used procedures, the one that most closely reflects the conditions of immunostaining is the immunoblot. The immunoblot compares the reaction of your antibody against denatured versions of all proteins in the cells and in settings where the proteins are bound to a solid support. The major difference between immunostaining and immunoblotting is that the proteins are fully denatured for the immunoblot, whereas in immunostaining many of the proteins retain a much more native state. In addition, the immunostaining procedure retains a semblance of the natural architecture of the cells, and this is completely lost in the immunoblot. However, this is still the best comparison method available. To make this comparison, run, for example, a sample of total protein of 100–150 μg from the cells being used for the immunostaining on an immunoblot and develop with your antibody. The best result will be a single, easily detected band that is your antigen. This indicates that your cells do not contain large numbers of proteins that are recognized in their denatured state by your antibodies. However, it does not rule out cross-reactions following the fixation conditions used for immunostaining. Multiple bands suggest that cross-reactions are likely and indicate that other antibodies should be sought for localization studies.

### *Use multiple distinct antibodies*

If similar staining patterns can be seen from several independent antibodies that are shown to recognize independent regions of the antigen (antibodies raised to different regions or monoclonal antibodies that bind different epitopes, p. 381), the argument that the pattern is due to the antigen under study is greatly strengthened. Using two different antibodies provides a very strong argument; three are almost indisputable. Keep in mind that multiple antibody-binding sites can also be created by using fusion proteins with tags that are detectable with commercially available antibodies (p. 347).

### *Titrate*

Titrate the amount of antibody to the minimum level needed to give a useful signal. This keeps the chances of minor activities in the serum giving spurious results at a minimum.

### *Antigen-negative cells*

The ultimate test is to examine the pattern in genetically matched cells that differ only in the deletion of your antigen. A perfect version of this type of control would be a cell from a knock-out mouse. If the pattern is absent in these cells, while still present in samples of the wild-type cells prepared in parallel, then the pattern is at least due to the presence of your antigen. Keep in mind that if you have access to an antigen-negative cell line, your antigen can often be reintroduced by some method of gene transfer. In this case, be sure the final levels of your antigen are similar to those found in cells that express your antigen naturally.

### *GFP fusions*

If cells can be transfected with DNA or infected with retroviral vectors that express your antigen, then comparing the pattern of a fusion protein between the full-length version of your protein and green fluorescent protein (GFP) provides a second method of locating your antigen. Similar staining patterns strengthen your argument

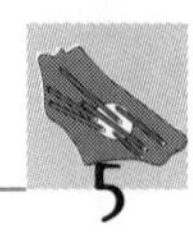



for specific localization, whereas different patterns are uninterpretable, but should raise worries in your preliminary localization data.

As discussed above, it is difficult to be completely certain that any staining pattern is due to localization of your antigen. Our recommendations would be to characterize the different antibody preparations by immunoblot, test them side by side in staining with the appropriate negative control antibodies, rely on multiple independent antibodies recognizing different epitopes or regions of the antigen, and, if at all possible, compare with a GFP fusion protein. A result that is supported by these careful controls is the best evidence available for confirming a subcellular localization.

## Cell staining with polyclonal versus monoclonal antibodies

Cell staining is commonly performed with either monoclonal or polyclonal antibodies. In general, polyclonal antibodies give stronger signals, whereas monoclonal antibodies provide less background. Both can be used effectively with the appropriate care.

### *Cell staining with polyclonal antibodies*

A good polyclonal serum contains multiple antibodies directed against different epitopes on the antigen. Although steric competition may prevent large numbers of antibodies from binding to the same antigen molecule, several antibodies often will bind, and a strong signal can be expected. The potential for generating a strong signal is the major advantage of using polyclonal antibodies for cell staining.

In addition to the specific antibodies, polyclonal sera also contain relatively high concentrations of irrelevant antibodies of unknown specificity. These include the entire repertoire of antibodies in the animal when the serum was collected. These antibodies create the most troublesome problems for cell staining. Satisfactory cell-staining experiments can be conducted using polyclonal antibodies, but their use requires careful control. This should include careful titration of the primary antibody to minimize the signal from spurious antibodies in the serum and careful comparisons with control sera.

Even sera from unimmunized animals give an intense background when used at high concentrations. Part of this background is from antibodies binding nonspecifically to the fixed cells, and part are specific interactions arising from spurious activities in the serum. Because these antibodies are normally not the major activities in the serum, their binding can often be reduced below the levels of detection by careful titration of the polyclonal antibodies. A second method for lowering these types of background problems is to preadsorb the polyclonal sera with suitable acetone powders (p. 437). A third method used to circumvent these problems is to remove the nonspecific antibodies completely. Immunoaffinity purification of the antigen-specific antibodies (p. 77) can be used to prepare an excellent source of antibodies for cell staining. For some purposes, immunoaffinity purification of the antibodies is essential to obtain clear staining patterns.

Because polyclonal sera usually contain antibodies specific for a broad range of epitopes on the antigen, including denaturation-resistant epitopes, they often work well

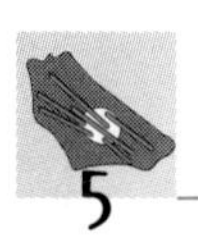


on heavily fixed samples and are the best source of antibodies for techniques such as the staining of paraffin sections of paraformaldehyde-fixed tissues (see Chapter 6).

### *Cell staining with monoclonal antibodies*

Monoclonal antibodies often work exceptionally well in cell-staining techniques, where their purity and specificity yield low backgrounds over a wide range of antibody concentrations. Most monoclonal antibodies work well on cells that have been fixed in organic solvents or by paraformaldehyde. However, some monoclonal antibodies do not give satisfactory results in cell staining. Presumably, this is due to one of two factors: Either the epitope is hidden within a cell structure or it is destroyed during fixation.

Occasionally, monoclonal antibodies show cross-reactions in cell-staining procedures. Some of these cross-reactions are specific and presumably reflect the presence of common epitopes on two cellular components. Cross-reactions with multimeric cellular proteins present in high concentrations, such as cytoskeletal filaments, are commonly observed. This usually results from weak cross-reactions that are enhanced by bivalent binding and by the high concentrations of such antigens. The location of an antigen should be confirmed, whenever possible, by using a panel of monoclonal antibodies directed to discrete epitopes on the same antigen.

### *Cell staining with pooled monoclonal antibodies*

Pooled monoclonal antibodies increase the signal strength for a given antigen provided the antibodies in the pool can bind to it noncompetitively. This increase in signal strength can mean the difference between successful detection and failure. Care in pooling must be exercised, however. Each antibody in the pool must be tested individually as part of a panel.

# Protocols for immunostaining of tissue culture cells



Immunostaining is a versatile technique and, if the antigen is highly localized, can be used to detect as few as a thousand antigen molecules in a cell. Recent improvements in antibody labeling methods, microscopes, cameras, and image analyzers continue to extend the sensitivity of immunostaining procedures and are making these techniques more quantitative. Even without these new improvements, immunostaining can yield important qualitative and semi-quantitative data.

## Overview of the basic immunostaining procedure

Immunostaining techniques can be divided into three steps:

1. cell preparation
2. fixation
3. antibody binding and detection

As a first step for most cases, the cells to be stained are attached to a solid support to allow easy handling in the subsequent procedures. This can be achieved by a number of methods. Adherent cells may be grown on microscope slides, coverslips, or optically suitable plastic. Suspension cells can be centrifuged onto glass slides or bound to slides using chemical linkers. Although it is more work, in some cases suspension cells are handled entirely by centrifugation and resuspension for each step. The second step for cell staining usually is to fix and permeabilize the cells to ensure free access of the antibody, although this step is omitted when examining cell-surface antigens. The cell preparations are then incubated with the primary antibody. Unbound primary antibody is removed by washing, and the bound antibody is detected indirectly by using a labeled secondary reagent.

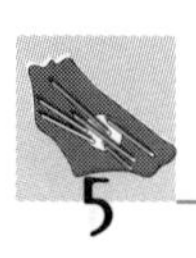



## Preparation of cells

Tissue culture cells for staining are usually prepared from one of two sources, adherent cells or suspension cells. Adherent cells normally are prepared for cell staining by growing on a suitable support. Suspension cells can be fixed directly or can be attached to a solid support by centrifugation or chemical capture.

### *Adherent cells*

Adherent cells are easily prepared for cell staining by growing on a suitable microscope slide, coverslip, or plastic tissue-culture dish. For high-resolution work and for studies that will be photographed, cells should be grown on coverslips or slides. For lower-resolution work or for large-scale screening procedures, the cells can be grown on plastic tissue-culture dishes.

The major advantage of staining adherent cells that are growing on solid supports is the ease with which all of the washing, fixing, permeabilization, and staining steps can be performed. Having cells bound to the solid supports allows large numbers of cell types, different antibodies, or various conditions to be done simultaneously with little extra effort.

### *Suspension cells*

Suspension cells can be prepared for staining by a number of different methods. For localization of internal antigens, the cells are normally centrifuged onto a glass microscope slide in a cytocentrifuge or attached to slides by using a coverslip coated with a charged cross-linker that will bind the cells to the surface. They then are handled just as for adherent cells.

In some cases, cells are stained in suspension. This is normally done because they will be processed in some further step in suspension; for example, for cell sorting. Handling cells in suspension is more tedious, because each washing step involves centrifugation and resuspension.

## Growing adherent cells on coverslips or multiwell slides



*One of the most useful methods to stain tissue culture cells is to grow the cells on coverslips in 24-well multiwell plates. This can be done simply by placing a round glass coverslip in the empty culture dish prior to adding the cells. The cells can be grown directly on the coverslips and normal culture procedures can be used. The washing, fixation, and permeabilization of the cells on the coverslips can be handled easily by flooding each well with the appropriate solution. The various buffers are removed easily by vacuum aspiration.*

Glass is an excellent substrate for most tissue-culture-adapted cells. Suitable carriers include glass coverslips or multiwell glass slides. The glass surface is compatible with all fixing and staining solutions.

For high-resolution studies, adherent cells should be grown on the highest available grade glass coverslips, because the controlled thickness, flatness, and good optical properties of a proper coverslip are required to produce the best images. Grade #1 or #1.5 coverslips are the appropriate thickness for most microscopes. Multiple coverslips can be added to most tissue-culture dishes, and the cells can be grown directly on the coverslips without further treatment.

If many antibodies, different dilutions, or various controls are to be tested on the same cell type, plating the cells onto multiwell slides can be helpful. Suitable Teflon-coated slides are available from a number of commercial sources. The hydrophobic nature of the Teflon allows different solutions to be added, with a careful hand, to the individual wells without flowing into adjacent sample wells.

### Thinking ahead

The coverslips (round) or slides (Teflon coated) can be sterilized and stored aseptically weeks or months in advance. See step 1 for these instructions. This will provide a useful store that can be accessed whenever a cell-staining experiment is needed.

### Needed solutions

All of the standard media to grow and maintain the cells under study

### Special equipment

An appropriate tissue-culture setup for the cells under study

### Caution

Ethanol, see Appendix IV.

**1** If you are using coverslips or slides, they must be sterilized prior to cell staining. These can be prepared well before use and stored in sterile conditions.

For small numbers of coverslips, dip them in 70% ethanol, and then flame. Hold them loosely with metal forceps, because holding them tightly will often lead to cracking. For convenience, coverslips can be stored in 70% alcohol prior to flaming.

*If the coverslips or slides are touching, do not use the steam cycle of an autoclave. The steam will cause stacked slides and coverslips to stick to one another.*

For sterilization of intermediate numbers of coverslips or slides, many manufacturers sell convenient metal racks to hold coverslips or slides for sterilization. With these racks, slides or coverslips can be autoclaved.

For large batches of coverslips, sterilize by placing them in a glass petri dish or other suitable heat-resistant container. Bake in an oven at 180°C for 2 hours.

2. Aseptically place the dry coverslips or slides in suitable tissue-culture dishes. Coverslips can be handled with sterile forceps or by using a sterile pasteur pipet connected to a vacuum line.

   A single round coverslip fits conveniently in each well of a 24-well tissue-culture plate. As many as 10–15 coverslips available in many convenient shapes can be added to a 90-mm-diameter tissue-culture dish (see Fig. 5.1). One standard-size microscope slide will fit conveniently in a 90-mm-diameter tissue-culture dish.

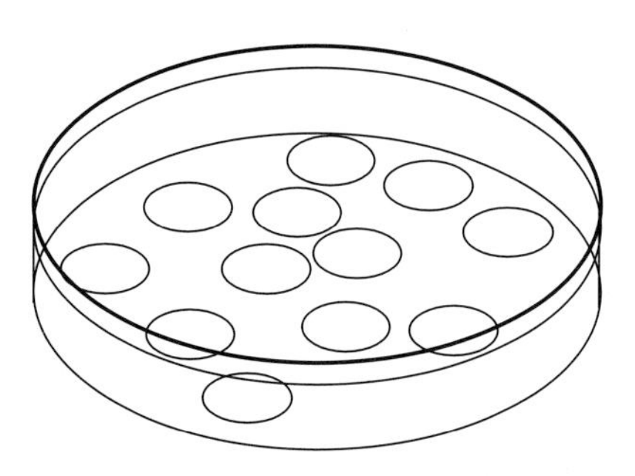

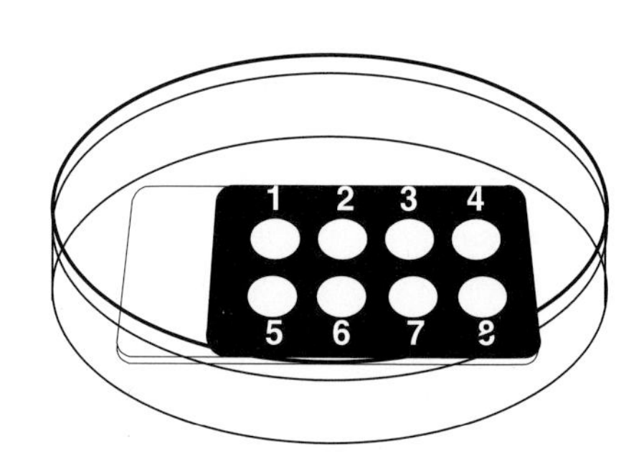


Figure 5.1
(*Left*) Coverslips in plate. (*Right*) Slide in plate.

*The subcellular localization of most antigens is improved by plating the cells at low density. This induces the cell to spread on the surface and allows the subcellular architecture to be seen more easily.*

3. Plate the cell suspension into the tissue-culture dish or well and let the cells adhere to the glass for at least 24 hours. For greater resolution of most antigens, plate the cells at a low density to avoid overcrowding.

4. If the number of cells is limited, drops of the cell suspension can be placed directly onto the coverslips or slides, left for 4 hours, and then the dish gently filled with medium. This way, most cells will be captured on the glass coverslips or slides. Cells still need approximately 24 hours to spread properly.

**Cells are now ready for fixing** (p. 120).

## Growing adherent cells directly on tissue culture dishes

PREPARING
FIXING, 120
STAINING, 126

For low-resolution work, cells to be used for staining can be grown directly on regular tissue-culture dishes. Because of the poorer optical properties of the plastic and the ease of scratching the surface, this method is not suitable for most photographic methods nor for any high-resolution work. Because cells are commonly grown on plastic tissue-culture dishes, this approach is a useful method that does not require much preparatory work.

This method of preparing cells for immunostaining is not appropriate for confocal examination.

*This approach is used by many labs to screen hybridoma tissue-culture supernatants for antibodies to antigens of known subcellular localization or for antibody titration.*

### Needed solutions

All of the standard media to grow and maintain the cells under study

### Special equipment

An appropriate tissue-culture setup for the cells under study

1. Plate the cell suspension into a fresh tissue-culture dish and let the cells adhere for at least 24 hours.

*The subcellular localization of most antigens is improved by plating the cells at low density. This induces the cell to spread on the surface and allows the subcellular architecture to be seen more easily.*

2. If the cells are in short supply, mark the bottom of the dish with small circles using a permanent ink marking pen (Fig. 5.2). Add the cell suspension dropwise above each circle and leave for 4 hours, then gently fill the dish with medium. This will allow the cells to attach only to the original area in the circle.

**Cells are now ready for fixing** (p. 120).

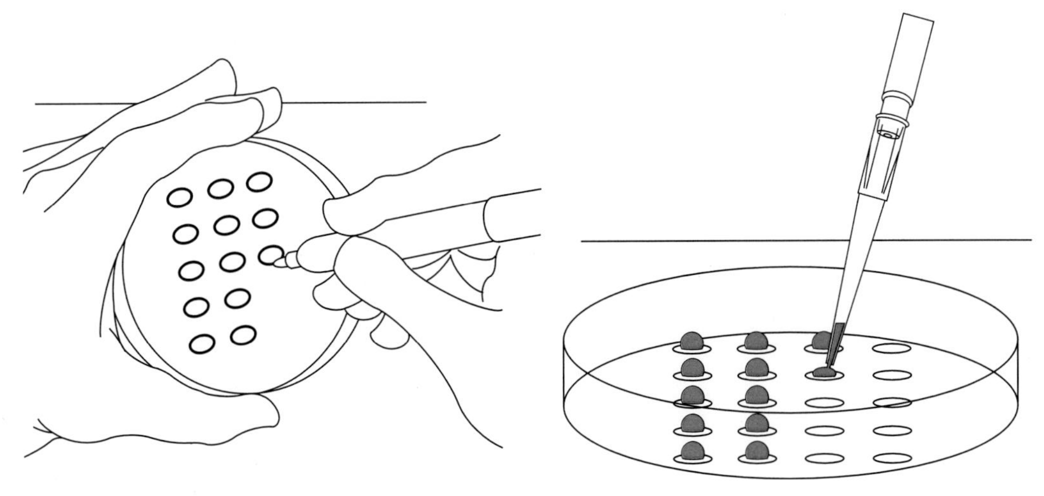

Figure 5.2
Marking tissue culture dishes.

## Common problems

The only problems that normally come from using this approach are caused by using the wrong types of fixative. The fixative must not contain more than 50% acetone, otherwise the dish will become crazed and optically opaque. If the resolution of the stained images is not sufficiently high, switch to glass coverslips.

# Attaching suspension cells to slides using a cytocentrifuge

PREPARING
FIXING, 120
STAINING, 126

A simple method for handling suspension cells is to attach the cells to a solid substrate before fixation. One method for binding suspension cells to a solid support is the use of the cytocentrifuge. This method uses a special centrifuge to spin cells onto a slide prior to fixation. One point to be aware of is that the centrifugal force also spreads the cells slightly, allowing better access of the antibodies to the internal structures but also distorting the normal cellular architecture.

Be sure to consult the operating instructions for any special features of your cytocentrifuge.

### Needed solutions

PBS

### Special equipment

Cytocentrifuge

1. Wash cells by centrifugation at 400*g* and resuspend in PBS. Resuspend at $1 \times 10^6$/ml to $2 \times 10^6$/ml.
2. Mount the microscope slides in a cytocentrifuge with card covers. Add 0.1–0.5 ml of cell suspension to the reservoir.
3. Accelerate rapidly to 1200*g*. Spin for 5–10 minutes.
4. *Optional:* Dry cell monolayer in air for 15–20 minutes.

**Cells are now ready for fixation** (p. 120).

## Attaching suspension cells to slides using chemical linkers

● PREPARING
○ FIXING, 120
○ STAINING, 126

A simple method for detecting intracellular antigens in cells that grow in suspension is to attach the cells to a solid substrate before fixation by chemical linkage to the solid substrate. For chemical linkage, a charged polymer that will bind to both the solid substrate and the cells can be used to keep the cells attached during staining steps. Chemical linkage is commonly done using poly-L-lysine or a commercial equivalent such as Vectabond. Lysine can be polymerized to any desired length, and poly-L-lysine binds to most solid supports through its charged side chains. The positively charged polymer provides a site for binding of cells, which carry an overall negative charge. Although this cross-link is not covalent, it is sufficiently strong for cell-staining techniques.

### Needed solutions

1 mg/ml poly-L-lysine (average MW 400,000) in distilled water (or commercial equivalent such as Vectabond)
PBS

1. Prior to cell staining, prepare a solution of 1 mg/ml poly-L-lysine (average MW 400,000) in distilled water. This solution should not be stored indefinitely but should be prepared fresh every week.

2. Coat clean glass slides, coverslips, or tissue-culture dishes with poly-L-lysine by dipping or incubating in this solution for 10 minutes.

3. Wash the slides, coverslips, or dishes with several changes of water. Allow to air-dry by placing in a rack. The poly-L-lysine-coated solid phase can be stored at room temperature after drying.

4. Wash the suspension cells by centrifugation at 400*g* for 5 minutes and resuspension in PBS. Repeat.

5. Resuspend the cell pellet in PBS at $10^5$ cells/ml. Add to the solid phase. Incubate for 10 minutes at room temperature.

**The cells are now ready for fixing** (p. 120).

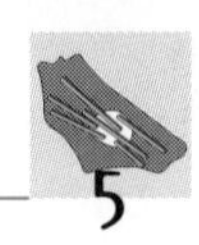


## Common problems

There are two major concerns in using this method. The first is the possibility of over cross-linking. If cross-linking is too extensive, the cells will be highly distorted, and this will confuse the visualization of the subcellular architecture. This problem can be lessened by lowering the concentration of cross-linker to the minimum needed to bind a suitable number of target cells. The second concern is that the background may be high, as the poly-L-lysine provides binding sites for many of the antibody reagents. If this becomes a problem, add a blocking step in which saturating amounts of nonspecific proteins have been incubated with the substrate after the cells have been bound.

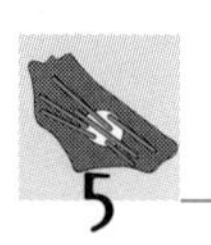



## Fixation

All fixation protocols must (1) prevent antigen leakage, (2) permeabilize the cells to allow access of the antibody, (3) keep the antigen in such a form that it can be recognized as efficiently as possible by the antibody, and (4) maintain the cell structure.

A wide range of fixatives are in common use, and the correct choice of method depends on the nature of the antigen being examined and on the properties of the antibody preparation. Fixation methods fall generally into two classes, organic solvents and cross-linking reagents. Organic solvents such as alcohols and acetone remove lipids and dehydrate the cells, precipitating the proteins on the cellular architecture. Cross-linking reagents form intermolecular bridges, normally through free amino groups, thus creating a network of linked antigens. Both methods partially denature protein antigens, and for this reason, antibodies recognizing denatured proteins may be more useful for cell staining. In some instances, anti-denatured protein antibodies are the only ones that can work.

Choosing between fixation in organic solvents or cross-linking agents is empirical. There are no general rules to decide between the two, although most workers find slightly better results using the chemical cross-linking approaches. Try both and choose the one that works better.

# Fixing attached cells in organic solvents

PREPARING, 112
FIXING
STAINING, 126

Organic solvents, most often alcohols or acetone, act as fixation agents by solubilizing the membrane lipids, washing away soluble molecules, and dehydrating the cell. This treatment removes the cytosol and nucleosol, and exposes the cellular architecture. All of the organic solvents used for cell fixation are also extremely hydrophilic and dehydrate and precipitate the cellular proteins. This decorates the local cellular structures with the proteins of the cells and gives a fairly accurate view of cell substructure.

The procedure is straightforward. The cells are washed briefly in an isotonic buffer and then flooded with the alcohol or acetone solution. After a brief incubation, the cells are washed with water and processed for antibody detection.

Cells attached to a solid support are simple to manipulate, because the slides, coverslips, or dishes are easily washed and placed in different fixatives or staining solution. When manipulating large numbers of slides or coverslips, it may be easier to place them in racks or staining jars.

## Needed solutions

PBS
Organic solvent (methanol, acetone, or a freshly prepared mixture of 50% acetone/50% methanol)

## Caution

Acetic acid, acetone, ethanol, methanol, see Appendix IV.

1. Rinse the coverslip, slide, or plate once with PBS.

   For individual slides or coverslips, hold them by a forceps and dip in a beaker of PBS.

   For batches of coverslips or slides, use racks that can hold large numbers of these samples. Many metal racks sold through commercial vendors are suitable for this.

   For plates, simply pour off the media and flood the plate with PBS.

2. Drain well, but do not allow the specimen to dry.

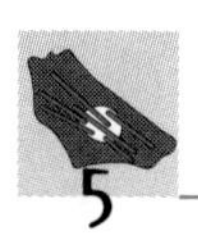



*Different antigens may be affected differently by the various solvents. If no previous data are available for your antigen, we recommend starting with the 50% acetone/50% methanol mix.*

3. Fix and permeabilize the cells by treating with an organic solvent. Possible solvents include methanol, acetone, or a freshly prepared mixture of 50% acetone/50% methanol (all at room temperature).

   For tissue-culture dishes, simply flood the plate with a freshly prepared mixture of 50% acetone/50% methanol at room temperature. Higher concentrations of acetone will destroy the integrity of the plastic.

4. Agitate gently and incubate for 2 minutes.

5. Drain off or remove from solvent and rinse with PBS.

*Some antigens give much better reactions after fixation in strongly acidified alcohol solutions, and this fixation method is favored by some laboratories. This technique has become the method of choice for detecting intracellular antibody in lymphoid cells. However, acid alcohol fixation can destroy the antigenicity of many antigens and should not be used as a first choice when examining a new antigen or antibody preparation. In place of the solvents listed above, incubate the sample in 5% glacial acetic acid, 95% ethanol at –20°C for 5 minutes. Wash as usual.*

**Antibodies can now be applied to the samples** (p. 126).

## Note

Coverslips, slides, and plates fixed in organic solvents can be stored at –70°C. After step 4 in the above protocol, the samples are removed from the solvent and air-dried without a PBS wash. The dry samples are then stored in a sealed container at –70°C. For most antigens, the samples must be carefully thawed to avoid damage. Transfer the specimen to a solution of 50% acetone/50% methanol in a beaker on dry ice. Remove the beaker from the dry ice and transfer with the samples to room temperature. When the acetone/methanol solution has reached room temperature, remove the specimens and rinse in PBS as in step 5. Antibodies can now be applied to the specimen.

## Common problems

The major problem encountered in this method is the distortion of the cell by treatment with the organic solvent. This fixation will destroy any membrane structure, will distort the structure of most proteins, and may destroy the authentic subcellular structure. This is a problem that is inherent in the methodology and cannot be fixed by any remedy other than switching to another fixative or another approach. Workers should be aware that all fixation methods suffer this problem to some degree, although trying both organic and paraformaldehyde methods and achieving the same result is helpful. An alternative approach to fixation and immunostaining is to create a fusion protein with green fluorescent protein and then reintroduce a construct to express the fusion into your test cells. Careful manipulation to achieve levels of the fusion protein that resemble the endogenous levels is important, and the fusion protein should always be considered a mutant version of your antigen. However, assignment of subcellular location by multiple methods is better than relying on a single method.

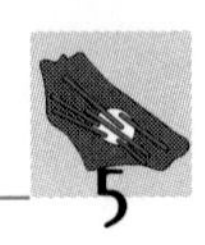


## Fixing attached cells in paraformaldehyde

PREPARING, 112

FIXING

STAINING, 126

When pure formaldehyde is dissolved in water, it forms long, self-assembling polymers of formaldehyde subunits. These can be of any length and undergo spontaneous assembly or disassembly in water. Formaldehyde is readily soluble in lipid and thus passes through the membrane to gain access to the cell. Treating cells with paraformaldehyde leads to the establishment of chemical cross-links between free amino groups. When the cross-links join different molecules, a latticework of interactions occurs that holds the overall architecture of the cell together.

Simple fixation with paraformaldehyde does not allow access of the antibody to the specimen and therefore is followed by a permeabilization step using a nonionic detergent.

### Needed solutions

4% solution of paraformaldehyde (prepared fresh, see p. 465)
PBS

*We do not recommend the use of commercial formaldehyde solutions for immunostaining. Formaldehyde is actually a mixture of formaldehyde and an alcohol, most often methanol. The methanol acts to keep the formaldehyde from polymerizing and thus keeps it in its monomeric state. Treating cells with commercial formaldehyde solutions has two disadvantages: You will not get the advantages of using a variable-length polymer, and the cells will simultaneously be fixed with the methanol.*

### Caution

Paraformaldehyde, see Appendix IV.

1. Prior to the staining, prepare a fresh 4% paraformaldehyde solution in PBS as described on p. 465.

2. Rinse the coverslip, slide, or plate once with PBS.

   For individual slides or coverslips, hold them by a forceps and dip in a beaker of PBS.

   For batches of coverslips or slides, use racks that can hold large numbers of these samples. Many metal racks sold through commercial vendors are suitable for this.

   For plates, simply pour off the media and flood the plate with PBS.

3. Drain well, but do not allow the specimen to dry.

4. For paraformaldehyde, incubate in a 4% solution for 10 minutes at room temperature.

5. Wash the cells twice with PBS.

6. Permeabilize the fixed cells by incubating in 0.2% Triton X-100 or NP-40 in PBS for 2 minutes at room temperature. Some preparations may need as long as 15 minutes. Check this for each antigen.

7. Rinse gently in PBS with four changes over 5 minutes.

**The sample is now ready for the application of antibodies** (p. 126).

## Common problems

Fixation in protein cross-linking reagents such as paraformaldehyde preserves cell structure better than organic solvents but may reduce the antigenicity of some cell components. Any antibody that binds to a free amino group may be unable to recognize the antigen after paraformaldehyde treatment. If antibodies work well in other procedures but fail to work in cell staining, try titrating the levels of paraformaldehyde to lower concentrations. This may achieve a low level of cross-linking, but the cell architecture will be maintained and the antibody will have access to at least some of the antigen-binding domains.

Remember that paraformaldehyde fixation is not stable. If the paraformaldehyde fixation is followed by nonionic detergent lysis, long incubations in aqueous buffers will reverse the cross-linking and thus should be avoided.

## Fixing suspension cells with paraformaldehyde

PREPARING, 112
FIXING
STAINING, 126

Staining of suspension cells after fixation is normally used only to detect cell-surface antigens. Because the cells are in suspension, the washing steps are tedious, and care should be taken not to centrifuge for long durations or at high speeds.

### Needed solutions

4% solution of paraformaldehyde (prepared fresh, p. 465)
PBS

### Caution

Paraformaldehyde, see Appendix IV.

1. Prior to the staining, prepare a 4% solution of paraformaldehyde (see p. 465).

2. Wash the suspension cells twice with PBS by centrifugation at 200*g* for 5 minutes and resuspend.

3. Carefully resuspend the cell pellet in 4% paraformaldehyde/PBS at approximately $10^6$ cells/ml. Incubate at room temperature with occasional mixing for 15 minutes.

4. Wash the cells by centrifugation at 200*g* for 5 minutes and resuspend in PBS. Repeat the wash twice.

5. Permeabilize the fixed cells by incubating in 0.2% Triton X-100 or NP-40 in PBS for 2 minutes at room temperature. Some preparations may need as long as 15 minutes. Check this for each antigen.

6. Wash the cells by centrifugation at 200*g* for 5 minutes and resuspend in PBS. Repeat the wash twice.

**The samples are now ready for the addition of antibodies** (p. 126).

## Antibody binding and detection

Three major decisions need to be made before starting this stage of the process. The underlying approach is simple. The antibodies are added to the cells, allowed to bind to the displayed antigens, and then located by following an easily detected label that has been added to some component of the binding reagents to determine the position of the antigen. The questions that need to be determined are:

1. **Where should the label be placed?** Here, as in many other immunochemical techniques, the antibodies can be labeled directly or they can be detected indirectly by using a labeled secondary reagent that will bind specifically to the primary antibody. For cell staining, we recommend the use of indirect detection in almost all cases. The reasons for this recommendation are discussed below.
2. **If indirect detection will be used, what secondary reagent should be used?** Through the development of immunochemical techniques, many different secondary reagents have been discovered that will bind to antibodies. These include the bacterial cell-wall proteins, protein A and protein G, as well as specific secondary antibodies that have been raised in other animals and will specifically bind to the primary antibody. Several of the secondary reagents make good choices. The uses of these reagents are discussed below, but for most procedures we recommend the use of labeled secondary antibodies that have been purchased from a commercial supplier.
3. **What will the label be?** There is a wide choice of detection methods. For cell staining, we recommend either horseradish peroxidase- or fluorochrome-conjugated reagents. Both have specific advantages that make them appropriate for specific applications.

### *Where should the label be placed? Direct versus indirect detection*

For direct detection methods, the antibodies that are specific for your antigen are purified and labeled with an easily detected label. These antibodies are added directly to the samples from the fixation step above, and their location in the cell is determined by detection of the label. For the indirect method, the antibodies are not labeled but are added to the samples without further steps. After binding and removal of unbound antibodies, a secondary reagent is added that will bind to the primary antibody. This secondary reagent is tagged with an easily detected label, and the location of the antigen/primary antibody/secondary antibody complex is determined by locating this label.

In general, we recommend the use of indirect methods. The method is versatile, cost effective, and saves the time needed to purify and label each preparation of primary antibody. Good secondary labeled reagents can be purchased from many different commercial suppliers, and this approach allows a wide array of different primary antibodies to be tested with a common labeled secondary reagent. This approach also normally produces a stronger signal, because two or more labeled secondary reagents will bind to the antibodies.

There still are some instances when direct labeling of the primary antibody will be an important approach, however. Direct labeling will produce cleaner signals with lower background, although with some loss of signal strength. With direct labeling it is also easier to compare the location of two (or more) antigens in the same cell. The purification and labeling of antibodies are discussed in Chapter 4.

### *What secondary reagent should be used?*

Three common reagents can be used to bind with high affinity and good specificity to the primary antibodies. These are protein A, protein G, and anti-immunoglobulin antibodies (secondary antibodies). All are useful and perform well in most cell-staining applications. We have a slight preference for the use of secondary antibodies. Secondary antibodies have been used for many years successfully, so there is an excellent record of their application. They provide the opportunity to bind to multiple sites on the primary antibodies and thus can give a stronger signal. In addition, secondary antibodies are available from a wide number of commercial suppliers in all possible forms. Protein A- and protein G-labeled reagents also fit many of the same qualifications. The only two minor disadvantages with their use is that they bind to only one site on the primary antibodies, and protein A and G do not bind equally well to all species and isotypes of primary antibodies. So although they bind with high affinity and with excellent specificity, some care is needed in using these reagents.

### *What will the label be? Detection methods*

Two methods are used to detect antigens in cultured cells by immunostaining. These use fluorochromes and enzymes. The properties of each detection method are summarized in Table 5.2. Both are covalently coupled to the anti-immunoglobulin, protein A, or protein G secondary reagents. Enzyme-linked detection works by modifying a chemical agent that is included in the reaction mixture so that it becomes colored and insoluble. The insoluble product precipitates at the site of the coupled antigen/antibody/secondary reagent complex. Fluorochromes can be excited by characteristic wavelengths of light to emit a second wavelength. Detection is made by looking for the location of the emitted light. The decision between enzyme- and fluorochrome-labeled reagents should be made on the basis of the needed sensitivity and resolution, as well as available equipment. Both choices provide useful applications.

**Enzyme-labeled reagents.** Enzyme-labeled antibodies provide extremely sensitive antigen detection and require only a suitable substrate and a light microscope for their detection. Because the signal is detected by differential absorption rather than by emission of light, and because the insoluble colored product of the chromogenic substrate is deposited on a small area around the site of enzyme localization, this detection method can never approach the resolution of fluorescent techniques.

Enzyme-labeled reagents are detected using soluble chromogenic substrates that precipitate following enzyme action, yielding an insoluble colored product at the site of enzyme localization (Avrameas and Uriel 1966; Nakane and Pierce 1967a,b; Avrameas 1972). A range of enzymes and substrates is available, but over the last several years horseradish peroxidase with the substrate diaminobenzidine (DAB) has become the combination of choice for staining of tissue-culture cells.

Table 5.2 *Cell-staining detection methods*

| Method | Advantages | Disadvantages | Recommended for |
|---|---|---|---|
| Fluorescence | High resolution<br>Double labeling possible<br>Staining live cells possible<br>Cell sorting possible | Requires special microscope | High resolution studies<br>Double labeling |
| Enzyme | High sensitivity<br>Only need light microscope<br>Permanent | Low resolution<br>Endogenous enzyme activities<br>Double staining difficult<br>Some substrates toxic | Low resolution studies<br>Rapid antigen screens |

A wide range of conjugated reagents is available commercially. The commercial products are cost effective and generally of high quality. Horseradish peroxidase can be coupled to anti-immunoglobulin antibodies, protein A, protein G, avidin, or streptavidin, and any of these secondary reagents can be used to detect the location of the primary antibody bound to the antigen under study.

**Fluorochrome-linked reagents.** For this type of detection, samples are examined under light of a specific wavelength. Absorbing radiation of the appropriate wavelength causes the electrons of the fluorochrome to be raised to a higher energy level. As these electrons return to their ground state, light of a characteristic wavelength is emitted. This emitted light forms the fluorescent image seen in the microscope.

The resolution of subcellular structures using fluorochrome-labeled antibodies exceeds that of the transmitted light microscope due to the visualization of an expanding cone of emitted light from the excited fluorochrome in the specimen. For example, excellent information on the cellular localization of filamentous structures of 5-nm diameter can be obtained by this method using a fluorescent microscope. This is well beyond the resolving power of even the best light microscopes. The major limitation on the sensitivity of this method has been the relatively weak emission from the fluorochrome coupled with the effect of quenching of the fluorescence emission after relatively short periods of exposure to exciting radiation. Thus, good images have been traditionally obtained only for antigens present in relatively high local concentrations. However, the field is progressing rapidly with the introduction of more efficient fluorochromes, confocal scanning microscopes, and low-light-level camera systems coupled to image analyzers.

Individual fluorochromes have discrete and characteristic excitation and emission spectra. Filters are used to ensure that the specimen is irradiated only with light at the correct wavelength for excitation. By placing a second set of filters in the viewing light path that only transmit light of the wavelength emitted by the fluorochrome, images are formed only by the emitted light. This produces a black background and a high-resolution image.

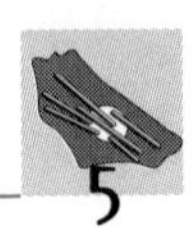


Because some fluorochromes have emission spectra that do not overlap, two fluorochromes can be observed on the same sample. This allows the study of two different antigens in the same specimen even when they have identical subcellular distributions. The most commonly used fluorochromes are fluorescein, rhodamine, and Texas Red. The properties of the commonly used fluorochromes are listed in Table 5.3.

To detect fluorochrome-labeled reagents, a specially equipped microscope is required. There are two general classes of microscopes that can be used. The cheaper alternative, but still reaching into the $20,000 to $50,000 range, is a fluorescence microscope. The low levels of fluorescence produced in cell-staining experiments mean that this microscope should be equipped for epifluorescence in which the sample is illuminated with light that passes through the objective. The second microscope that is appropriate for examining immunofluorescence is a confocal. There are several versions of confocal microscopes available on the market at this time, and they range in price from $100,000 to $400,000. The principle in these microscopes is that the very highly focused light is used to illuminate the sample on different focal planes. The cell is viewed in each of these different planes, and the images are captured digitally. Then the cell can be examined later either in each individual plane or by reassembling the entire image into a view of the whole cell. Both microscopes work well for cell staining.

**Fluorescence versus enzyme.** Both of these detection methods are useful for cell staining. In terms of ease of use and ability to look at many samples in one setting, enzyme-linked detection is by far the best choice. If maximum resolving power is needed, fluorescence-linked detection is superior, with confocal far surpassing the use of an epifluorescence microscope. For sensitivity, the best choice would again be the confocal microscope followed by enzyme-linked detection; less sensitive would be epifluorescence. If price is important, enzyme-linked detection is clearly the only alternative.

Table 5.3 *Properties of fluorochromes used in cell staining*

| Fluorochrome | Excitation (nm) | Emission (nm) | Color |
|---|---|---|---|
| DAPI | 358 | 461 | Blue |
| Hoechst 33258 | 352 | 461 | Blue |
| Fluorescein | 495 | 525 | Green |
| Rhodamine | 552 | 570 | Red |
| Texas Red | 596 | 620 | Red |
| Allophycocyanin | 650 | 660 | Red? |
| B-phycoerythrin | 546,565 | 575 | Orange, red |
| R-phycoerythrin | 480,546,565 | 578 | Orange, red |
| CyDyes (Amersh.) | 489→743 | 506→767 | Green→near-IR |
| BODIPY dyes (M.P.) | 500→589 | 506→617 | Green→red |
| Oregon green (3)(M.P.) | 496→511 | 522→530 | Green |
| Cascade blue (M.P.) | 400 | 420 | Blue |

**Caution:** DAPI, fluorescein, see Appendix IV.

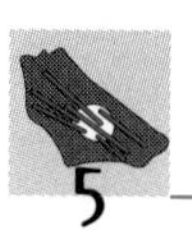



## Controls

Specific cell-staining reactions should always be compared with control reactions. To assess a staining pattern accurately, two antibodies from the same species should be compared. The best control will be a prebleed from the same animal used to prepare the specific antibodies, but nonimmune sera from the same species are acceptable in most cases. For monoclonal antibodies, the control must be from the same source as the specific antibody, i.e., supernatant versus supernatant, ascites versus ascites, or pure antibody versus pure antibody. If possible, the control antibodies should be of the same class and subclass as the specific antibody. Tissue-culture supernatants from the parental myeloma are never appropriate controls, because they do not contain antibodies. Suitable control hybridoma cell lines are available from the American Type Culture Collection and the European Collection of Animal Cell Cultures.

If possible, a control against a known positive should be included. In addition, if using indirect detection, the secondary reagent should be tested on its own. Finally, when using enzyme-linked detection, the enzyme reaction should be done on the specimen without the addition of any antibodies. This will demonstrate the presence and location of any endogenous enzyme activities.

# Indirect detection using horseradish peroxidase-labeled reagents

PREPARING, 112

FIXING, 120

STAINING

Indirect detection using unlabeled primary antibodies and horseradish peroxidase-coupled secondary reagent involves a simple series of incubations followed by an enzyme reaction. Binding primary antibodies to the antigens in the cell requires nothing more than adding the antibodies directly to cells. Each coverslip or well of a multiwell slide will be used for a different antibody or antibody dilution. The antibodies are allowed to find their cognate antigens in the cell and then unbound material is removed by washing. Labeled secondary reagents are then added and the procedure is repeated. Finally, a horseradish peroxidase enzyme reaction is performed that produces a brown precipitate at the site of the antibody–antigen complex.

## Horseradish peroxidase-labeled reagents

Horseradish peroxidase-linked secondary reagents are best used for low-resolution studies that are aimed at the rapid detection of the presence or the localization of the antigen. The major advantages of using this detection method are the sensitivity and the ability to observe the results with just a light microscope.

Dozens of possible enzyme and substrate combinations are available linked to secondary reagents. Of the commercially available choices, we recommend horseradish peroxidase with the substrate diaminobenzidine (DAB) for cell staining. The horseradish peroxidase enzyme is relatively robust and the enzyme reaction is linear for a relatively longer incubation. Of the many possible substrates, DAB is the most commonly used for horseradish peroxidase development, and it is one of the most sensitive as well. It yields an intense brown product that is insoluble in both water and alcohol. The DAB substrate for horseradish peroxidase can be made more sensitive by adding metal salts such as cobalt or nickel to the substrate solution. This reaction product is slate gray to black, and again the products are stable in both water and alcohol. These products also are easy to photograph or scan to allow reproduction for publication.

When using horseradish peroxidase-labeled reagents, the buffers for dilution and washing must not contain sodium azide, because even small levels of residual azide will kill the enzyme activity of horseradish peroxidase. Azide added to the starting primary antibodies is normally diluted sufficiently by the washes that it will not affect the enzyme detection step.

### Controls

Each assay should include at least two controls: (1) An irrelevant antibody from the same species and type as the primary antibody to determine the specificity of the staining. (2) A sample with no primary antibody to test for the background of the labeled secondary antibody. (3) If possible, a control against a known positive should be included.

## Thinking ahead

The most important preparation for antibody binding and observation is the titering of the primary and secondary antibody preparations. Starting points for the amounts of antibodies to be added are suggested in the technique below, but the single biggest problem in immunostaining is to adjust the input of the primary and secondary antibodies to levels that are sufficient to give strong robust signals, but still below levels that promote nonspecific staining. This is best achieved by doing serial dilutions of each antibody preparation (normally in a protein-containing buffer such as 3% BSA/PBS) and doing text observations on the target cell line. One-in-three dilutions (1 volume into 2 volumes) will approximate half-log steps and will quickly give a reasonable measure of the desired input. These titering tests should be repeated for each preparation of primary antibodies. However, once these dilutions have been established for the secondary reagents, they can be used as a standard for that antibody lot.

## Needed solutions and chemicals

Primary antibody solution
Secondary antibody solution (most often commercial horseradish peroxidase-coupled anti-immunoglobulin antibodies)
3% BSA/PBS
Diaminobenzidine tetrahydrochloride
0.05 M Tris buffer (pH 7.6)
0.3% weight/volume stock solution of nickel chloride in water
30% Hydrogen peroxide
DPX

## Special equipment

Light microscope (most often with a camera to record the results)

## Caution

Diaminobenzidine tetrahydrochloride, DPX, hydrogen peroxide, nickel chloride, see Appendix IV.

---

Place coverslips, slides, or plates on a flat surface.

For short incubations of 1 hour or less, humidification will not be needed and the coverslips or slides can be placed right on the benchtop. If a small number of coverslips are needed, they can be placed on a layer of Parafilm. This helps to stop the antibody solution from rolling off the edge of the coverslip and makes it easy to pick up the coverslips with fine forceps, because the Parafilm is compressible. For larger numbers of round coverslips, it may be best to leave them in the 24-multiwell plates in which the cells were grown and fixed.

*If incubations longer than 1 hour will be used, a useful trick is to place the antibody solution on a piece of Parafilm and invert the coverslip or slide onto the antibody solution (specimen side down). Samples can be removed using PBS.*

For incubations over 1 hour, it is convenient to array them directly in a dish or chamber that will be used for humidification. There are several methods to array slides or coverslips to allow easy handling and humidified incubations, and any method that suits your personal needs is fine. For example, slides can be placed in a petri dish containing a water-saturated filter paper. Coverslips can be handled similarly. If you are using 24-well multiwell plates, a damp filter paper can be placed in the lid to provide a humid atmosphere.

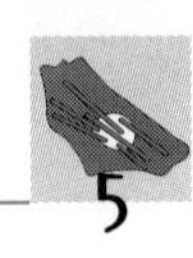

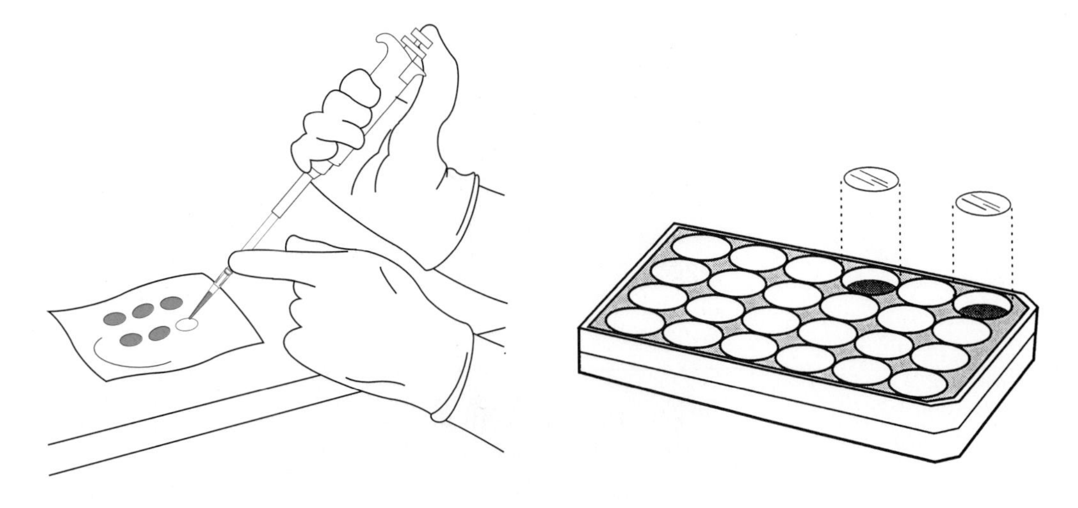

Figure 5.3
Using coverslips on Parafilm (*left*) or in a 24-well plate (*right*).

**2** Add the first antibody solution. Add sufficient volume to cover the desired area of the cells, but not enough to push beyond the edge of the coverslip or the well of the slide. Volumes as small as 10 μl are often sufficient. All dilutions must be carried out in protein-containing solutions. For example, use PBS containing 3% BSA.

Monoclonal antibodies are often applied as tissue-culture supernatants (specific antibody concentration of 20–50 μg/ml, use undiluted).

Ascites fluids, purified monoclonal and polyclonal antibodies, and crude polyclonal sera should be tested at a range of dilutions. If the specific antibody concentration of the antibody sample is unknown, prepare and test 1/10, 1/100, 1/1000, and 1/10,000 dilutions of the starting material.

**3** Incubate the coverslips, slides, or plates for a minimum of 30 minutes at room temperature. Incubations over 30 minutes should be done in a humidified atmosphere or using the technique in the sidebar next to step 1.

*For some reactions, prolonged incubations of up to 12 hours can increase sensitivity.*

**4** Wash in three changes of PBS over 5 minutes. This buffer may be supplemented with 0.5% Triton X-100 or NP-40 to help with any background problems.

5. Apply the horseradish peroxidase-coupled anti-immunoglobulin antibodies. These should be purchased from a reputable commercial source. Be sure to select a secondary antibody that is specific for the source of your antibodies. For example, goat anti-rabbit IgG would be a good choice for a primary antibody raised in rabbits.

   Secondary antibodies should be diluted in a protein-containing solution such as 3% BSA/PBS. The supplier may suggest appropriate dilutions, but if not, test dilutions of the secondary antibodies between 1/10 and 1/1000.

*An excellent protein competitor to add to the diluent would be nonimmune antibodies purified from the same species as the labeled secondary antibodies. For example, if you are using labeled goat anti-rabbit immunoglobulins for the detection step, the diluent would contain 1% nonimmune goat immunoglobulins. These should be isolated from nonimmunized animals and can be purified as described on p. 74.*

6. Incubate with the labeled secondary reagent for a minimum of 20 minutes at room temperature. Incubation times of greater than 1 hour should be avoided.

7. Wash in three changes of PBS over 5 minutes.

8. During the last wash, prepare the diaminobenzidine tetrahydrochloride/metal substrate. Dissolve 6 mg of diaminobenzidine tetrahydrochloride in 10 ml of 0.05 M Tris buffer (pH 7.6). Add 1 ml of a 0.3% wt/vol stock solution of nickel chloride in water (the same amount of cobalt chloride can be used as an alternative).

   Add 0.1 ml of a 3% solution of hydrogen peroxide in water. Hydrogen peroxide generally is supplied as a 30% solution and should be stored at 4°C, at which it will last about 1 month.

   If a precipitate appears, filter through Whatman No. 1 filter paper (or equivalent).

9. Apply to specimen. Observe the specimen and stop the reaction when a suitable black precipitate is seen and before the background has begun to change. This commonly will be between 1 and 20 minutes. The reaction is stopped by simply washing the cells several times in water.

10. Mount in DPX and observe under a light microscope.

## Common problems

The two most common problems are weak signals and bad backgrounds. Potential methods to reduce background problems are discussed in the box on p. 140.

Weak signals can be countered by several methods. The first is to extend the time of incubation with the substrate in the enzymatic detection step. This will allow more deposition of substrate and will increase the signal. The second method to increase the sensitivity is to increase the primary and/or secondary antibody concentrations. This should be done by testing various titrations of antibody concentrations. A third method is to increase the binding incubation times for both the primary and secondary antibodies. Because the antigen in cell staining will be fixed to a solid phase, the time needed for the antibody to find the antigen will be longer than if both molecules are in solution. The incubation times can be adjusted for the experimental design, but seldom will times less than 30 minutes yield efficient binding. In the first three suggestions, some compromise will need to be reached between achieving a good signal and keeping the background to an acceptable level. This will need to be determined by trial and error, because each group of antibodies and each antigen will pose different problems. The fourth method to increase the strength of the signal is to switch to fluorochrome-linked secondary reagents and examine the samples with a confocal microscope, greatly extending the sensitivity.

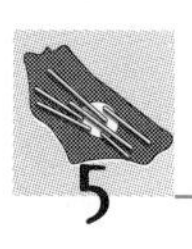



# Indirect detection using fluorochrome-labeled reagents*

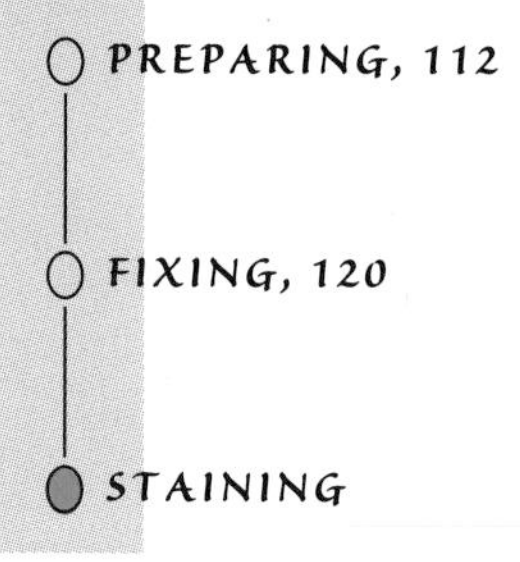


Indirect detection using unlabeled primary antibodies and fluorochrome-coupled secondary reagents involves a simple series of incubations. Binding primary antibodies to the antigens in the cell requires nothing more than adding the antibodies directly to cells. Each coverslip or well of a multiwell slide is used for a different antibody or antibody dilution. The antibodies are allowed to find their cognate antigens in the cell, and unbound material is removed by washing. Labeled secondary reagents are added and the procedure is repeated. Then the samples are examined using either a fluorescence or confocal microscope.

## Choosing the correct fluorochrome

The choice of fluorochromes is limited primarily by filter sets that are available for microscopy. Most filter sets are best matched to the properties of rhodamine or fluorescein. Texas Red can be used with rhodamine filter sets, but its emission spectra are not matched exactly by these filters. The increasing availability of phycobiliproteins, which are theoretically about 30 times or more brighter, is going to have substantial influence on the design of immunofluorescence experiments over the next few years as other filter sets become available (Oi et al. 1982).

Fluorescein and rhodamine are the most frequently used. Fluorescein emits a yellow-green light that is detected well by the human eye and by most films. However, fluorescein is prone to rapid photobleaching, and bleaching retardants such as DABCO should be added to the mounting medium. Rhodamine emits a red color and is not as prone to fading as fluorescein, but the rhodamine conjugates are more hydrophobic and therefore yield higher backgrounds than fluorescein. Texas Red also emits a strong red light, and its emission spectra are farther from the emissions of fluorescein than rhodamine. It is the least likely to produce problems of fading, and when available, is the best choice for a red emitter.

When using double labels, fluorescein is best when compared to either Texas Red or rhodamine conjugates.

### Controls

Each assay should include at least two controls: (1) An irrelevant antibody from the same species and type as the primary antibody to determine the specificity of the staining. (2) A sample with no primary antibody to test for the background of the labeled secondary antibody. (3) If possible, a control against a known positive.

*Adapted from Coons et al. (1942).

## Thinking ahead

The most important preparation for antibody binding and observation is the titering of the primary and secondary antibody preparations. Starting points for the amounts of antibodies to be added are suggested in the technique below, but the single biggest problem in immunostaining is to adjust the input of the primary and secondary antibodies to levels that are sufficient to give strong robust signals, but still below levels that promote nonspecific staining. This is best achieved by doing serial dilutions of each antibody preparation (normally in a protein-containing buffer such as 3% BSA/PBS) and doing test observations on the target cell line. One-in-three dilutions (1 volume into 2 volumes) will approximate half-log steps and will quickly give a reasonable measure of the desired input. For each preparation of primary antibodies, these titering tests should be repeated. However, once these dilutions have been established for the secondary reagents, they can be used as a standard for that antibody lot.

## Needed solutions

Primary antibody solution
Fluorochrome-conjugated anti-immunoglobulin antibody (normally purchased commercially)
3% BSA/PBS; PBS
Gelvatol or Mowiol
Glycerol

## Special equipment

Fluorescence microscope equipped with epifluorescent illumination or a confocal microscope. The use of these microscopes is described in detail in Spector et al. (1998).

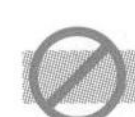

## Caution

DABCO, fluorescein, see Appendix IV.

1. Place coverslips, slides, or plates on a flat surface.

For short incubations of 1 hour or less, humidification will not be needed and the coverslips or slides can be placed right on the benchtop. If a small number of coverslips are needed, they can be placed on a layer of Parafilm. This helps to stop the antibody solution from rolling off the edge of the coverslip and makes it easy to pick up the coverslips with fine forceps, as the Parafilm is compressible. For larger numbers of round coverslips, it may be best to leave them in the 24-multiwell plates in which the cells were grown and fixed.

For incubations over 1 hour, it is convenient to array them directly in the dish or chamber that will be used for humidification. There are several methods to array slides or coverslips to allow easy handling and humidified incubations, and any arrangement that suits your personal needs is fine. For example, slides can be placed in a petri dish containing a water-saturated filter paper. Coverslips can be handled similarly. If you are using 24-well multiwell plates, a damp filter paper can be placed in the lid to provide a humid atmosphere.

*If incubations longer than 1 hour will be used, a useful trick is to place the antibody solution on a piece of Parafilm and invert the coverslip or slide onto the antibody solution (specimen side down). Samples can be removed using PBS.*

2. Add the primary antibody. Use a sufficient volume to cover the desired area of the cells, but not enough to push beyond the edge of the coverslip or the well of the slide. Volumes as small as 10 μl are often sufficient. All dilutions should be made with protein-containing solutions. For example, use PBS containing 3% BSA.

   Monoclonal antibodies are often applied as tissue-culture supernatants (specific antibody concentration of 20–50 μg/ml, used undiluted).

   Ascites fluids, purified monoclonal and polyclonal antibodies, and crude polyclonal sera should be tested at a range of dilutions. If the specific antibody concentration of the antibody sample is unknown, prepare and test 1/10, 1/100, 1/1000, and 1/10,000 dilutions of the starting material.

*For some reactions, prolonged incubations of up to 12 hours can increase sensitivity.*

3. Incubate the coverslips, slides, or plates for a minimum of 30 minutes at room temperature.

*This buffer may be supplemented with 0.5% Triton X-100 or NP-40 to help with any background problems.*

4. Wash in three changes of PBS over 5 minutes.

5. Apply the fluorochrome-conjugated anti-immunoglobulin antibody. These should be purchased from a reputable commercial source. Be sure to select a secondary antibody that is specific for the source of your antibodies. For example, goat anti-rabbit IgG would be a good choice for a primary antibody raised in rabbits.

   Secondary antibodies should be diluted in a protein-containing solution such as 3% BSA/PBS. The supplier may suggest appropriate dilutions, but if not, test dilutions of the secondary antibodies between 1/10 and 1/1000.

*An excellent protein competitor to add to the diluent would be nonimmune antibodies purified from the same species as the labeled secondary antibodies. For example, if you are using labeled goat anti-rabbit immunoglobulins for the detection step, the diluent would contain 1% nonimmune goat immunoglobulins. These antibodies should be isolated from nonimmunized animals and can be purified as described on p. 74.*

6. Incubate with the labeled secondary reagent for a minimum of 20 minutes at room temperature. Incubation times of greater than 1 hour should be avoided.

7. Wash in three changes of PBS over 5 minutes.

8. Mount the specimens in glycerol with a quenching agent such as Gelvatol or Mowiol, as described on p. 183. Observe and photograph under the fluorescence or confocal microscope.

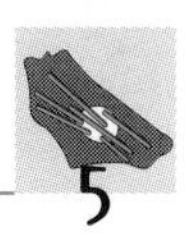



## Common problems

**Fluorescent quenching.** One of the most serious problems when using fluorochrome-conjugated secondary reagents is quenching. Each fluorochrome has a limited capacity for excitation and emission, so over time the emitted light will decline. The problems caused by fading can be minimized in two ways: first by limiting the exposure of the specimen to exciting radiation, and second by including specific antifade reagents in the mounting media.

The specimen should always be located under phase-contrast illumination with the UV light source shielded. An initial assessment of the staining reaction should be made and a photograph taken as soon as possible. To limit the amount of irradiation of the fluorochrome, it is a good idea to focus and scan the specimen initially using phase-contrast optics with transmission from the UV source blocked. Another approach is to use a second fluorescent probe that emits light at another wavelength. Some of the DNA-intercalating agents such as Hoechst 33258 or DAPI (4′, 6-diamidino-2-phenylindole) are useful in this respect. Nuclei can be stained with these dyes by including a few microliters of dye (to 0.002%) in the second antibody incubation or in a subsequent wash buffer. The absorption and emission curves of these dyes do not overlap the narrow band filters for fluorescein or rhodamine. Filters for DAPI and Hoechst 33258 are relatively inexpensive.

A wide range of antifade reagents can be used. They appear to work by scavenging free radicals liberated by excitation of the fluorochromes. The free radicals attack unexcited fluorochromes and damage them, thus producing exponential fading. The most useful antifade compound is 1,4-diazobicyclo-[2.2.2]-octane (DABCO), because of its solubility and chemical stability. For use of *p*-phenylenediamine, see Johnson and Nogueria Araujo 1981; Johnson et al. 1982; for use of *n*-propyl gallate, see Giloh and Sedat 1982.

**Weak signals or bad backgrounds.** The two most common problems are weak signals and bad backgrounds. Potential methods to reduce background problems are discussed in the box on p. 140.

Weak signals can be countered by several methods. The first is to increase the primary and/or secondary antibody concentrations. This should be done by testing various titrations of antibody concentrations. A second method is to increase the binding incubation times for both the primary and secondary antibodies. Because the antigen in cell staining will be fixed to a solid phase, the time needed for the antibody to find the antigen will be longer than if both molecules are in solution. The incubation times can be adjusted for the experimental design, but seldom will times less than 20 minutes yield efficient binding. In the first two suggestions, some compromise will need to be reached between achieving a good signal and keeping the background to an acceptable level. This will need to be determined by trial and error, because each group of antibodies and each antigen pose different problems. A third approach to produce a stronger signal is to switch detection methods. Examining the samples with a confocal microscope greatly extends the sensitivity.

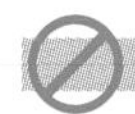

## Caution

DABCO, DAPI, *p*-phenylenediamine (antifade), UV light, see Appendix IV.

## Troubleshooting for bad backgrounds

Background problems in cell staining come primarily from two sources, nonspecific sticking and specific cross-reactions. To identify the source of background problems, compare control samples that omit each of the various stages of the staining protocol. Controls should include a nonimmune antibody, no primary antibodies, and no antibodies at all.

**Nonspecific sticking.** Nonspecific background problems are not caused by antigen binding. They are due to either the primary antibodies or secondary reagents binding to the specimen through interactions that do not involve the antigen combining site.

- Spin all antibody preparations or secondary reagents at 100,000*g* for 30 minutes to remove any protein aggregates.
- Titrate the concentration of the primary antibody and detection reagents to the minimum needed to produce a suitable signal.
- After fixation, soak the specimen in saturating amounts of nonspecific proteins that will not be recognized by the detecting agent. Useful blocking solutions include 5% serum derived from the same species as the labeled secondary antibody, 3% BSA, and 3% nonfat dry milk.
- Dilute the antibody and detection reagents in one of the above blocking solutions.
- After fixation, add 0.2% Tween-20 to all buffers and wash solutions.
- Reduce the incubation time of the primary antibody or the labeled reagent.
- Increase number and duration of washes.
- Switch detection methods.

**Specific backgrounds.** Specific background problems arise from three sources. These are contaminating antibodies with spurious reactions, cross-reacting antibodies, and immunoglobulin-binding proteins in the sample.

- If using polyclonal antibodies, titrate the antibody (spurious reactions).
- If using polyclonal antibodies, affinity-purify the antigen-specific antibodies (p. 77, spurious reactions).
- If using polyclonal antibodies, block the spurious activities with an appropriate acetone powder (p. 437).
- Try a different antibody preparation (cross-reaction or spurious).

Incubate the specimen with normal serum derived from the same species as the labeled antibody. Also dilute specific antibody in 1% normal serum from the same species as the labeled antibody (immunoglobulin-binding proteins in the sample).

# Variations on the immunostaining procedure

Immunostaining is a versatile and powerful method for identifying and characterizing the expression of an antigen. Part of its power comes from the large number of variations that can be used to characterize antigens. Discussed below are the more commonly used variations.

## Double staining

Double-labeling experiments are used to detect two different antigens in the same cell. This is performed by using two different fluorochromes, each linked to the detection of different antigens. To use two fluorochromes on the same specimen, each antigen must be recognized by only one of the labeled reagents. There are three ways to achieve this distinction.

The surest is to label each primary antibody directly. For example, when using two purified monoclonal antibodies specific for different antigens, one could be labeled with fluorescein and the other with Texas Red. This would give excellent results as long as the antibodies themselves were good for immunofluorescence.

A second method to locate two antigens in the same specimen is to use two detection reagents that are species-, class-, or subclass-specific. For example, a polyclonal rabbit antibody and a mouse monoclonal antibody specific for two different antigens could be studied using a fluorescein-conjugated goat anti-mouse immunoglobulin antibody and a Texas Red-conjugated goat anti-rabbit immunoglobulin antibody. In these protocols, the species specificity of the anti-rabbit immunoglobulin antibodies must be checked rigorously. In our example, the goat anti-rabbit immunoglobulin antibodies must not recognize any epitopes on the mouse monoclonal antibodies, and vice versa, the goat anti-mouse immunoglobulin antibodies must not cross-react with any epitopes on the rabbit antibodies. This is made somewhat easier because several companies sell reagents that have been tested for this property. Another way to ensure this does not affect your results is to choose secondary antibodies that are prepared in the same species as the other primary antibody. For example, a potential combination would be to stain cells with a mouse and a rabbit primary antibody. Then for detection, use two different fluorochromes coupled to a mouse anti-rabbit immunoglobulin antibody and a rabbit anti-mouse immunoglobulin antibody. In these cases, the animals will not make antibodies against their own antibodies and no cross-reactions should be seen.

The third, and least preferred, method is to perform the staining reactions sequentially. Particular care must be used in this approach to ensure that no dissociation and reassociation are possible. Fixing between the steps will stop this problem, but it adds extra time to the protocol.

Extreme care in all three approaches must be used in choosing double-labeling reagents to ensure that no cross-reaction between the labeled detection reagents is possible. This should always be tested in control reactions.

## Immunostaining compared with autoradiography

Any cellular event or location that can be determined by autoradiography can be compared to the location of an antigen by combining autoradiography and immunostaining. The procedure here is straightforward. Cells are radiolabeled by the appropriate method for the type of autoradiography you are using. Next they are fixed and stained as standard for any immunostaining method, taking care to handle the samples and washes with the appropriate methods for radioactive disposal that are required by your institute. Then the cells are processed for autoradiography and examined simultaneously for the location of the grains and the stain of the antibodies.

The most common use of autoradiography and immunostaining is the comparison between DNA synthesis and antigen localization. Here cells are labeled with [$^3$H]thymidine followed by immunostaining and autoradiography. This is a sensitive and accurate method to compare localization of an antigen in cells undergoing DNA synthesis. However, in most cases, we suggest trying double labeling for these comparisons. Cells are grown in the presence of BrdU to label newly synthesized DNA. Then two-color immunostaining with antibodies to BrdU (available commercially) and your antigen can be done using the methods described above for double staining.

## Caution

BrdU, radioactive substances, see Appendix IV.

## Staining proteins on the cell surface

Immunostaining techniques can be used to detect many proteins on the cell surface by minor variations in the fixation steps. There are two important points to change to visualize cell-surface antigens. The first concerns access of the antibodies and the second is how to increase the sensitivity of staining antigens on the cell surface.

One goal of this variation is to avoid lysing the cells. This will ensure that antibodies do not have access to intracellular compartments, where unprocessed antigens or potential cross-reacting antigens are found. This is done by using the paraformaldehyde fixation method, but skipping the detergent lysis. This should keep the cells intact and allow staining only on the surface. This is a useful approach for many of the abundant cell-surface proteins.

One important point to keep in mind, however, is that many cell-surface antigens are found in relatively low concentrations, some as low as 1,000 molecules per cell. Therefore, it may be necessary to take advantage of some of the optical properties of viewing spheres to stain for these antigens. The problem with visualizing low numbers of antigens on the cell surface when examining adherent cells is the low relative number of molecules that are found at any one location. A strategy to overcome this problem is to view the staining pattern on cells in suspension. This technique helps because when you view the outer ring of the rounded cell, the focal plane at the surface actually includes many layers of surface antigens. So, even in settings where the antigen is equally distributed throughout the cell surface, an antigen-positive cell will appear as a ring of staining. In the center, only one layer of the antigen is stained, whereas the edge is made up of many layers, all adding to the intensity of the staining.

Both suspension cells and adherent cells can be viewed in the manner described above. Cells growing in suspension pose no problem; they can be handled as normal. Adherent cells need special handling. Removing these cells with trypsin or other proteolytic enzymes is likely to destroy the surface proteins. Cells should be removed by treating them with EDTA or EGTA only. This frees most adherent cells and allows them to be processed just as suspension cells.

## Immunostaining for cell selection

One of the most powerful variations of the immunostaining procedure is to use the binding of antibodies as a method to mark cells for separation from nonlabeled cells. Separation from unlabeled cells is performed on a fluorescence-activated cell sorter, which examines individual cells for positive staining as they pass through a detector. A cell sorter can be used in an analytical mode to count the number of expressing cells and to characterize the level of expression in individual cells or in a preparative mode in which marked cells are isolated from nonstaining cells. This approach has become even more powerful as cell sorters have been developed that can simultaneously examine the presence of more than one marker. Now, you can examine the presence of several markers simultaneously and compare their relative levels of expression or isolate cells on the basis of multiple parameters.

Immunostaining can be used for many different approaches. In its simplest form it can identify cells that express an endogenous protein under study. It can be used to identify transected from nontransfected cells by including in the transfection cocktail a plasmid that expresses a well-characterized antigen. Another example is the identification of cells in S phase by labeling with BrdU and staining with anti-BrdU antibodies, and in turn, the timing of S phase can be compared with any other antigen expression.

Obviously, this is an extremely versatile and powerful technology. It is impossible to cover all of the techniques needed to operate a cell sorter in this short section, because cell sorters are complicated machines that normally are run by experienced technicians. Workers should contact their local experts for further information on the use of these machines. However, the methodology for preparing samples for cell sorting is generally the same as preparing samples for any of the cell-staining techniques discussed above. In these cases, the cells need to be in single-cell suspension for analysis on the sorter, but the methods for staining are identical to those for preparation for any microscopic viewing.

## Quantitation using immunostaining

Accurate quantitation is not possible using immunostaining techniques, but it is possible to determine a relative measure of the number of accessible epitopes displayed after fixation. This will not give an absolute number of molecules present in the sample, but it can be used in well-controlled comparisons to give a relative value. The strength of staining will always be a reflection of the accessibility of the antigen to antibody binding. Perhaps the best example of why this approach must be carefully interpreted is shown by early studies on the subcellular localization of the proliferating cell nuclear antigen (PCNA; also known originally as cyclin for its cyclical appearance during the cell division cycle). PCNA was shown by several labs to be found in the nucleus at distinct foci during S phase. It was not seen earlier and later in the cell cycle, leading researchers to suggest that PCNA levels were regulated during the cell cycle. However, when immunoblotting techniques were developed and used to look at the levels of PCNA, it was found that the levels were approximately equal throughout the cell cycle. In this case, what was changing was the accessibility of PCNA to binding with the primary antibody. In more recent experiments other fixation methods have been used and now PCNA staining levels can be shown not to vary extensively during the cell cycle, although its subcellular localization does change.

Even given these caveats, it is still important in some circumstances to compare the relative levels of a given antigen. To gain the most accurate information, it is important to make sure you are in the linear portions of the antibody concentration curve. For example, consider the situation in which two cells have tenfold different levels of a given antigen. If the amount of primary antibody that is added is sufficient to bind to only the amount of antigen found in the cell with the lower amount, assuming the antibody-binding step goes to completion, the levels of staining would appear similar. One might conclude that the cells have similar amounts of antigen, yet the levels are really tenfold different. Problems such as this one and many others that are not discussed as examples here can be avoided by using a range of primary antibody concentrations, being sure to use concentrations that bridge the spectrum from undetectable to saturating amounts. The comparison of antigen levels is best established by determining the dilution of primary antibody that gives a relative value equal to 50% of the highest staining. Then the various 50% points of different cells can be compared. By choosing to compare points that are still in the linear range of reactivity, you can ensure that other factors, such as the concentration of the secondary reagent or some factor in the detection system, are not limiting.

Overall, we do not recommend the use of immunostaining to determine quantitative values. Immunoblotting or immunoassays are more accurate and much less prone to errors in interpretation. However, if the samples are precious or if the cells are in a mixed population, immunostaining may be the only alternative.

## Biotin and streptavidin

An alternative labeling and detection method that is very useful for cell staining is the biotin/streptavidin system. The primary antibody is purified and conjugated with biotin. For detection, labeled streptavidin or avidin is added and allowed to bind. Streptavidin or avidin can be labeled with enzymes or fluorochromes. These labeled reagents can be purchased commercially. In general, streptavidin reagents are recommended over avidin because of their more favorable pI. The biotin/streptavidin detection methods are recommended only when large numbers of samples must be tested with the same primary antibody. This is due to the extra step needed to purify and label the primary antibody. When many different antibodies are to be tested, the purification and labeling steps for each antibody make this variation too tedious for general use.

## Caution

Biotin, see Appendix IV.

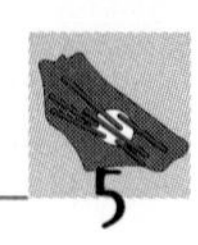


## References


Avrameas S. 1972. Enzyme markers: Their linkage with proteins and use in immunohistochemistry. *Histochem. J.* **4:** 321–330.

Avrameas S. and Uriel J. 1966. Methode de marquage d'antigen et danticorps avec des enzymes et son application en immunodiffusion. *C.R. Acad. Sci. D* **262:** 2543–2545.

Coons A.H., Creech H.J., Jones R.N., and Berliner E. 1942. The demonstration of pneumococcal antigen in tissues by the use of fluorescent antibody. *J. Immunol.* **45:** 159–170.

Giloh H. and Sedat J.W. 1982. Fluorescence microscopy: Reduced photobleaching of rhodamine and fluorescein protein conjugates by *n*-propyl gallate. *Science* **217:** 1252–1255.

Hansen P.A. 1967. Spectral data of fluorescent tracers. *Acta Histochem.* (suppl. 1) **7:** 167–180.

Johnson G.D. and Nogueira Araujo G.M. 1981. A simple method of reducing the fading of immunofluorescence during microscopy. *J. Immunol. Methods* **43:** 349–350.

Johnson G.D., Davidson R.S., McNamee K.C., Russell G., Goodwin D., and Holborow E.J. 1982. Fading of immunofluorescence during microscopy: A study of the phenomenon and its remedy. *J. Immunol. Methods* **55:** 213–242.

Nakane P.K. and Pierce G.B., Jr. 1967a. Enzyme-labeled antibodies for the light and electron microscopic localization of tissue antigens. *J. Cell Biol.* **33:** 307–318.

———. 1967b. Enzyme-labeled antibodies: Preparations and applications for the localization of antigens. *J. Histochem. Cytochem.* **14:** 929–930.

Oi V.T., Glazer A.N., and Stryer L. 1982. Fluorescent phycobiliprotein conjugates for analyses of cells and molecules. *J. Cell Biol.* **93:** 981–986.

Spector D.L., Goldman R.D., and Leinwand L.A. 1998. *Cells: A laboratory manual*, vol. 2: *Light microscopy and cell structure.* Cold Spring Harbor Laboratory Press, Cold Spring Harbor, New York.

# Staining cells growing on coverslips

Detection limit is approximately 1,000–10,000 molecules/cell if the antigen is localized.

## Summary

Rapid and easy
Detects antigen presence and localization
Qualitative to semi-quantitative
Sensitivity dependent on minimal level and localization of antigen
High local concentration of antigen, so lower affinity antibody OK

## Caution

Ethanol, FITC, fluorescein, paraformaldehyde, see Appendix IV.

1. Sterilize glass coverslips prior to cell staining. Place round coverslips (grade #1 or #1.5) in 70% ethanol. Remove individually and flame to sterilize.

2. Aseptically transfer the coverslips into a sterile tissue-culture dish by using a sterile pasteur pipet connected to a vacuum line. A light vacuum flow through the pipet will allow the coverslips to be picked up and moved easily.

3. Plate the cell suspension in the tissue-culture dish at low density. Grow overnight.

4. Remove the tissue-culture media by aspiration and wash the coverslips once with PBS. Sterility is not needed at this or later steps.

5. Aspirate the wash buffer and fix the cells by adding 4% paraformaldehyde (made fresh, p. 466). Incubate for 10 minutes at room temperature.

6. Remove the paraformaldehyde by aspiration and wash the cells twice with PBS.

7. Aspirate the last wash buffer and permeabilize the cells by adding 0.2% Triton X-100 in PBS. Incubate for 5 minutes at room temperature.

8. Remove the detergent solution by aspiration. Wash the coverslips in 0.2% Triton X-100 in PBS with three changes over 5 minutes. Drain well but do not allow the specimens to dry. Move each coverslip to the well of a 24-well tissue-culture plate.

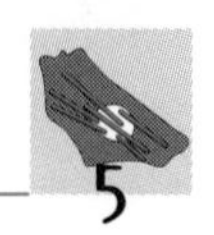



**9** Add the primary antibody solution to the coverslip. Use 25 µl to cover the entire coverslip. Make sure the coverslip does not touch the side of the well.

Monoclonal antibodies are most often used as undiluted tissue-culture supernatants. Ascites fluids, purified monoclonal and polyclonal antibodies, and crude polyclonal sera need to be checked for the proper dilution prior to use. To determine the proper titration of the antibody to use, test 1/10, 1/100, 1/1000, and 1/10,000 dilutions of the starting antibody solution. All dilutions should be done in 0.2% Triton X-100 in PBS containing 3% BSA.

Each assay should include three controls: (1) An irrelevant antibody from the same species and type as the primary antibody to determine the specificity of the staining. (2) A sample with no primary antibody to test for the background of the labeled secondary antibody. (3) If possible, a known control against a positive.

Incubate for 60 minutes at room temperature.

**10** Wash the coverslips in three changes of 0.2% Triton X-100 in PBS over 5 minutes. After the last wash, drain well but do not allow the specimens to dry.

**11** Apply the labeled secondary reagent. Add 25 µl.

A useful secondary reagent is anti-immunoglobulin antibodies conjugated to FITC. All labeled secondary reagents need to be checked for the proper dilution prior to use. To determine the proper titration of these reagents to use, test 1/10, 1/100, 1/1000, and 1/10,000 dilutions of the starting material. All dilutions should be done in 0.2% Triton X-100 in PBS containing 3% BSA.

Incubate for 20 minutes at room temperature.

**12** Wash the coverslips in three changes of 0.2% Triton X-100 in PBS over 5 minutes. Drain well.

**13** On a clean and labeled microscope slide place a drop (approximately 50 µl) of mounting medium (p. 183.)

Remove the coverslip from the dish using fine-tipped forceps and drain the last of the wash buffer by touching the edge of the coverslip to a clean paper towel. Invert the coverslip and place on the drop of mounting medium with the cell side down. Gently lower the coverslip, touching one edge to the slide next to the drop. Then allow the coverslip to fall on the drop. This will push any bubbles ahead of the falling coverslip. Allow to air dry for at least 30 minutes prior to observing.

**14** Observe and photograph under the fluorescence microscope.

# Staining Tissues

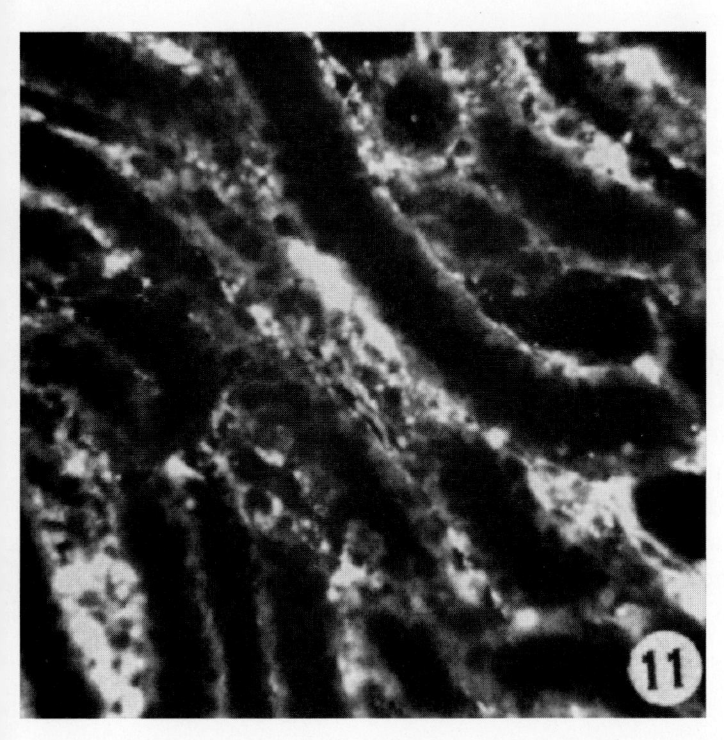

From Kaplan M.H., Coons A.H., and Deane H.W. 1949. Localization of antigen in tissue cells III. Cellular distribution of pneumococcal polysaccharides types II and III in the mouse. *J. Exp. Med.* **91:** 15–30. (Reprinted with permission [copyright The Rockefeller University Press].)

Fig. 11. Kidney medulla from mouse 91 (4 mg. polysaccharide type II: killed after 4 days). Fixed in picric acid-alcohol-formalin. Granules of polysaccharide occur in the walls of the capillary plexuses surrounding the loops of Henle as well as in several macrophages. × 300.

Combining immunochemical localization of an antigen with the examination of tissue structure was one of the prime motives in the design of all of the early developments of immunolocalization. As shown in this early staining figure, the original intent was to identify the location of pathogens; here bacteria, but in other settings viruses, were often the immunological targets. After checking for the presence of infectious agents, antibody staining became a useful marker of other pathologic events. As antibody production began to yield good reagents for important proteins in development, these methods have become important experiments for the characterization of many antigens. It now is common to check for tissue localization as an important early step in the analysis of any newly identified protein, no matter the experimental species.

Immunostaining of tissues or whole organisms can be used to examine the localization of antigens in physiological settings. Using these methods, you can follow an antigen's distribution during development, mark the location of a particular cell type in a multicellular in vivo setting, or determine the presence of an antigen in a diseased tissue. The protocols normally require multiple steps over several days as well as extensive knowledge of the architecture of the tissues being studied. These procedures demand methods to preserve the structure of tissues, which unfortunately are often damaging to the antigens. Therefore, many antibodies that work beautifully in other immunomethods may be ineffective in tissue staining. Careful choice of antibodies is essential, and comparison with the correct controls is needed to reach accurate conclusions.

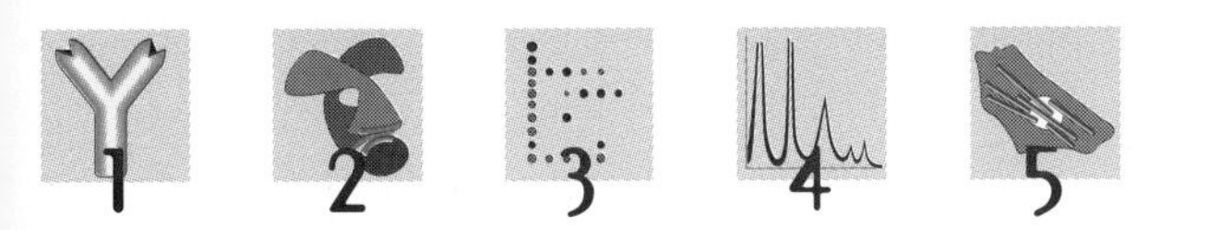

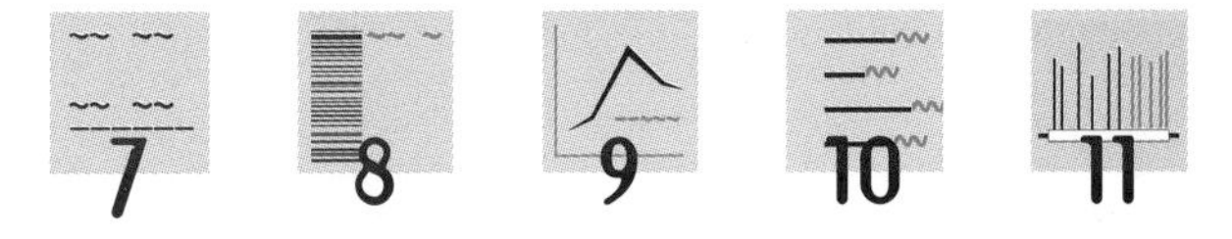


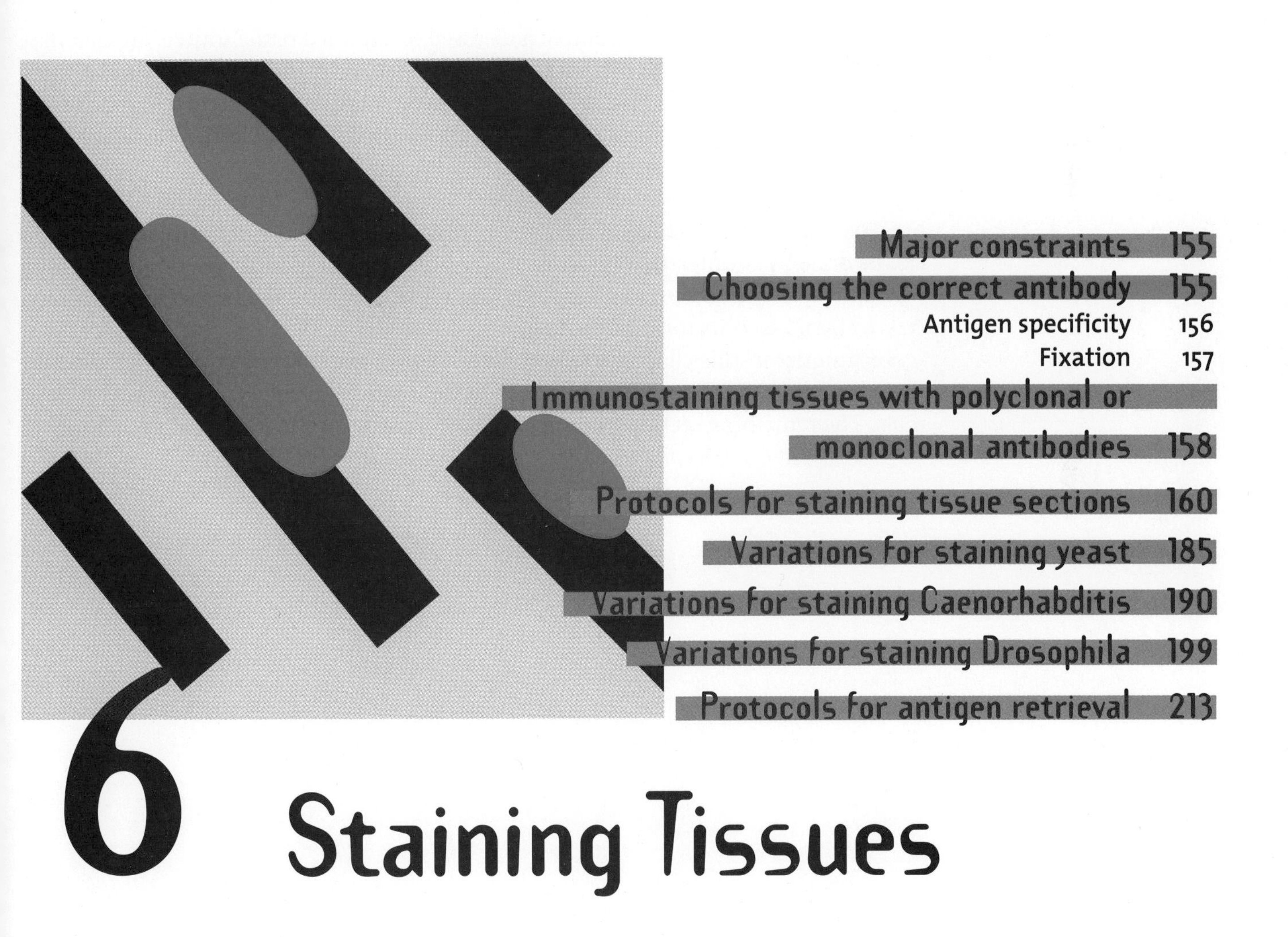



# 6 Staining Tissues

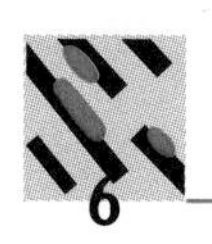



The immunostaining techniques discussed in this chapter rely on the ability of specific antibodies to bind to their cognate antigens in the natural setting of a tissue or whole organism. The techniques are designed to preserve key aspects of the tissue architecture, so that cell types and tissue structures can be identified, and to allow access of the antibodies to the local environment in which the antigen sits. Once the antibodies are bound, they are located by using a labeling secondary reagent that interacts with the immobilized antibody.

When labeled antibodies are used to detect antigens in tissues or organisms, several characteristics of an antigen can be readily determined. The most important aspect of this type of approach is to find and localize an antigen in its physiological environment. Staining of tissues is used extensively in two manners. First, it is used during the first stages of characterizing an antigen when little is known about its potential role. This immediately gives the researcher a clue as to the type of cell in which the antigen functions and a potential role to test for the antigen activity. The second key use of staining tissues is the examination of a diseased or mutated tissue source. Here, it may be possible to learn whether the antigen is mislocalized or misexpressed due to these changes. Cell staining can also be used in pathology studies for determining such variables as the type of infectious organism, the progenitor of a neoplastic cell, or the presence of an inflammatory response.

It is particularly important for this type of staining that the tissue architecture is well preserved to be able to confirm the types of cells that are expressing your antigen. This can be done by counterstaining with conventional histological stains, double staining with known secondary markers, or comparing with other methods to locate known cells or tissue architectural landmarks.

Techniques in this chapter are first described for the staining of tissue sections or tissue smears taken from sources of biological material ranging from plants to animals. The remaining sections are variations of these techniques applied specifically to staining yeast, *Caenorhabditis elegans*, and *Drosophila*.

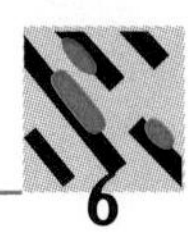


## Major constraints

There are four major constraints that determine how easily an antigen is detected using tissue staining. These are (1) the local antigen concentration and its configuration, (2) how the fixative modifies the antigen, (3) how easy it is for the antibody to gain access to the antigen, and (4) the specificity of the antibody used.

The major factor that influences the strength of the signal in tissue staining is how the antigen is displayed in its local environment, which depends on the local antigen concentration and configuration of the epitope display. The antigens that are easiest to detect have a characteristic structure and present a large number of identical antibody-binding sites in a small local environment, thus allowing multiple interactions to take place and making detection simple (see Chapter 2). Diffuse antigens, even when present at high concentrations, are difficult to detect or distinguish from background signals.

The second factor that determines how easy an antigen is to detect in tissue staining is how severe the problems of fixation are. Fixation for tissue-staining methods is often highly destructive to antigenic structure. Perfect fixation would immobilize the antigens, while retaining authentic cellular and subcellular architecture and creating no change in epitope structure. No fixation method reaches this ideal. Many epitopes are masked or altered by certain fixatives.

The third factor that affects the success of immunostaining of tissues is how easily the antibody can reach the antigen. Immunostaining only succeeds if the preparation of the tissue permits unhindered access of antibodies to all cells and subcellular compartments. Following fixation, the structural features of tissues often make antibody access more difficult than in cells fixed in culture. In some cases, hidden epitopes may be unmasked by limited protease treatment or heating, but many may not.

The fourth factor that determines the success of tissue staining is the specificity of the antibodies. Tissue staining places exceptional demands on antibody specificity. Antibody preparations that are satisfactory for other techniques such as immunoprecipitation or immunoblotting may show spurious cross-reactions in cell staining. This is particularly vexing because these cross-reactions are difficult to identify. Therefore, you need to be exceptionally careful in deciding whether the detected signal is due to the presence of the antigen or a spurious and unwanted cross-reaction.

## Choosing the correct antibody

As discussed above, the problems encountered in staining of tissues and organisms can be severe. Therefore, choosing the best antibody to use in tissue staining is very important. Antibodies that work well in immunoblotting, immunoprecipitations, or even in staining of cells in culture, may fail in tissue staining. The problems that are encountered in immunostaining stem primarily from the difficulties of observing your antigen in situ. This means that the antigen must be fixed in its local environment, providing ample opportunities for epitope damage, blockage of antibody ac-

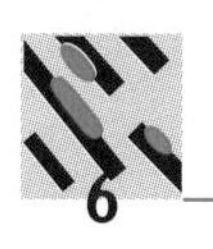



cess, and enhancement of low-affinity interactions. It also means that the antigen presence is difficult to confirm by independent criteria. The inability to confirm the identity of your antigen by a second criterion, for example by protein size as in immunoprecipitations or immunoblots, means that special care must be used in choosing your antibodies and in designing experimental controls.

## Antigen specificity

A first feature to test when choosing antibodies for tissue staining is the specificity of antigen binding. None of the techniques commonly used in immunology perfectly reflects the conditions found in immunostaining of tissues. Therefore, there is no straightforward method to determine whether your antibody will cross-react with other antigens in your specimen. As a preliminary step, test your antibody in immunoblotting and immunoprecipitations using samples from the same tissues that will be used for staining. These tests will detect major cross-reactions that might be shared with fully denaturation-resistant epitopes (immunoblots) and native epitopes (immunoprecipitations). Detection of any major bands should preempt the use of this antibody in immunostaining, unless there are clear methods to distinguish the correct signal from a cross-reaction.

When performing the immunostaining technique, you can gain some measure of specificity by comparing the staining pattern with controls. These controls should include a negative antibody that is matched by species, and, if using a monoclonal antibody, by isotype, with your antibody. Be sure to include a sample in which the primary antibody has been omitted to distinguish your signal from any background that might arise from the secondary reagent.

Another useful approach to testing for antigen specificity is to use two or more antibodies that are raised against separate portions of your antigen and that can be shown to be entirely distinct (see Chapter 11). If multiple antibodies recognizing distinct regions of the antigen give the identical staining pattern, this result suggests that the signal arises from your antigen. One caveat, however, is that your antigen might share extensive structural features with a related molecule, for example another protein of the same protein family, and you might be examining the location of this molecule rather than your antigen. If this is a protein antigen, it is likely that such a cross-reaction would also appear in the immunoblotting or immunoprecipitation controls.

An excellent test for specificity is to examine the staining pattern seen with your antibody on a sample from a wild-type animal and from an animal that carries a homozygous deletion (or other nonexpressing alleles) for your gene. The loss of a signal indicates at the very least that the signal you have observed is due in part to the expression of your protein.

Other excellent controls for specificity include comparing the pattern of your antigen staining with green fluorescent protein (GFP) or fusions or epitope-tagged versions of your protein-coding region (Chapter 10). This will not be possible in many cases, but if this approach is available to you, it does provide an excellent control.

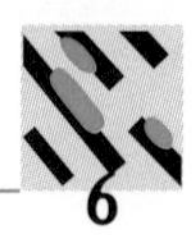


## Fixation

Problems caused by the severe conditions often used to fix tissues are probably the most common reason that an antibody fails in staining of tissue, a result that is often true even with antibodies that work well in staining of cells in culture (Chapter 5).

Several events can cause fixation to block the ability of an antibody to bind to the antigen. First, the fixation method can modify amino acid side chains and, if they are part of the epitope, the antibodies will not interact. This is most often seen when using formaldehyde or paraformaldehyde, which react with the primary amines of lysine to establish a cross-link that stabilizes the antigen display. The fixation method frequently denatures the antigen and causes the loss of many denaturation-sensitive epitopes.

The second problem brought about by fixation is the hindrance of antibody access to the antigen, which may be caused by the cross-linking of proteins in the local cellular environment by the fixation method and may create stable structures that do not allow antibody access. Also, if the fixative contains organic solvents such as alcohols or acetones, all of the proteins in the local environment will be precipitated, thus blocking antibody access.

These types of fixation problems are difficult to control, but researchers should be aware of these problems because they greatly influence the success of a particular antibody in the staining process. Many different antibodies may need to be tested to find one that is not severely affected by fixation problems. It is important to keep in mind that if tissue staining is the major goal of an antibody that you are preparing, it may be worthwhile to consider modifying the antigen source by passing it through the fixation process before immunization. This will not remove the problems associated with hindrance of the antibody by local structures, but it will provide antibodies against an antigen that has been modified as in the fixation regime.

### Perfused tissues

For laboratory animals, perfusion of tissue or organs with fixative solutions in situ is often used to preserve tissue and cell architecture. This technique is particularly useful for soft tissues. Once preserved, tissue samples can be prepared for cell staining using either of the methods listed (frozen sections or paraffin-embedded sections). A wide range of different fixative solutions and perfusion methods are used. The best choice of fixative and technique depends on the tissue, antigen, and animal. For suggestions, see Meek (1976), Sternberger (1979), Bullock and Petrusz (1982), and Polak and Van Noorden (1983).

Regulations governing perfusion vary. Consult your local authorities for the proper procedures.

# Immunostaining tissues with polyclonal or monoclonal antibodies

Tissue staining is commonly performed with both monoclonal and polyclonal antibodies. In general, polyclonal antibodies give stronger signals, whereas monoclonal antibodies provide less background and better specificity. Either can be used effectively with the appropriate care.

## Cell staining with polyclonal antibodies

A good polyclonal serum contains multiple antibodies directed against different epitopes on the antigen. Because polyclonal sera usually contain antibodies specific for a broad range of epitopes on the antigen, including denaturation-resistant epitopes, they often work well on heavily fixed samples and are the best source of antibodies for techniques such as the staining of sections cut from paraffin-embedded tissue samples. In addition, it is possible to have more than one antibody bind to the antigen when using polyclonal antibodies; therefore, the signal may be stronger when using polyclonal antibodies for tissue staining.

In addition to the specific antibodies, polyclonal sera also contain relatively high concentrations of irrelevant antibodies of unknown specificity. These include the entire repertoire of antibodies in the animal when the serum was collected, and they create the most troublesome problems for tissue staining. Satisfactory cell-staining experiments can be conducted using polyclonal antibodies, but their use requires careful control. This should include careful titration of the primary antibody to minimize the signal from spurious antibodies in the serum and careful comparisons with control sera.

Even sera from unimmunized animals give an intense background when used at high concentrations. Part of this background is from antibodies binding nonspecifically to the fixed cells, and part is from specific interactions arising from spurious activities in the serum. Because these antibodies are normally not the major activities in the serum, their binding can often be reduced below the levels of detection by careful titration of the polyclonal antibodies. A second method for lowering these types of background problems is to preadsorb the polyclonal sera with suitable acetone powders (p. 437). A third method used to circumvent these problems is to remove the nonspecific antibodies completely. Immunoaffinity purification of the antigen-specific antibodies (Chapter 9) can be used to prepare an excellent source of antibodies for tissue staining. For some purposes, immunoaffinity purification of the antibodies is essential to obtain clear staining patterns. Finally, great improvements in background can be achieved by simply purifying the IgG fraction of the serum using protein A or G affinity methods (see Chapter 4).

## Tissue staining with monoclonal antibodies

When appropriate monoclonal antibodies are available, they often work exceptionally well in tissue-staining techniques, where their purity and specificity yield low backgrounds over a wide range of antibody concentrations. However, most monoclonal antibodies do not work well in heavily fixed tissues, so finding antibodies for tissue staining is more difficult than for cell staining.

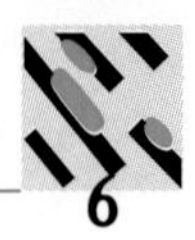


Like other antibody sources, monoclonal antibodies may show cross-reactions in tissue-staining procedures. Some of these cross-reactions are specific and presumably reflect the presence of common epitopes on two cellular components. Cross-reactions with multimeric cellular proteins present in high concentrations, such as cytoskeletal filaments, are the most commonly observed background. This usually results from weak cross-reactions that are enhanced by bivalent binding and by the high concentrations of such antigens. The location of an antigen should be confirmed, whenever possible, by using a panel of monoclonal antibodies directed to discrete epitopes on the same antigen.

## Tissue staining with pooled monoclonal antibodies

Pooled monoclonal antibodies increase the signal strength for a given antigen provided the antibodies in the pool can bind to it noncompetitively. Such an increase in signal strength can mean the difference between successful detection and failure. Care in pooling must be exercised, however. Each antibody in the pool must be tested individually before being added as part of a panel. Because of the difficulty in finding even one antibody that works well in tissue-staining methods, it is not common to be able to pool monoclonal antibodies for this method; however, when they are available they provide an excellent choice.

Table 6.1 *Antibody choice*

| | Polyclonal antibodies | Monoclonal antibodies | Pooled monoclonal antibodies |
|---|---|---|---|
| **Signal strength** | Excellent | Fair | Excellent |
| **Specificity** | Good, but some background | Excellent, but some cross-reactions | Excellent |
| **Good features** | Signal strength | Specificity<br>Unlimited supply | Signal strength<br>Specificity<br>Unlimited supply |
| **Bad features** | Nonrenewable<br>Background<br>Need to titer | Seldom available | Seldom available |

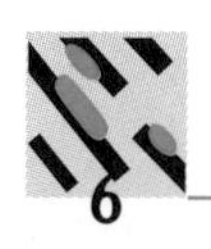



# Protocols for staining tissue sections



Four methods commonly are used to prepare tissue for staining. These are sectioning of frozen tissues; sectioning of paraformaldehyde-fixed, paraffin-embedded tissues; sectioning of tissues prepared from perfused animals; and preparing cytological smears. All these procedures ultimately yield fixed specimens bound to a glass microscope slide ready for the addition of antibody.

## Overview of the staining procedure for tissue sections

Staining techniques for tissue sections can be divided into three steps:

1. tissue preparation and sectioning
2. antibody binding
3. detection

After the specimens are attached to glass slides, the antibodies are applied. Antibodies bind to their cognate antigen, and unbound antibodies are removed by washing. The location of the bound antibodies is determined by adding labeled secondary reagents that interact specifically with the primary antibody. After washing, the location of the antigen is determined by the location of the labeled secondary reagent.

## Preparation of tissue specimens

Histological material for immunostaining can be derived from two types of sources. First, investigators may obtain and fix the material themselves. Consequently, all steps can be optimized and carefully controlled. Although this is the optimal situation, many investigators will wish to apply their reagents to the second source of histological material, that derived from archives stored in pathology departments or other repositories. Here, the samples are almost always stored as paraffin blocks. The wealth of information based on the histochemical analysis of these tissues is enormous and is a major resource for anyone trying to localize his antigen. However, it is essential to realize that when these samples are collected (1) fixation times and conditions are rarely standardized and (2) the nature of the fixatives differs between repositories and may differ with the time within the same repository. In the case of some antigen/antibody combinations, these issues are not of major significance, because they are not particularly sensitive to fixation differences. For other combinations, they are of major significance, and as yet there is no rational basis for this. Methods for antigen retrieval are discussed on p. 213.

Repositories now frequently collect samples of flash-frozen tissues. These are also valuable sources of material for staining. Here the problems of standardization are less, but the wealth of histochemical information is more limited. However, frozen sections generally yield specimens that work better with most sources of antibodies.

The methods below are divided into the major sources of tissue samples. We have not included instructions for the use of the various microtomes or cryostats needed to cut these sections, because they vary so much. Consult manufacturers' instructions for the use of this equipment.

# Preparing frozen tissue sections



Immunostaining studies on mammalian tissue are often carried out on frozen sections. This is the gentlest method for the preparation of samples and gives good preservation of tissue structure and antigens. The principal disadvantages are that the specimens must be stored frozen, and a special microtome, known as a cryostat, is required. Also, many clinical specimens are not available in this form and most classic histological descriptions of tissue structure and pathology are based on the use of paraffin-embedded sections of formalin-fixed material.

## Thinking ahead

Before starting, it is often valuable to prepare a stock of gelatin-coated slides (step 3). These can be prepared in advance and stored in a cool dry place for several weeks.

## Needed solutions

Freezing agent, such as isopentane or OCT (see step 2)

1% Gelatin with 0.02% sodium azide

4% Paraformaldehyde (freshly prepared, see p. 466) or other fixative (see step 5)

1% NP-40 in PBS

PBS

## Special equipment

Cryostat

## Cautions

Acetone, hydrogen peroxide, isopentane, methanol, OCT, paraformaldehyde, phenylhydrozine hydrochloride, sodium azide, see Appendix IV.

1. Dissect a small sample, no bigger than approximately 1 $cm^2 \times 0.4$ cm, of undamaged tissue.

*The tissue samples can be stored at –70°C for up to 1 year. Long-term storage should be done in airtight containers.*

2. **Either:** If the tissue is very dense and compact (such as skin or muscle), place the specimen on one end of a strip of card and submerge the specimen in liquid nitrogen. After 60 seconds in the liquid nitrogen, remove the sample and place it on dry ice. Trim the card to just larger than the size of tissue and transfer it to a precooled (–70°C), labeled freezing vial. Alternatively, freeze the samples in isopentane, precooled to liquid nitrogen temperature. Isopentane will not bubble as the sample is immersed, thus shortening the time needed for freezing. Transfer to a precooled (–70°C), labeled freezing vial.

   **Or:** If the tissue has little intrinsic strength (such as spleen or lymph nodes), place the specimen in a gelatin capsule containing OCT. (OCT is a mixture of polyvinyl alcohol, polyethylene glycol, and dimethyl benzyl ammonium chloride, sold by BDH and other commercial outlets. Another useful freezing solution is Lipshaw Number 1.) Freeze the capsule gradually in liquid nitrogen as follows: Immerse the bottom of the capsule first, allow to freeze, and then submerge the whole capsule. Transfer the capsule to a precooled (–70°C), labeled freezing vial. Alternatively, place a puddle of

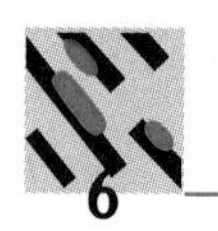



OCT on a flat piece of dry ice. As the OCT begins to freeze, slide the piece of tissue into the solution. Allow to freeze completely, wrap in foil, and label.

3. Prior to sectioning, coat clean glass slides with 1% gelatin. Dissolve gelatin in water by heating to 50°C, cool, and add sodium azide to 0.02%. Dip the slides in the solution for 30 seconds, remove, and allow to air-dry.

4. Prepare sections of frozen tissues by standard techniques. The thickness of the sections will depend on the tissue being studied. In general, thinner sections are better for staining. Sections between 5 and 10 μm commonly are used. Collect the sections on the coated slides. (Consult the manufacturers' instructions on the proper use of a cryostat.)

5. Depending on the type of tissue and the nature of the antigen, several different steps can be used next.

   **Either:** Allow the section to air-dry. Dip in freshly prepared paraformaldehyde (see p. 466) for 2 minutes. Wash with several changes of PBS, and place in 1% NP-40, PBS for 5 minutes.

   **Or:** Fix the section in acetone at room temperature for 30 seconds.

6. Rinse in several changes of PBS.

**Antibodies can now be applied to the samples (p. 166).**

## Common problems

If peroxidase- or alkaline phosphatase-labeled detection methods are to be used, it may be necessary to block or inhibit endogenous enzyme activity within the specimen before the application of antibody. Because the blocking procedures may harm some antigens, it may be easier to change the detection reagent rather than block endogenous enzyme activities.

To block endogenous peroxidase activity, incubate the specimen with a solution of 4 parts of methanol to 1 part of 3% hydrogen peroxide for 20 minutes. Hydrogen peroxide is generally supplied as a 30% solution and should be stored at 4°C, at which temperature it will last about 1 month. For specimens such as spleen or bone marrow containing high peroxidase activities, better results may be obtained by using a solution of 0.1% phenylhydrazine hydrochloride in PBS. Although some sources suggest the simple application of 3% hydrogen peroxide to the specimen, this should not be done because violent reactions and bubble formation can destroy the specimen.

To block endogenous alkaline phosphatase activity, include 0.1 mM Levamisole in the substrate solution. This inhibitor does not diminish the activity of intestinal alkaline phosphatase used to prepare the labeled antibody but does inhibit the activity of other tissue phosphatases. Alkaline phosphatase-labeled antibodies should not be used to stain specimens containing endogenous intestinal alkaline phosphatase.

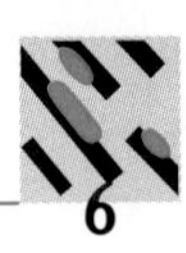

## Preparing paraffin tissue sections



*When asking for archival material, remember to follow the standards of scientific courtesy. Many of these repositories are the lifeblood of histological research and have been painstakingly prepared and maintained over decades.*

Most histological studies are carried out on paraformaldehyde-fixed, paraffin-embedded tissue samples. Therefore, there is an extensive atlas of most tissues and organs prepared from these sources, and comparing the location of antigens to these data is immediately informative. Histologists and pathologists have extensive experience with tissues, and their input is often valuable in the interpretation of patterns of antigen expression.

The fixation and embedding procedures are harsh, and many antigens are not well preserved. Duration of fixation is an important variable, because prolonged fixation diminishes the ability of antibodies to work. In pathology laboratories, the duration and other details of fixation are rarely standardized. Furthermore, because the rate of penetration of fixative into tissues is constant at a given temperature (about 1 mm per hour at room temperature), not all parts of a sample will be fixed in the same way. Consequently, there may be heterogeneity in fixation with consequent variation in immunostaining properties. Ideally, an investigator will attend to specimen collection and fixation personally, thus optimizing the ability to identify the antigens under study.

**Avoid mercury-containing fixative absolutely.**

### Thinking ahead

Paraffin blocks can be prepared well in advance, and sections can be cut beginning at step 5. Many pathology or other reference labs have large stores of archival material for study.

*To prepare 1 liter of Bouin's fixative, dissolve 2 g of picric acid in 500 ml of deionized $H_2O$. Filter through a Whatman No. 1, or equivalent. Add 20 g of paraformaldehyde, and heat to 60°C in a fume hood. Add a few drops of 1 N NaOH to dissolve. Cool and add 500 ml of 2× PBS.*

### Needed solutions

4% Paraformaldehyde (prepared fresh, see p. 466) or Bouin's fixative, see step 2

Xylene
Absolute ethanol
95% Ethanol

### Special equipment

Microtome
Paraffin embedding equipment

### Cautions

Acetic acid, chloroform, ethanol, hydrogen peroxide, methanol, sodium hydroxide, paraformaldehyde, phenylhydrazine hydrochloride, picric acid, xylene, see Appendix IV.

1. Cut small blocks of tissue approximately 1 $cm^2$ × 0.4 cm.

*Methocarn is a mixture of methanol, chloroform, and glacial acetic acid prepared in a 6:3:1 ratio. When using methocarn, the first step of the sectioning procedure must use* ***anhydrous*** *ethanol.*

2. Place the tissue blocks in fixative. If the samples are being prepared solely for immunochemical localization either directly or with counter or double stains, we recommend the use of freshly prepared 4% paraformaldehyde (see p. 466). However, standard pathological methods effectively use any of a broad range of fixatives, including Bouin's or methocarn.

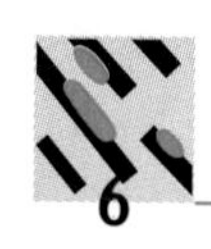



*Fixatives penetrate tissues at a rate of about 1 mm per hour. You can use this estimate to judge the minimum for your fixation incubation.*

3. Incubate the samples for 2 hours to overnight.

4. Follow standard paraffin embedding procedures as suggested by the makers of your microtome.

*Paraffin blocks at this stage (step 4) are often archived and stored for later examinations. Paraffin blocks are a stable storage setting and are known to be useful for many years.*

5. Collect 4-μm sections onto clean glass slides.

6. Incubate the sections at 37°C overnight.

7. Dewax the sections in xylene. Change two times, 3 minutes each.

8. Rehydrate by passing through graded alcohols (two changes, absolute ethanol, 3 minutes each; followed by two changes, 95% ethanol, 3 minutes each).

*Higher temperatures (step 6) are suggested for most histochemistry procedures, but these temperatures tend to cause loss of many epitopes and should be avoided if possible.*

9. Rinse in water.

**Antibodies can now be applied to the specimen (p. 166).**

*Because of the harsh fixation, embedding, and preparation conditions, tissue staining of paraffin-embedded tissue sections usually requires sensitive detection methods and may need amplification using multiple-layer techniques.*

## Common problems

If peroxidase- or alkaline phosphatase-labeled detection methods are to be used, it may be necessary to block or inhibit endogenous enzyme activity within the specimen before the application of antibody. Because the blocking procedures may harm some antigens, it may be easier to change the detection reagent rather than block endogenous enzyme activities.

To block endogenous peroxidase activity, incubate the specimen with a solution of 4 parts methanol to 1 part 3% hydrogen peroxide for 20 minutes. Hydrogen peroxide is generally supplied as a 30% solution and should be stored at 4°C, at which temperature it will last about 1 month. For specimens containing high peroxidase activities, such as spleen or bone marrow, better results may be obtained by using a solution of 0.1% phenylhydrazine hydrochloride in PBS. Although some sources suggest the simple application of 3% hydrogen peroxide to the specimen, this should not be done because violent reactions and bubble formation can destroy the specimen.

To block endogenous alkaline phosphatase activity, include 0.1 mM Levamisole in the substrate solution. This inhibitor does not diminish the activity of intestinal alkaline phosphatase used to prepare the labeled antibody, but it does inhibit the activity of other tissue phosphatases. Alkaline phosphatase-labeled antibodies should not be used to stain specimens containing endogenous intestinal alkaline phosphatase.

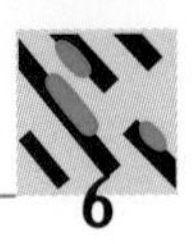


## Preparing cell smears from tissue samples

PREPARATION

BINDING, 166

DETECTION, 170

Staining of tissues can be carried out on cell smears prepared from biopsy samples, such as needle aspirates, tissue scrapings, or freshly dissected tissues. In these protocols, a thin layer of cells is deposited on a dry slide by physical methods. The most important factor in obtaining good staining patterns is that the smear be only a single cell thick. Tissue smears do not preserve tissue architecture, but they are useful for identifying pathological changes and infectious organisms in tissue samples.

### Needed solutions

Acetone, methanol, or a 50/50 mix of acetone and methanol
PBS

### Cautions

Acetone, methanol, see Appendix IV.

1. For tissues or organs that have internal fluid spaces (e.g., spleen or liver), cut a small block of unfixed tissue and dab directly onto a clean, dry, glass slide.

   For tissue scrapings and needle aspirates, deposit the tissue sample at one end of the slide. For well-dispersed samples, touch a second slide to the sample and use it to push the sample across the first slide. For denser samples, use the second slide to pull the sample across the first slide, helping to break up the tissue.

2. Allow the sample to air-dry.

3. Dip the slide into any organic fixative. Most often this is acetone, but methanol or 50% acetone/50% methanol are also used.

4. Incubate the sample for 2 minutes at room temperature.

5. Rinse twice in PBS.

**The sample is now ready for the addition of antibodies (p. 166).**

## Binding

Once tissues are fixed and permeabilized, the antibodies are added. Here, as in many other immunochemical techniques, the antibodies can be labeled directly or they can be detected by using a labeled secondary reagent that will bind specifically to the primary antibody. In general, direct labeling of the primary antibody produces cleaner signals with lower background. The major disadvantage of direct detection is the time needed to purify and label each preparation of primary antibody. This makes direct detection much more difficult for tissue staining and, except in unusual cases, we recommend indirect methods where the secondary detection reagent can be purchased from one of the many commercial sources.

For indirect detection, any reagent that binds specifically to the primary antibody can be "tagged" and used to locate the antibody. The possible reagents include anti-immunoglobulin antibodies, protein A or G, or, if the first antibody is labeled with biotin, streptavidin (p. 83). The major advantage of indirect detection is that one set of labeled reagents can be used for a number of primary antibodies. Indirect methods normally give stronger signals, but the backgrounds may be worse, and so, appropriate controls are essential.

Detection reagents for tissue staining are most often labeled with enzymes or with gold (Table 6.2). Each of the labels has advantages and disadvantages that vary between different experimental designs. The choice of label is discussed in the detection section below (p. 170).

Table 6.2 *Detection methods for tissue and organism staining*

| Method | Advantages | Disadvantages | Recommended for |
|---|---|---|---|
| Fluorescence | High resolution<br>Double labeling possible | Requires special microscope<br>Fades over time | High resolution studies<br>Double labeling<br>Best choice for yeast and worm staining |
| Enzyme | High sensitivity<br>Only need light microscope<br>Permanent | Low resolution<br>Endogenous enzyme activities<br>Double staining difficult<br>Some substrates toxic | Low resolution studies<br>Rapid antigen detection |
| Gold | High resolution<br>Double labeling possible<br>Only need light microscope | Less widely used so less experience | Good alternative for tissue staining |

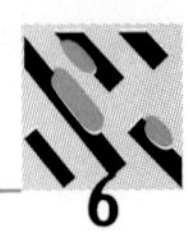

## Binding antibodies to tissue sections

PREPARATION, 160

BINDING

DETECTION, 170

Because the antigen in cell staining will be fixed to a solid phase, the time needed for the antibody to find the antigen is longer than if both molecules are in solution. The incubation times can be adjusted for the experimental design, but seldom do times less than 30 minutes yield efficient binding. The incubation times can be lowered by increasing the concentration of the secondary reagents. Usually, some compromise needs to be reached between these two variables. Higher amounts promote stronger signals but also larger background problems. Lower concentrations reduce the backgrounds but lower the signal strength. In general, our recommendations are to pick a relatively short and convenient time for the incubation with the labeled secondary reagent (for example, 30 or 60 minutes), then titrate the amount of the labeled secondary reagent to a level that gives low background with an acceptable signal strength. In all cases, the antibodies should be diluted in buffers containing high concentrations of nonspecific proteins. Proteins that are commonly used are bovine serum albumin (BSA), fetal bovine serum (FBS), nonfat dry milk, or serum from the same species as the labeled antibody.

### Controls

Specific staining reactions should always be compared with control reactions. To assess a staining pattern accurately, two antibodies from the same species should be compared. For polyclonal antibodies, the best control is a prebleed from the same animal used to prepare the specific antibodies, but nonimmune serum from the same species is acceptable in most cases. For monoclonal antibodies, the control must be from the same source as the specific antibody; i.e., supernatant versus supernatant, ascites versus ascites, or pure antibody versus pure antibody. If possible, the control antibodies should be of the same class and subclass as the specific antibody. Tissue-culture supernatants from the parental myeloma are never appropriate controls, because they do not contain antibodies. Suitable control hybridoma cell lines are available from the American Type Culture Collection.

In addition, if using indirect detection, the secondary reagent should be tested on its own. Finally, when using enzyme-linked detection, the enzyme reaction should be done on the specimen without the addition of any antibodies. This will demonstrate the presence and location of any endogenous enzyme activities.

### Thinking ahead

The most important preparation for antibody binding and observation is the titering of the primary and secondary antibody preparations. Although starting points for the amounts of antibodies to be added are suggested in the technique below, the single biggest problem in immunostaining is to adjust the input of the primary and secondary antibodies to levels that are sufficient to give robust signals, but still below levels that promote nonspecific staining. This is best achieved by doing serial dilutions of each antibody preparation (normally in a protein-containing buffer such as 3% BSA/PBS) and doing test observations on the target cell line. One-in-three dilutions (1 volume into 2 volumes) approximate half-log

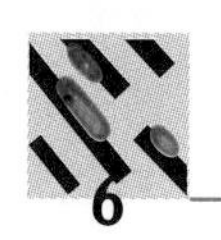



steps and quickly give a reasonable measure of the desired input. For each preparation of primary antibodies, these titering tests should be repeated. However, once these dilutions have been established for the secondary reagents, they can be used as a standard for that antibody lot.

### Needed solutions and reagents

Primary antibody solution
Secondary antibody (most often purchased from a commercial source)
PBS
3% BSA/PBS

1. Place slides with the tissue sections or cell smears in a humidified chamber.

2. Add the first antibody solution. All dilutions must be carried out in protein-containing solutions. For example, use PBS containing 3% BSA.

   Monoclonal antibodies are normally applied as tissue-culture supernatants (specific antibody concentration of 20–50 μg/ml; use neat). Ascites fluids, purified monoclonal and polyclonal antibodies, and crude polyclonal sera should be tested at a range of dilutions aimed at producing specific antibody concentrations between 0.1 and 10 μg/ml. If the specific antibody concentration of the antibody sample is unknown, prepare and test 1/10, 1/100, 1/1000, and 1/10,000 dilutions of the starting material.

3. Incubate the slides for a minimum of 30 minutes at room temperature in the humidified chamber. For some reactions, prolonged incubations of up to 24 hours can increase sensitivity.

4. Wash in three changes of PBS over 5 minutes. This buffer may be supplemented with 1% Triton X-100 or NP-40 to help with any background problems.

5. Apply the labeled secondary reagent. It is essential to carry out all dilutions in a protein-containing solution such as 3% BSA/PBS or 1% immunoglobulin/PBS (prepared from the same species as the detection reagent). Useful secondary reagents include anti-immunoglobulin antibodies, protein A, or protein G (see Chapter 4). They can be labeled with enzymes or gold. Labeled secondary reagents can be purchased from several suppliers.

   **For enzyme-labeled reagents:** If using a commercial preparation, test dilutions of the secondary antibodies 1/50 to 1/1000. Alkaline phosphatase-labeled reagents should be handled using Tris-buffered saline, not PBS.

   **For gold-labeled reagents:** Wash the gold particles once in PBS. Dilute in PBS containing 1% gelatin and add to the specimen.

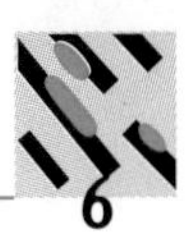


6. Incubate with the labeled secondary reagent for a minimum of 20 minutes at room temperature in the humidified chamber. For gold-labeled reagents, observe periodically under the microscope until a satisfactory signal is obtained.

7. Wash in three changes of PBS over 5 minutes.

**The specimen is now ready for the detection step (p. 170).**

## Common problems

If background problems are seen, the nonspecific binding can often be inhibited by preincubating the specimen with protein. Commonly used proteins are BSA at 3%, FBS at 10% (use fetal and not calf, as fetal bovine serum has lower amounts of IgGs), 10% dry milk, or purified antibodies (used at 1%) from the same species as the detection reagent. The blocking protein can be added to each antibody preparation and/or can be used to incubate the samples before the addition of antibody.

## Detection

Two types of methods are used in tissue staining to label the detecting reagent. These are enzymes and gold. The properties of each detection method are summarized in Table 6.1. Enzyme-labeled antibodies provide extremely sensitive antigen detection and require only a suitable substrate and a light microscope for their detection. Importantly, they are compatible with the counterstains commonly used in classic histology.

Gold-labeled reagents are relatively new for detection at the level of light microscopy, but they have been used widely for electron microscopy. When gold-labeled reagents are used with silver enhancement, they offer some excellent advantages.

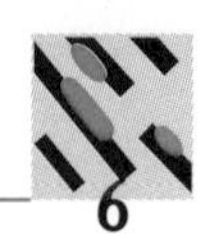


## Troubleshooting for bad backgrounds

Background problems in cell staining come primarily from two sources, nonspecific sticking and specific cross-reactions. These problems are discussed separately below. Other problems are encountered with particular detection methods and include autofluorescence and endogenous enzyme activities. Resolution of these problems is covered for each detection method within its particular section.

To identify the source of background problems, compare control samples that omit each of the various stages of the staining protocol. Controls must include a nonimmune antibody, no primary antibodies, and no antibodies at all (see p. 130).

*Nonspecific sticking* Nonspecific background problems are not caused by antigen binding. They are due to either the primary antibodies or secondary reagents binding to the specimen through interactions that do not involve the antigen combining site.

- Spin all antibody preparations or secondary reagents at 100,000*g* for 30 minutes.
- Titrate the concentration of the primary antibody and detection reagents to the minimum needed to produce a suitable signal.
- After fixation, soak the specimen in saturating amounts of nonspecific proteins that will not be recognized by the detecting agent. Useful blocking solutions include 1% serum derived from the same species as the labeled antibody, 3% BSA, and 10% nonfat dry milk.
- Dilute the antibody and detection reagents in one of the above blocking solutions.
- After fixation, add 0.2% Tween-20 to all buffers and wash solutions.
- Reduce the incubation time of the primary antibody or the labeled reagent.
- Increase number and duration of washes.
- Switch detection methods.

*Specific backgrounds* Specific background problems arise from three sources. These are contaminating antibodies with spurious reactions, cross-reacting antibodies, and immunoglobulin-binding proteins in the sample.

- If using polyclonal antibodies, titrate the antibody (spurious reactions).
- If using polyclonal antibodies, affinity-purify the antigen-specific antibodies (p. 77, spurious reactions).
- If using polyclonal antibodies, block the spurious activities with an appropriate acetone powder (p. 437).
- Try a different antibody preparation (cross-reaction or spurious).
- Incubate the specimen with normal serum derived from the same species as the labeled antibody. Also dilute the specific antibody in 1% normal serum from the same species as the labeled antibody (immunoglobulin-binding proteins in the sample). When using horseradish peroxidase-labeled reagents, the buffers used for dilution and washing should not contain sodium azide.

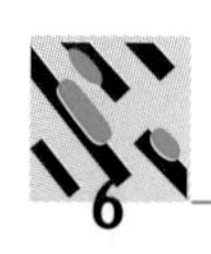



## Detection using enzyme-labeled reagents

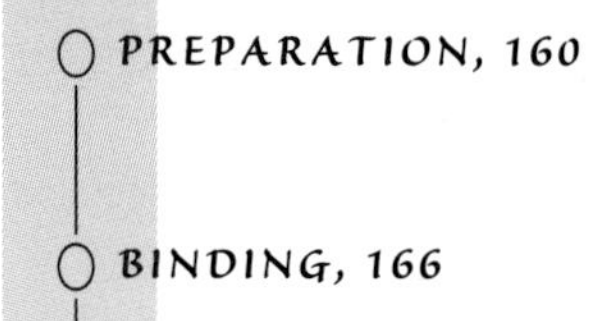

PREPARATION, 160
BINDING, 166
DETECTION

Enzyme-labeled reagents are detected using soluble chromogenic substrates that precipitate following enzyme action, yielding an insoluble colored product at the site of enzyme localization (Avrameas and Uriel 1966; Nakane and Pierce 1967a,b; Avrameas 1972). A range of substrates is available for each enzyme, and the following protocols represent some of the most useful alternatives. A wide range of conjugated reagents are available commercially. Enzymes can be coupled to anti-immunoglobulin antibodies, protein A, protein G, avidin, or streptavidin.

Table 6.2 summarizes the various detection methods that are in common use and the advantages and disadvantages of each. Extra sensitivity can be found using enzyme-labeled reagents by observing the precipitated enzyme products by interference reflection microscopy. Carefully note the cautions for the chromogenic substrates, which may be carcinogenic, used in the following protocols.

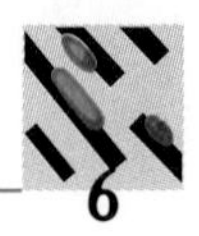


# Horseradish peroxidase-labeled reagents

PREPARATION, 160
BINDING, 166
DETECTION

A range of substrates are useful, including diaminobenzidine (DAB), chloronaphthol, and aminoethylcarbazole.

## Diaminobenzidine/metal

DAB is the most commonly used substrate and one of the most sensitive for horseradish peroxidase. It yields an intense brown product that is insoluble in both water and alcohol. In most cases, we recommend including the variation of metal addition to DAB. The DAB substrate for horseradish peroxidase can be made more sensitive by adding metal salts such as cobalt or nickel to the substrate solution. These reaction products are slate gray to black, and the products are also stable in both water and alcohol. DAB/metal staining is compatible with a wide range of common histological stains.

### Solutions needed

Diaminobenzidine tetrahydrochloride (DAB)
0.05 M Tris buffer (pH 7.6)
0.3% wt/vol stock solution of nickel chloride in water
30% Hydrogen peroxide
DPX (p. 183)

### Specialized equipment

Light microscope (most often with a camera to record the results)

### Cautions

DAB, DPX, hydrogen peroxide, nickel chloride, see Appendix IV.

1. Dissolve 6 mg of DAB in 9 ml of 0.05 M Tris buffer (pH 7.6).

2. Add 1 ml of a 0.3% wt/vol stock solution of nickel chloride in water (the same amount of cobalt chloride can be used as an alternative).

3. Add 0.1 ml of a 3% solution of hydrogen peroxide in water. Hydrogen peroxide generally is supplied as a 30% solution and should be stored at 4°C, at which temperature it will last about 1 month.

4. If a precipitate appears, filter through Whatman No. 1 filter paper (or equivalent).

5. Apply the solution to the specimen and incubate for 1–20 minutes. Stop the reaction by washing in water.

6. **Optional:** Counterstain if necessary (see p. 181).

7. Mount in DPX (p. 183).

## Chloronaphthol

Chloronaphthol gives a blue-black product. It is less sensitive than DAB, and the products are soluble in alcohol. It can be used when the DAB reaction gives too high a background, or if the alternate product colors are required.

### Solutions needed

0.03% Chloronaphthol in absolute ethanol (store at –20°C)
0.05 M Tris (pH 7.6)
Hydrogen peroxide
Gelvatol or Mowiol (p. 183)

### Specialized equipment

Light microscope (most often with a camera to record the results)

### Cautions

Chloronaphthol, ethanol, hydrogen peroxide, see Appendix IV.

1. Prepare a stock solution of chloronaphthol by dissolving 0.3 g of chloronaphthol in 10 ml of absolute ethanol and storing at –20°C.

2. Add 100 µl of chloronaphthol stock with stirring to 10 ml of 0.05 M Tris (pH 7.6).

3. Add 0.1 ml of 3% hydrogen peroxide, in water. Hydrogen peroxide generally is supplied as a 30% solution and should be stored at 4°C, at which temperature it will last about 1 month.

4. A white precipitate forms that is removed by filtering through Whatman No. 1 filter paper (or equivalent).

5. Apply the solution to the specimen and incubate for 10–40 minutes at room temperature. Stop the reaction by washing in water.

6. **Optional:** Counterstain if necessary. Only aqueous stains can be used (see p. 181).

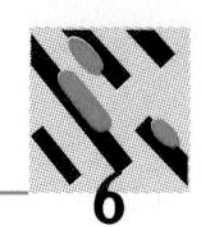

7. Mount in Gelvatol or Mowiol (p. 183).

## Aminoethylcarbazole

Aminoethylcarbazole (AEC) yields a red product. It is less sensitive than DAB, but can be used if the DAB reaction gives too high a background or if the alternate product colors are required. The products are soluble in alcohol, but not in water.

### Needed solutions

0.4% AEC in *N,N*-dimethylformamide (DMF)
0.1 M Sodium acetate buffer (pH 5.2)
Hydrogen peroxide
Gelvatol or Mowiol

### Specialized equipment

Light microscope (most often with a camera to record the results)

### Cautions

AEC, DMF, hydrogen peroxide, see Appendix IV.

1. Dissolve 4 mg of AEC in 1 ml of *N,N*-dimethylformamide (DMF). AEC is stable in DMF, so a stock can be prepared by dissolving 0.4 g in 100 ml of DMF.

2. Add 1.0 ml of the AEC solution to 15 ml of 0.1 M sodium acetate buffer (pH 5.2) with stirring.

*The AEC product fades if oxidized. Take special care to avoid air bubbles on mounting.*

3. Add 0.15 ml of 3% hydrogen peroxide, in water. Hydrogen peroxide generally is supplied as a 30% solution and should be stored at 4°C, at which temperature it will last about 1 month.

4. Filter through Whatman No. 1 filter paper (or equivalent).

5. Apply the solution to the specimen and incubate for 10–40 minutes at room temperature. Stop the reaction by washing in water.

6. **Optional:** Counterstain if necessary. Only aqueous stains can be used (see p. 181).

7. Mount in Gelvatol or Mowiol (p. 183).

# Alkaline phosphatase-labeled reagents

PREPARATION, 160
BINDING, 166
DETECTION

Bromochloroindolyl phosphate/nitro blue tetrazolium (BCIP/NBT) is the most commonly used of the chromogenic substrates for alkaline phosphatase. Coupled reagents should be prepared with eukaryotic alkaline phosphatase, because this enzyme is readily inactivated with EDTA. The bacterial enzyme is difficult to stop and will cause overdevelopment, leading to high background.

The BCIP/NBT substrate generates an intense black-purple precipitate at the site of enzyme binding. The reaction proceeds at a steady rate, thus allowing accurate control of the development of the reaction. This allows the relative sensitivity to be controlled by the length of incubation.

## Needed solutions

Alkaline phosphatase buffer: 100 mM sodium chloride, 5 mM magnesium chloride, 100 mM Tris (pH 9.5) NBT solution (0.5 g of NBT in 10 ml of 70% DMF, store at 4°C)
BCIP solution (0.5 g of BCIP [disodium salt] in 10 ml of 100% DMF, store at 4°C)
20 mM EDTA in PBS
DPX (p. 183)

## Specialized equipment

Light microscope (most often with a camera to record the results)

##  Cautions

BCIP, DMF, DPX, NBT, see Appendix IV.

---

1. Prior to developing the cell staining, prepare the three stock solutions. (1) NBT: Dissolve 0.5 g of NBT in 10 ml of 70% DMF. (2) BCIP: Dissolve 0.5 g of BCIP (disodium salt) in 10 ml of 100% DMF. (3) Alkaline phosphatase buffer: 100 mM sodium chloride, 5 mM magnesium chloride, 100 mM Tris (pH 9.5). All stocks are stable at 4°C for at least 1 year.

2. Just prior to developing, prepare fresh substrate solution. Add 66 μl of NBT stock to 10 ml of alkaline phosphatase buffer. Mix well and add 33 μl of BCIP stock. Use within 1 hour.

3. Place the washed slides in a suitable container. Add enough substrate solution to cover the slides (3–5 ml is appropriate for a 100-mm dish). Develop at room temperature with agitation until the stain is suitably dark. Periodic monitoring under the microscope may be necessary for some antigens. A typical incubation would be approximately 30 minutes.

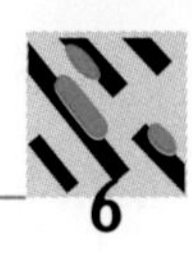


4. To stop the reaction, rinse with PBS containing 20 mM EDTA, chelating the $Mg^{++}$ ions.

5. **Optional:** Counterstain if necessary (see p. 181).

6. Wash in water and mount in DPX (p. 183).

# β-Galactosidase-labeled reagents

PREPARATION, 160
BINDING, 166
DETECTION

β-Galactosidase has been used extensively as a label in enzyme immunoassays, but has only recently become popular for immunocytochemistry. One good substrate is 5-bromo-4-chloro-3-indolyl-β-D-galactopyranoside (BCIG), which gives an intense blue product. The product is stable and insoluble in alcohol as well as in water.

## Needed solutions and reagents

5-Bromo-4-chloro-3-indolyl-β-D-galactopyranoside
*N,N*-Dimethylformamide
1 mM magnesium chloride, 3 mM potassium ferrocyanide in PBS
DPX (p. 183)

## Specialized equipment

Light microscope (most often with a camera to record the results)

## Cautions

BCIG, DMF, DPX, potassium ferrocyanide, see Appendix IV.

1. Dissolve 4.9 mg of BCIG in 0.1 ml of DMF.
2. Add 0.1 ml of the BCIG solution to 10 ml of PBS containing 1 mM magnesium chloride, 3 mM potassium ferrocyanide.
3. Filter through Whatman No. 1 filter paper (or equivalent).
4. Apply the solutions to the specimen, and incubate for 10–40 minutes at room temperature. Stop the reaction by washing with water.
5. **Optional:** Counterstain if necessary (see p. 181).
6. Mount in DPX (p. 183).

# Detecting the gold-labeled reagents*

Colloidal gold particles bind tightly but not covalently to proteins at pH values around the protein's pI. Colloidal gold particles conjugated with a wide range of anti-immunoglobulin antibodies, protein A, or streptavidin are available commercially. Because some of the bound protein may slowly dissociate from the gold particles, the colloid should be washed before use to remove free protein.

Gold labels were developed originally for electron microscopy studies (see, e.g., Roth et al. 1978), but they also work well at the level of the light microscope. They give higher resolution than enzyme-based methods and avoid the problems of substrate preparation and endogenous enzyme activity. Until recently, the gold labels lacked sensitivity at the level of light microscopy, but the recent development of the photochemical silver method of amplification has overcome this problem.

Unamplified gold labels can be detected under the light microscope using bright-field illumination where the label ranges from pale pink to deep red, depending on the strength of reaction. Nomarski differential interference contrast microscopy makes the label appear dark red to black. With the silver enhancement method, the gold particles become coated in metallic silver and yield a black-brown label, best detected by bright-field optics. Gold-labeling methods are compatible with many histochemical stains. Gold-labeling reactions are very readily controlled, because the appearance of staining can be monitored directly and continuously under the microscope.

### Needed solutions

0.5 M Sodium citrate (pH 3.5)
5.6% Hydroxyquinone (store in the dark)
0.73% Silver lactate (store in the dark)
1% Acetic acid
Standard photographic fixative

### Specialized equipment

Darkroom for developing
Light microscope (most often with a camera to record the results)

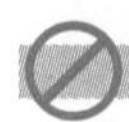

### Cautions

Acetic acid, DPX, silver lactate, see Appendix IV.

---

1. Rinse the specimen in distilled water briefly. The samples can be examined directly or can be processed for silver enhancement. For direct observation mount in Gelvatol or Mowiol (p. 183).

---

*Several companies have introduced silver enhancement kits that do not require using a darkroom, permitting development to be monitored under the microscope.*

2. For silver enhancement, transfer the sample to a darkroom equipped with a safe light. To prepare the developer, mix two parts of 0.5 M sodium citrate (pH 3.5) with three parts of 5.6% hydroxyquinone and 12 parts of water. Immediately before use, add three parts of 0.73% silver lactate.

---

*Danscher (1981); Danscher and Nörgaard (1983); Holgate et al. (1983).

3. Immerse the slides with the gold-labeled specimens into this developer. Incubate for 2–3 minutes at room temperature.

4. Rinse briefly in 1% acetic acid and fix in a standard photographic fixative for several minutes.

5. **Optional:** Counterstain if necessary (see p. 181).

6. Samples are now ready for mounting in DPX (p. 183).

## Counterstains

PREPARATION, 160

BINDING, 166

DETECTION

Counterstains are used to help differentiate the various cell types or subcellular structures seen in cell staining. They are essential for tissue sections, allowing the identification of the cell types, but also may be helpful in other staining reactions. Counterstains should not be used with fluorochromes, because the commonly used counterstains autofluoresce. To choose an appropriate counterstain, first determine whether the cell-staining detection reagent (often a chromogenic substrate) is soluble in alcohol.

### Cautions

Acetic acid, ammonium hydroxide, DPX, ethanol, see Appendix IV.

### Alcohol insoluble

1. Wash the slide gently with water.
2. Add a few drops of Harris' Hematoxylin (available commercially) to the specimen. Incubate for approximately 5 minutes. The length of time will determine the intensity of the stain.
3. Wash the slide gently in water.
4. Dip the slide in 0.5% glacial acetic acid/99.5% ethanol for 10 seconds.
5. Wash the slide gently in water.
6. Mount in DPX (p. 183).

### Alcohol soluble

1. Wash the slide gently with water.
2. Add a few drops of Mayer's Hematoxylin (available commercially) to the specimen. Incubate for approximately 5 minutes. The length of time will determine the intensity of the stain.

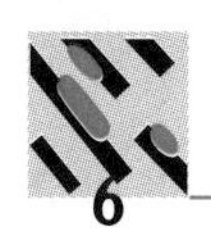



3. Wash the slide gently in water.

4. Dip the slide repeatedly into 30 mM ammonium hydroxide. Continue until the stain turns blue.

5. Wash the slide gently in water.

6. Mount in Gelvatol or Mowiol (p. 183).

| Counterstain | Recommended usage | Preparation | Advantages | Disadvantages |
|---|---|---|---|---|
| **Hematoxylin** | Use with black or brown chromagens<br>Can use with nuclear or cytoplasmic antigen | Purchase | Enormous archival information<br>Largely nuclear | Stain darkly<br>Do not use with weak antigen signal |
| **Methyl green** | Use with black or brown stains<br>Use with nuclear antigen | Stock solution = 1% (wt/vol) in 100 mM sodium acetate (pH 5.5)<br>Working solution is 0.1% of stock | Stains lightly<br>Use with weak antigen signal<br>Largely cytoplasmic | Limited tissue or cellular detail |
| **Fast red** | Use with blue chromagens or LacZ detection<br>Can use with nuclear or cytoplasmic antigen | Purchase | | Very light<br>Limited tissue or cellular detailed |

For more information about stains and counterstains, see Sheehan and Hrapchak (1987).

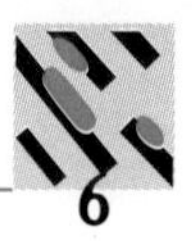

# Mounting

PREPARATION, 160
BINDING, 166
DETECTION

Mounting media for immunohistology must be compatible with the detection method used. There are two classes of mounting media, the aqueous and nonaqueous. Suitable aqueous media are made from Gelvatol or Mowiol. If these are not available, glycerol can be substituted, but permanent mounts are not possible. A suitable nonaqueous mounting medium is DPX, which is available commercially from Electron Microscopy Sciences. DPX is named for its components, 10 g of Distyrene 80, 5 ml of dibutyl phthalate, and 35 ml of xylene.

## DPX

### Caution

DPX, ethanol, see Appendix IV.

1. Samples for mounting in DPX must be dehydrated by passing through graded alcohols. Incubate twice for 3 minutes each in 75% ethanol, twice for 3 minutes each in 95% ethanol, and twice for 3 minutes each in absolute ethanol. Air-dry. Alternately, air-dry directly without passing through the ethanol washes.

2. Add a small drop of DPX to the specimen. If the sample is on a slide or tissue culture dish, carefully place a coverslip on the drop, avoiding air bubbles. If the sample is on a coverslip, invert the coverslip on a clean glass slide (sample side down).

3. Remove any excess mount with a paper towel.

DPX will set almost immediately and the samples can then be observed or photographed.

## Gelvatol or Mowiol*

### Cautions

DABCO, see Appendix IV.

1. To prepare Gelvatol or Mowiol: Add 2.4 g of Gelvatol 20–30 (Air Products, Monsanto Chemicals) or Mowiol 4–88 (Calbiochem, Hoechst) to 6 g of glycerol. Stir to mix. Add 6 ml of water and leave for several hours at room

*Heimer and Taylor (1974); Osborn and Weber (1982).

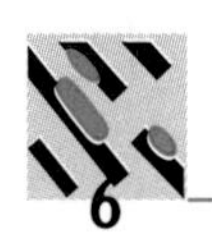



temperature. Add 12 ml of 0.2 M Tris (pH 8.5) and heat to 50°C for 10 minutes with occasional mixing. After the Mowiol or Gelvatol dissolves, clarify by centrifugation at 5000*g* for 15 minutes. For fluorescence detection, add 1,4-diazobicyclo-[2,2,2]-octane (DABCO) to 2.5% to reduce fading. Aliquot in airtight containers and store at –20°C. Stocks of these mounts are stable at room temperature for several weeks after thawing.

2. Gelvatol and Mowiol can be used directly on the washed specimen.

3. Add a small drop of mounting medium to the specimen. If the sample is on a slide or tissue-culture dish, carefully place a coverslip on the drop, avoiding air bubbles. If the sample is on a coverslip, invert the coverslip on a clean glass slide (sample side down).

4. Remove any excess mount with a paper towel.

The mounting medium will set overnight. To observe immediately, secure the coverslip to the slide by placing a small drop of nail polish at the edges of the coverslip. The samples can be observed and photographed. The results of tissue-staining experiments should be stored on film or videotape. Photography of enzyme- or gold-labeled samples presents no special difficulties.

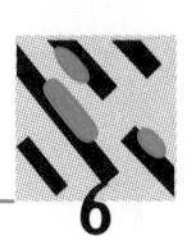

# Variations for staining yeast

In principle, the factors that control the success of staining tissue sections apply to using yeast as the antigen source. However, staining yeast cells for the presence and location of antigens has been particularly challenging because of several additional factors. The yeast cells are small, making the resolution of any antigen difficult; they have a thick cell wall that antibodies cannot penetrate and that is difficult to remove; and they grow in suspension, making handling difficult. Background problems can also be especially severe, particularly with polyclonal antibodies, because many antisera contain antibodies to yeast cell-wall components. Nonetheless, with care, the problems encountered in localizing antigens in yeast can be overcome by simple variations in the staining procedures.

### *Small size*

The relatively small size of yeast cells demands that the highest-resolution detection methods must be used. In practice, this means that the more sensitive methods of enyzyme-labeled secondary reagents cannot be used because of their lower resolving power. The better choice is the use of fluorochrome-labeled secondary antibodies. Because the presence of these reagents is due to their light emissions, they are highly localized. With abundant antigens, good localization can be achieved with good high-power epifluorescent microscopy. When more minor antigens are studied, the enhanced sensitivity of confocal microscopy is necessary.

### *Cell wall*

The presence of a cell wall in yeast is probably the most severe limitation for handling yeast for immunostaining. The cell wall poses an impermeable barrier for antibody passage and so must be removed prior to the addition of antibodies. There are several possible approaches to this removal, but the only one that has been broadly useful is enzymatic removal. This presents its own serious hurdles, because the quality of enzyme preparations varies, as do the size and composition of the cell wall in different strains. Therefore, the enzymatic removal of the cell wall needs to be controlled carefully to allow its efficient removal without inducing artifactual changes in the remaining antigenic display.

### *Handling*

To make the processing of the yeast cells simple, they are frequently bound to a solid phase so that the cells can be handled just as adherent culture.

In the method below, adapted from the work of J. Kilmartin (see Kilmartin and Adams 1984), the yeast cells are fixed, the cell wall is removed by enzyme treatment, the spheroplasts are attached to poly-L-lysine-coated slides, and then the cells are stained as per normal. Except in unusual circumstances, the detection reagent should be fluorochrome labeled. We have not included all of the background information of many of the individual steps (for example, in regard to indirect detection with fluorescent-labeled secondary reagents), and the reader is referred to those sections above and in Chapter 5 for more detailed discussions.

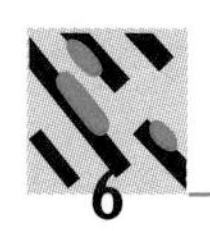



## Controls

Specific staining reactions should always be compared with control reactions. To assess a staining pattern accurately, two antibodies from the same species should be compared. For polyclonal antibodies, the best control is a prebleed from the same animal used to prepare the specific antibodies, but nonimmune serum from the same species is acceptable when this is not available. For monoclonal antibodies, the control must be from the same source as the specific antibody; i.e., supernatant versus supernatant, ascites versus ascites, or pure antibody versus pure antibody. The control antibodies should be of the same class and subclass as the specific antibody. Tissue-culture supernatants from the parental myeloma are never appropriate controls, because they do not contain antibodies. Suitable control hybridoma cell lines are available from the American Type Culture Collection or the European Collection of Animal Cell Cultures. In addition, the secondary reagent should be tested on its own.

Finally, whenever possible, yeast that carry a deletion of the gene for the antigen under study should be stained. This provides an excellent genetic control for the specificity of the antibody.

### Thinking ahead

The most important preparation for antibody binding and observation is the titering of the primary and secondary antibody preparations. Although starting points for the amounts of antibodies to be added are suggested in the technique below, the single biggest problem in immunostaining is to adjust the input of the primary and secondary antibodies to levels that are sufficient to give strong robust signals but are still below levels that promote nonspecific staining. This is best achieved by doing serial dilutions of each antibody preparation (normally in a protein-containing buffer such as 1% IgG/PBS) and doing test observations on the target cells. One-in-three dilutions (1 volume into 2 volumes) will approximate half-log steps and will quickly give a reasonable measure of the desired input. These titering tests should be repeated for each preparation of primary antibodies. However, once these dilutions have been established for the secondary reagents, they can be used as a standard for that antibody lot.

### Needed solutions and reagents

Primary antibody solution
Secondary antibody (most often purchased from a commercial source)
1 mg/ml Poly-L-lysine (average MW 400,000) in distilled water
4% Paraformaldehyde (see p. 466 for preparation, but rather than dilute with 2 × PBS, use 0.1 M potassium phosphate, pH 6.5)
0.1 M Potassium phosphate, (pH 6.5)
1.2 M Sorbitol, 0.12 M potassium phosphate, 33 mM citric acid (pH 5.9)
β-Glucuronidase (crude solution from *Helix pomatia*, 10,000 units/ml final concentration) and 1/100 volume Zymolyase
Methanol
Acetone
PBS
1% BSA in PBS
1% Goat IgG in PBS
Gelvatol or Mowiol (as described on p. 183)

### Specialized equipment

Light microscope equipped with epifluorescence or a confocal microscope

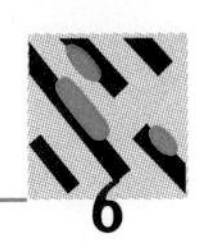

## Cautions

Acetone, β-glucuronidase, methanol, paraformaldehyde, see Appendix IV.

1. Prior to cell staining, prepare a solution of 1 mg/ml poly-L-lysine (average MW 400,000) in distilled water. Coat clean glass slides or coverslips with poly-L-lysine by incubating them in this solution for 15 minutes. Wash the solid phase with water. The poly-L-lysine-coated solid phase can be stored at room temperature after drying.

2. Establish a culture of early log-phase yeast cells. Remove a sample of the growing culture.

3. Add the yeast culture to 5× volume of a fresh solution of 4% paraformaldehyde (see p. 466 for preparation, but rather than PBS, use 0.1 M potassium phosphate, pH 6.5).

4. Incubate for 90 minutes at room temperature with occasional mixing.

5. Wash the cells by centrifugation three times in 0.1 M potassium phosphate (pH 6.5).

6. Resuspend the final pellet in 1.2 M sorbitol, 0.12 M potassium phosphate, and 33 mM citric acid (pH 5.9).

*The length of time for the enzymatic removal of the cell wall may need to be adjusted for each batch of glucuronidase and, in some cases, may need to be adjusted for different strains or species of yeast.*

7. Add 1/10 volume of β-glucuronidase (crude solution from *Helix pomatia*, ~10,000 units/ml final concentration) and 1/100 volume Zymolyase (or lyticase, 50 units/ml final concentration) to digest the cell wall. Incubate for 90 minutes at 30°C.

8. Wash three times in the sorbitol buffer.

9. Apply the cell suspension to poly-L-lysine-coated slides or coverslips by incubating for 15 minutes at room temperature.

10. Immerse the slides in methanol for 6 minutes at –20°C.

11. Transfer the slides to acetone for 30 seconds at – 20°C.

12. Rinse the slides for 5 minutes in 1% BSA in PBS.

13. Incubate the slides for 1 hour in 1% goat IgG in PBS.

*Throughout this protocol, goat IgG isolated from a nonimmune animal has been used as a blocking agent. This can be prepared by a simple protein G purification procedure from serum collected from a normal goat. This blocking reagent has been chosen because we have recommended labeled secondary reagents prepared from goat anti-immunoglobulin antibodies. If you are using another source of labeled secondary reagents, the blocking protein should be altered; for example, to 3% BSA.*

14. Wash the slides once in PBS.

15. Place coverslips, slides, or plates on a flat surface.

16. Add the primary antibody. Use a sufficient volume to cover the desired area of the cells. Volumes as small as 10 ml are often sufficient. All dilutions should be made with protein-containing solutions. For example, use PBS containing 1% goat IgG.

    Monoclonal antibodies are often applied as tissue-culture supernatants (specific antibody concentration of 20–50 μg/ml).

    Ascites fluids, purified monoclonal and polyclonal antibodies, and crude polyclonal sera should be tested at a range of dilutions. If the specific antibody concentration of the antibody sample is unknown, prepare and test 1/10, 1/100, 1/1000, and 1/10,000 dilutions of the starting material.

17. Incubate the coverslips, slides, or plates for a minimum of 30 minutes at room temperature.

    For short incubations of 1 hour or less, humidification is not needed, and the slides can be placed right on the benchtop.

    For some reactions, prolonged incubations of up to 12 hours can increase sensitivity. For these longer reactions, the samples must not dry out. A simple method to ensure this is to place a small volume of the antibody solution on a piece of parafilm that has been put on a flat surface. Lower the slide onto the antibody solution, specimen-side down. Note that longer reactions require lower concentrations of the primary antibodies.

*This buffer may be supplemented with 1% Triton X-100 or NP-40 to help with any background problems.*

18. Wash in three changes of PBS over 5 minutes.

19. Apply the fluorochrome-conjugated anti-immunoglobulin antibody. These reagents should be purchased from a reputable commercial source. Be sure to select a secondary antibody that is specific for the source of your antibodies. For example, goat anti-rabbit IgG would be a good choice for a primary antibody raised in rabbits.

    Secondary antibodies should be diluted in a protein-containing solution such as 1% goat IgG. The supplier may suggest appropriate dilutions, but if not, test dilutions of the secondary antibodies between 1/10 and 1/1000.

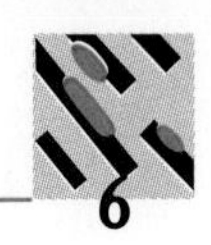


20. Incubate with the labeled secondary reagent for a minimum of 20 minutes at room temperature. Incubation times of more than 1 hour should be avoided.

21. Wash in three changes of PBS over 5 minutes.

22. Mount the specimens in Gelvatol or Mowiol as described on p. 183. Observe and photograph under the fluorescent or confocal microscope.

# Variations for staining Caenorhabditis

Immunolocalization of antigens in *Caenorhabditis* is still a comparatively new methodology. Although the basic theory follows all of the same principles on which staining of tissue sections relies, the added problem of permeabilizing the worm's cuticle makes these approaches much more difficult. The problems of the cuticle have been overcome by a series of harsh fixation and permeabilization steps, but because of the relatively short time that investigators have been concentrating on immunohistochemistry in the worm, there are only a few reliable methods for gaining antibody access. Presumably, as more researchers deal with the problems of antibody staining, more variations will be discovered and more concise protocols will be established.

### *Defeating the cuticle*

Staining worms is a difficult procedure almost entirely because of their cuticle. This problem is particularly difficult in young larval stages, especially in the L1 stage where the worms are much more resistant to permeabilization. Access is gained by a thorough fixation followed by freeze-thawing the animals and reduction of disulfides in the cuticle. In some cases, collagenase treatment is included to attack the cuticle enzymatically. The procedures are harsh and often destructive of the antigenic structure. The formation of ice crystals during any freeze-thaw is extremely destructive, and in many other systems, for example, in mammalian tissues, freeze-thaw is not recommended because of the problems of tissue and cell destruction. In the worm, the number of cycles of freeze-thaw should be kept to a minimum. The use of collagenase is equally difficult. Each lot of collagenase behaves differently, and each worm developmental stage is differentially sensitive. Therefore, some care needs to be used for immunostaining of worms to adjust the conditions of either method to the needed output for your antibody–antigen combination.

## Overview of the procedure

The general outline of the procedure is to fix the worms in either paraformaldehyde or Bouin's fixative, permeabilize by freeze-thawing and in some cases by collagenase treatment, treat with reducing agents to open the cuticle, and then proceed to the antibody additions. Detection for immunostaining of the worm is done almost completely with fluorochrome-labeled secondary reagents.

The procedures discussed below are divided into two sections. The first lists two procedures for fixation, and the second considers the antibody addition and detection steps that are common to all worm staining procedures. In the first section, methods for Bouin's and paraformaldehyde fixation are presented. If there is no history to suggest against it, we recommend the Bouin's method as a good starting point.

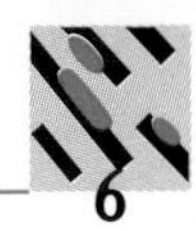

## Fixing worms in Bouin's*

Bouin's fixative has been used for decades in the preparation of paraffin sections for mammalian tissues. It penetrates dense tissues well and is extremely good for fixing antigens. It is a particularly good choice for worms because of these properties. Like all strong fixatives, however, it is not useful for all antibody–antigen pairs. In these cases, the length of time in the Bouin's fixative can be shortened, or paraformaldehyde fixation method can be tried.

### Needed solutions and reagents

Bouin's fixative (75 ml of saturated picric acid, 25 ml of formalin, 5 ml of glacial acetic acid; store at 4°C)
Methanol
1 M Dithiothreitol (DTT) (stored at –20°C)
0.5% NP-40 in PBS
0.05% NP-40 in PBS
0.5% NP-40, 200 mM DTT
20 mM Sodium borate

### Cautions

Picric acid, formalin, acetic acid, DTT, methanol, see Appendix IV.

1. Remove the worms from their growth media by washing the surface of the plates with 0.05% NP-40 in PBS. Transfer to a 15-ml conical tube.
2. Spin at 200*g* for 60 seconds. Remove the supernatant and transfer the worms to a 1.5-ml conical tube in 1 ml of 0.05% NP-40 in PBS.
3. Spin at 2,000*g* for 5 seconds. Remove the supernatant as completely as possible.
4. Add 400 μl of Bouin's fixative, 400 μl of methanol, and 200 μl of 1 M DTT.
5. Rock at room temperature for 30 minutes.
6. Snap-freeze by immersing the tube in liquid nitrogen. Remove the tube from the liquid nitrogen and thaw by holding the tube in running lukewarm water.

*Fixed worms can be removed from the liquid nitrogen and stored at this stage at −70°C for at least 1 year*

*Adapted from Iwasaki et al. (1997).

*If using first larval stage animals, freeze–thaw (as in step 6) two additional times during this 30-minute incubation to improve permeabilization.*

7. Rock at room temperature for 30 minutes.

8. Spin at 200*g* for 10 seconds. Remove the supernatant as completely as possible.

9. Wash the worms three times by resuspension in 0.5% NP-40, 200 mM DTT, 20 mM sodium borate (pH 9.6) and centrifugation at 200*g* for 10 seconds.

*At this stage, the yellow from the picric acid should be essentially gone. If not, repeat step 9.*

10. Add 1.0 ml of 0.5% NP-40, 200 mM DTT, 20 mM sodium borate (pH 9.6). Mix gently and rock for 2 hours at room temperature. Spin at 2,000*g* for 5 seconds. Remove the supernatant as completely as possible.

**The specimens are now ready for antibody addition (p. 195).**

## Common problems

These procedures are sufficiently harsh that many of the worms that go through these steps will be broken. These broken worms will not hurt the next steps of antibody addition, and they can easily be identified and ignored in the final examination.

## Fixing worms in paraformaldehyde

The second common method for fixing worms is to use paraformaldehyde. This method provides a gentler fixation than the Bouin's listed above, but often requires the use of collagenase. This method is particularly good for examining adult worms.

### Needed solutions and reagents

4% Paraformaldehyde (prepared fresh, p. 466)
PBS
1% NP-40, 200 mM dithiothreitol (DTT), in 20 mM sodium borate (pH 9.6)
1% NP-40 in PBS
50% methanol, 20 mM EGTA, 10 mM spermidine HCl in PBS

### Cautions

DTT, paraformaldehyde, see Appendix IV.

1. Remove the worms from their growth media by washing the surface of the plates with 0.05% NP-40 in PBS (4°C). Transfer to a 15-ml conical tube.

*The length of time in the fixative affects the ability of different antibody–antigen combinations to work. Be prepared to try different times to establish the best fixation time for your setting.*

2. Spin at 200*g* for 1 minute. Remove the supernatant. Transfer the worms to a 1.5-ml conical tube in 1 ml of 0.05% NP-40 in PBS (4°C).

3. Spin at 200*g* for 10 seconds. Remove the supernatant as completely as possible.

*Fixed worms can be removed from the liquid nitrogen and stored at this stage at –70°C for at least 1 year.*

4. Add 50 µl of 50% methanol, 20 mM EGTA, 10 mM spermidine HCl in PBS, and 500 µl of 4% paraformaldehyde (prepared fresh, p. 466). Snap-freeze by immersing the tube in liquid nitrogen. Remove the tube from the liquid nitrogen and thaw by holding the tube in running lukewarm water. Just as the ice melts, return the tube to the liquid nitrogen. Thaw under running water as above.

5. Incubate at 4°C for 1–24 hours.

6. Wash the worms two times in 0.05% NP-40 in PBS (4°C).

*If using first larval stage animals, freeze–thaw (as in step 4) two additional times during this incubation to improve permeabilization.*

7. Spin the worms and discard the final wash. Resuspend in 1% NP-40, 100 mM DTT, in 20 mM sodium borate (pH 9.6). Incubate at room temperature for 2 hours.

8. Wash the worms three times with 0.05% NP-40 in PBS (4°C).

9. Incubate in 0.3% hydrogen peroxide in 20 mM sodium borate (pH 9.6), made fresh, for 15 minutes.

10. Wash the worms three times in 0.05% NP-40 in PBS (4°C).

**The worms are now ready for antibody addition (p. 195).**

# Antibody addition and detection for staining worms

The procedures of antibody binding and detection are common for whichever method of fixation was used. The methodology and theory of antibody addition and detection are similar to the staining of any complex tissue source. Extreme care should be used to identify and verify positive reactions, because cross-reactions are common. The sections in the tissue-staining section above should be consulted for general procedures regarding selection of antibodies and potential methods for ensuring the correct interpretation of the localization. One major advantage for immunolocalization in the worm is the potential to examine a genetic null. If possible, it will be extremely useful to stain animals either that carry a mutation or are RNAi treated, which does not allow the synthesis of the antigen under study. This would provide a useful control for confirming a staining pattern. Obviously, this will not be possible in cases where the loss of gene function is lethal, but whenever possible, this control should be employed.

The most common method of detection for staining worms is to use fluorochrome-labeled reagents. Enzyme-linked secondary reagents are not commonly used in the study of antigens in worms. The reason for this high reliance on fluorochromes is primarily the desire for high resolution of the antigen location.

### *Background*

One serious problem that affects staining of worms is the chance for high backgrounds due to specific and nonspecific interactions. In addition to all of the problems encountered when examining antigens in a complex tissue, the staining of worms introduces some special problems that need special consideration.

The first consideration is the problems introduced by the harsh fixation and permeabilization methods. Many epitopes are destroyed by these methods, greatly limiting the number of antibodies that will recognize your antigen. In addition, the fixation exposes many new epitopes, increasing the possibilities of cross-reactions. In practice, this means that you may need to examine many antibodies to find the one that will be successful in the detection of your antigen.

One serious problem with worm immunostaining concerns the use of polyclonal antibodies. Polyclonal antisera almost always contain antibodies against bacteria found in the host animal used for antibody production. These are commonly bacteria found either in the gut or skin or against an infection. Because worms are commonly fed on bacteria such as *E. coli*, these antibodies can confuse the staining patterns. If possible, monoclonal antibodies should be used in place of polyclonal sera. If polyclonal antibodies are used, two strategies can be applied. Either the desired antibodies can be specifically purified on an antigen-affinity column (Chapter 9), or the undesired antibodies can be preabsorbed by the use of acetone powders (Appendix II).

### *Counterstains for worms*

Counterstaining is essential for examining worms by immunofluorescence and is used to identify the exact cell in which your antigen appears. Two general methods are used. In the first, all cells are labeled by using a fluorescent dye that is specific for nucleic acids. This is commonly DAPI for epifluorescence or propidium iodide for confocal work. These dyes are simply added to the wash buffers. The second commonly used counterstain is to use GFP driven by tissue-specific promoters. These transgenes are injected as expression plasmids, and their expression can be used to identify the cells that promote expression of the chosen promoter. GFP expression is normally followed by using GFP fluorescence or, if needed, by commercial available antibodies to GFP (Chapter 10).

## Controls

Specific staining reactions should always be compared with control reactions. To assess a staining pattern accurately, two antibodies from the same species should be compared. For polyclonal antibodies, the best control will be a prebleed from the same animal used to prepare the specific antibodies, but nonimmune serum from the same species is acceptable when this is not available. For monoclonal antibodies, the control must be from the same source as the specific antibody; i.e., supernatant versus supernatant, ascites versus ascites, or pure antibody versus pure antibody. The control antibodies should be of the same class and subclass as the specific antibody. Tissue-culture supernatants from the parental myeloma are never appropriate controls, because they do not contain antibodies. Suitable control hybridoma cell lines are available from the American Type Culture Collection or the European Collection of Animal Cell Cultures. In addition, the secondary reagent should be tested on its own. Finally, whenever possible, worms that carry a deletion of the gene for the antigen under study should be stained. This provides an excellent genetic control for the specificity of the antibody.

### Thinking ahead

The most important preparation for antibody binding and observation is the titering of the primary and secondary antibody preparations. Although starting points for the amounts of antibodies to be added are suggested in the technique below, the single biggest problem in immunostaining is to adjust the input of the primary and secondary antibodies to levels that are sufficient to give strong robust signals, but still below levels that promote nonspecific staining. This is best achieved by doing serial dilutions of each antibody preparation (normally in a protein-containing buffer such as 1% IgG/PBS) and doing test observations on the target cells. One-in-three dilutions (1 volume into 2 volumes) will approximate half-log steps, and this will quickly give a reasonable measure of the desired input. For each preparation of primary antibodies, these titering tests should be repeated. However, once these dilutions have been established for the secondary reagents, they can be used as a standard for that antibody lot.

### Needed solutions and reagents

Primary antibody solution
Secondary antibody (most often purchased from a commercial source)
PBS
1% BSA in PBS
1% Goat IgG in PBS
Gelvatol or Mowiol (as described on p. 183)

### Specialized equipment

Light microscope equipped with epifluorescence or a confocal microscope

## Cautions

DAPI, fluorescein, propidium iodide, see Appendix IV.

1. After the final wash, resuspend the worms in 1% goat IgG, 0.5% NP-40 in PBS. Incubate for 1 hour at room temperature.

*The use of double-labeling procedures is common in the analysis of antigens in the worm. See p. 142 for these considerations. FITC and Texas Red make a good comparison, but remember the FITC-conjugated antibodies, because of their more intense fluorescent emission, should be used to stain the antigen that is more difficult to detect.*

2. Add a dilution of the primary antibody made in 1% goat IgG in 0.5% NP-40 in PBS. Incubate the specimens for a minimum of 2 hours at room temperature.

   Monoclonal antibodies are often applied as 1-in-5 or 1-in-10 dilutions of tissue-culture supernatants. Ascites fluids, purified monoclonal and polyclonal antibodies, and crude polyclonal sera should be tested at a range of dilutions. If the specific antibody concentration of the antibody sample is unknown, prepare and test 1/100, 1/1000, and 1/10,000 dilutions of the starting material.

   For most reactions, prolonged incubations of up to overnight are preferred. The longer incubation times allow the primary antibodies time to penetrate and react with the immobilized antigens.

3. Wash in three changes of 0.5% NP-40 in PBS over 5 minutes.

4. Apply the fluorochrome-conjugated anti-immunoglobulin antibody. This reagent should be purchased from a reputable commercial source. Be sure to select a secondary antibody that is specific for the source of your antibodies. For example, goat anti-rabbit IgG would be a good choice for a primary antibody raised in rabbits.

   Secondary antibodies should be diluted in a protein-containing solution such as 1% goat IgG. The supplier may suggest appropriate dilutions, but if not, test dilutions of the secondary antibodies between 1/10 and 1/1000.

*If using propidium iodide as a counterstain, include 200 μg/ml of RNase A in the secondary antibody solution.*

5. Incubate with the labeled secondary reagent for a minimum of 20 minutes at room temperature. Incubation times of greater than 1 hour should be avoided.

*If using a DNA intercalating dye as a counterstain, it should be included in the secondary antibody dilution. Use DAPI at 1 µg/ml and propidium iodide at 1 µg/ml.*

6. Wash in three changes of PBS over 5 minutes.

7. Mount the specimens in Gelvatol or Mowiol as described on p. 183. Observe and photograph under the fluorescent or confocal microscope.

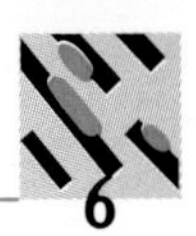


# Variations for staining Drosophila

The standard procedures for tissue staining can be applied to locate antigens in flies. In general, successful staining of flies relies on the principles discussed in the beginning of this chapter and in Chapter 5. One serious complication in staining flies is the presence of several different protective coatings that appear at different developmental stages of the fly. These organismal "coats" include such structures as the chorion, vitelline membrane, and cuticle. They are important stage-specific environmental barriers that serve essential roles in development and survival, but for immunochemical methods they must be removed to allow antibody penetration. The procedures to remove these structures are harsh for the antigens that you will be studying. Therefore, protocols for staining *Drosophila* are designed to include steps to keep backgrounds to a minimum. As would be expected, the choice of antibodies is particularly critical to the success of these methods.

## Overview of the procedure

The procedure for staining *Drosophila* specimens can be divided into two steps. The first step in handling specimens is to fix and permeabilize the tissue or whole organism. This requires strong conditions to remove the protective coating of the fly, fix the antigens in place, and allow access of the antibodies. The choice of fixation and permeabilization methods for examining flies depends on the stage of development. Early embryos at the stage before the cuticle is laid down are treated with a mixture of organic solvents, formaldehyde, and alcohols to fix and permeabilize the tissues for antibody access. The cuticle is normally opened by sonication. In this chapter, we have included methods to fix either early or late whole-mount embryos. Tissues from later stages of development are normally dissected by hand and then fixed and stained in a standard paraformaldehyde/detergent combination.

The second step for staining flies is the addition of the primary antibody and its detection. The steps for addition of the primary antibodies and detection are straightforward, and only change depending on the type of resolution needed in the final stain. Here, the key decision is the type of detection that will be used. Most localization experiments are done using enzyme-linked secondary reagents. This approach gives excellent sensitivity, and its use does not require a confocal microscope. When more resolution is required or when two antigens will be observed in the same specimen, fluorochrome-linked secondary reagents are used. Because of the thickness of the fly specimens, this detection method requires the use of a confocal microscope for observation. The results are superior, but rely on the access to a good confocal facility. Techniques for both are provided below.

## Preparing early whole-mount embryos*

### Needed solutions

Bleach
Heptane
3.7% Formaldehyde in 2 mM EGTA, 1 mM magnesium sulfate, 100 mM PIPES (pH 7.0)
Methanol
PBS

### Specialized equipment

Dissecting microscope

### Cautions

Bleach, formaldehyde, heptane, methanol, see Appendix IV.

*Most drosophilists prefer to rinse the embryos on a fine nylon mesh filter.*

1. Collect the embryos on apple or grape juice plates. Rinse with water.

2. Transfer the embryos to a 50-ml Erlenmeyer flask or an equivalent glass container that will allow easy agitation without spilling. Add 25 ml of 50% bleach to remove the chorion. Swirl occasionally. After 3 minutes, wash thoroughly with several changes of water. Use a dissecting microscope to observe the embryos. If the chorion has not been completely removed, repeat the bleach treatment.

*The correct length of time in the heptane/fixative mix will depend on the particular antibody–antigen combination being studied. Try removing embryos at 5, 10, 20, and 40 minutes to test for the best time.*

3. Remove as much of the water as possible by aspiration. Add 10 ml of heptane and swirl a couple of times. Then add 10 ml of 3.7% formaldehyde in 2 mM EGTA, 1 mM magnesium sulfate, 100 mM PIPES (pH 7.0). Mix gently to combine the phases for 10–60 minutes.

   The heptane will punch some holes in the vitelline membrane and allow the formaldehyde to penetrate and fix the embryos. The embryos will remain at the heptane/aqueous interface.

4. Stop the agitation and allow the phases to separate. Using aspiration, remove as much of the aqueous (bottom) phase as possible, being careful to avoid the embryos, which will be in the heptane near the organic/aqueous interface. If any embryos have fallen into the aqueous phase, they should be removed as well.

5. Add 10 ml of methanol. Shake vigorously for 60 seconds. The vitelline membrane will swell in the methanol and the embryos will drop out and fall into the methanol phase (bottom).

*0–17 hours or until cuticle formation.

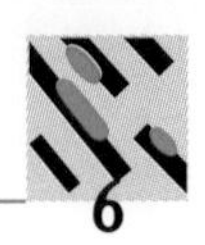


*Embryos can be transferred to a plastic tube and stored frozen at –20°C in methanol for several years.*

6. Remove the heptane and as much of the methanol as possible. Wash the embryos by swirling in three changes of methanol over 5 minutes to remove the remaining heptane.

7. Wash the embryos with three changes of PBS over 5 minutes.

**The embryos are now ready for antibody additions. The use of enzyme-linked secondary reagents is found on p. 204 and fluorochrome-linked secondary reagents on p. 209.**

## Preparing late whole-mount embryos*

### Needed solutions

Bleach
Heptane
3.7% Formaldehyde in 2 mM EGTA, 1 mM magnesium sulfate, 100 mM PIPES (pH 7.0)
Methanol
PBS

### Specialized equipment

Dissecting microscope
Probe tip sonicator

### Cautions

Bleach, formaldehyde, heptane, methanol, magnesium sulfate, see Appendix IV.

---

1. Collect the embryos on apple or grape juice plates. Rinse with water.

*Most drosophilists prefer to rinse the embryos on a fine nylon mesh filter.*

2. Transfer the embryos to a 50-ml Erlenmeyer flask or equivalent glass container that will allow easy agitation without spilling. Add 25 ml of 50% bleach to remove the chorion. Swirl occasionally. After 3 minutes, wash thoroughly with several changes of water. Use a dissecting microscope to observe the embryos. If the chorion has not been completely removed, repeat the bleach treatment.

3. Remove as much of the water as possible by aspiration. Add 10 ml of heptane and swirl a couple of times. Then add 10 ml of 3.7% formaldehyde in 2 mM EGTA, 1 mM magnesium sulfate, 100 mM PIPES (pH 7.0). Mix gently to combine the phases for 10–60 minutes.

   The heptane will punch some holes in the vitelline membrane and allow the formaldehyde to penetrate and fix the embryos. Embryos that are close to hatching will have already shed their vitelline membrane and will drop to the bottom of the aqueous phase. The embryos that still have the vitelline membrane will remain at the heptane/aqueous interface.

*The correct length of time in the heptane/fixative mix depends on the particular antibody–antigen combination being studied. Try removing embryos at 5, 10, 20, and 40 minutes to test for the best time.*

4. Stop the agitation and allow the phases to separate. Using aspiration, remove as much of the aqueous (bottom) phase as possible, being careful to avoid the embryos both in the formaldehyde and at the organic/aqueous interface.

*Embryos can be transferred to a plastic tube and stored frozen at –20°C in methanol for several years.*

5. Add 10 ml of methanol. Shake vigorously for 60 seconds.

   The vitelline membranes that still are attached to embryos will swell in the methanol, and the embryos will drop out and fall into the methanol phase (bottom).

---

*17–22 hours or until hatching.

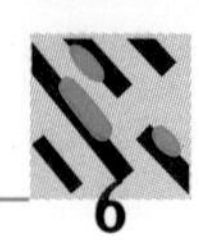


6. Remove the heptane and as much of the methanol as possible. Wash the embryos by swirling in three changes of methanol over 5 minutes to remove the remaining heptane.

7. Wash the embryos with three changes of PBS over 5 minutes.

8. Transfer the embryos to a small centrifuge tube. Remove the PBS and add 500 μl of PBS with no more than 100 μl of packed volume of embryo. To break the cuticle, sonicate with a probe tip set at lowest power output for 2–3 seconds. Observe the embryos. The time of sonication should not allow the embryos to show large numbers with morphological damage. Most antibodies will work after one cycle, but multiple cycles can be used until some embryos just begin to show damage. Between cycles, transfer the tubes to ice to keep heat to a minimum.

9. Wash the embryos with three changes of PBS over 5 minutes.

**The embryos are now ready for antibody additions. The use of enzyme-linked secondary reagents is found on p. 204 and fluorochrome-linked secondary reagents on p. 209.**

# Antibody addition to Drosophila specimens and detection using enzyme-linked reagents

Once the flies are fixed and permeabilized, the antibodies are added. Here, as in many other immunochemical techniques, the antibodies can be labeled directly or they can be detected by using a labeled secondary reagent that binds specifically to the primary antibody. In general, direct labeling of the primary antibody produces cleaner signals with lower background. The major disadvantage of direct detection is the time needed to purify and label each preparation of primary antibody. This makes direct detection much more difficult, and, except in unusual cases, we recommend indirect methods where the secondary detection reagent can be purchased from one of the many commercial sources.

There are two main choices for detection methods. Enzyme-linked reagents are recommended in most cases. They give excellent sensitivity and use a simple light microscope for detection. The next protocol discusses the use of fluorochrome-linked reagents. This method should be used when high resolution is needed or two antigens need to be localized simultaneously. Detection using fluorochrome-linked reagents requires access to a confocal microscope.

To counter the background problems commonly found when the preparation of the antigen source has been particularly harsh, as it is during the fixation of flies, workers in this field commonly use several approaches. One approach used in fly immunohistochemistry is the use of a preincubation of samples with normal goat serum. Most of the labeled secondary reagents are goat anti-mouse or anti-rabbit immunoglobulin antibodies. Because of this, using nonimmune goat antibodies to block nonspecific interaction sites becomes an excellent choice to lower background. In addition, lower concentrations of antibodies are commonly used and the incubations are allowed to go overnight. Both of these approaches are good ways to lower backgrounds.

## Enzyme-linked detection of Drosophila specimens

Enzyme-labeled reagents are detected using soluble chromogenic substrates that precipitate following enzyme action, yielding an insoluble colored product at the site of enzyme localization (Avrameas and Uriel 1966; Nakane and Pierce 1967a,b; Avrameas 1972). A range of substrates is available for each enzyme, but for staining in situ, horseradish peroxidase will suit most needs. A wide range of horseradish peroxidase-conjugated reagents are available commercially. Enzymes can be coupled to anti-immunoglobulin antibodies, protein A, protein G, avidin, or streptavidin.

## Horseradish peroxidase-labeled reagents

A range of substrates are useful, including diaminobenzidine (DAB), chloronaphthol, and aminoethylcarbazole, but the most useful substrate for immunolocalization in flies is the DAB/metal variation. DAB is the most commonly used substrate and one of the most sensitive for horseradish peroxidase. It yields an intense brown product that is insoluble in both water and alcohol. In most cases, we recommend including the variation of metal addition to DAB. The DAB substrate for horseradish peroxidase can be made more sensitive by adding metal salts such as cobalt or nickel to the substrate solution. The reaction product is slate gray to black, and the products are stable in both water and alcohol. DAB/metal staining is compatible with a wide range of common histological stains.

### Controls

Specific staining reactions should always be compared with control reactions. To assess a staining pattern accurately, two antibodies from the same species should be compared. For polyclonal antibodies, the best control is a prebleed from the same animal used to prepare the specific antibodies, but nonimmune serum from the same species is acceptable in most cases. For monoclonal antibodies, the control must be from the same source as the specific antibody; i.e., supernatant versus supernatant, ascites versus ascites, or pure antibody versus pure antibody. If possible, the control antibodies should be of the same class and subclass as the specific antibody. Tissue-culture supernatants from the parental myeloma are never appropriate controls, because they do not contain antibodies. Suitable control hybridoma cell lines are available from the American Type Culture Collection or the European Collection of Animal Cell Cultures.

In addition, the secondary reagent should be tested on its own. Finally, when using enzyme-linked detection, the enzyme reaction should be done on the specimen without the addition of any antibodies. This will demonstrate the presence and location of any endogenous enzyme activities.

### Thinking ahead

The most important preparation for antibody binding and observation is the titering of the primary and secondary antibody preparations. Although starting points for the amounts of antibodies to be added are suggested in the technique below, the single biggest problem in immunostaining is to adjust the input of the primary and secondary antibodies to levels that are sufficient to give strong robust signals, but still below levels that promote nonspecific staining. This is best achieved by doing serial dilutions of each antibody preparation (normally in a protein-containing buffer such as 1% goat IgG in PBS) and doing test observations. One-in-three dilutions (1 volume into 2 volumes) will approximate half-log steps, and this will quickly give a reasonable measure of the desired input. For each preparation of primary antibodies, these titering tests should be repeated. However, once these dilutions have been established for the secondary reagents, they can be used as a standard for that antibody lot.

Finally, whenever possible, flies that carry a deletion of the gene for the antigen under study should be stained. This provides an excellent genetic control for the specificity of the antibody.

### Needed solutions and reagents

Primary antibody solution
Secondary antibody (most often purchased from a commercial source) PBS
1% Normal goat IgG in PBS
Diaminobenzidine tetrahydrochloride (DAB)
0.05 M Tris buffer (pH 7.6)
0.3% wt/vol stock solution of nickel chloride in water
30% Hydrogen peroxide
50 : 50 Mixture of glycerol : PBS
70 : 30 Mixture of glycerol : PBS

### Specialized equipment

Dissecting microscope
Light microscope (most often with a camera to record the results)

### Cautions

DAB, ethanol, hydrogen peroxide, methyl salicylate, nickel chloride, see Appendix IV.

*Throughout this protocol, goat IgG isolated from a nonimmune animal has been used as a blocking agent. This can be prepared by a simple protein G purification procedure from serum collected from a normal goat. This blocking reagent has been chosen because we have recommended labeled secondary reagents prepared from goat anti-immunoglobulin antibodies. If you are using another source of labeled secondary reagents, the blocking protein should be altered, for example to 3% BSA.*

1. After the final wash (p. 203), the specimens are resuspended in 1% normal goat IgG in PBS. Keep the packed volume of embryos or other specimens to less than 50 μl in each 1.5-ml conical tube or 200 μl in a 5-ml snap-top tube. Incubate for 1 hour with rocking.

2. Wash the specimens twice with PBS.

3. Add the first antibody solution. All dilutions must be carried out in protein-containing solutions, such as goat IgG in PBS.

   Monoclonal antibodies are best applied as tissue-culture supernatants (specific antibody concentration of 20–50 μg/ml; use a 1-in-10 dilution as a good starting point). Ascites fluids, purified monoclonal and polyclonal antibodies, and crude polyclonal sera should be tested at a range of dilutions aimed at producing specific antibody concentrations between 0.01 and 1 μg/ml. If the specific antibody concentration of the sample is unknown, prepare and test 1/10, 1/100, 1/1000, and 1/10,000 dilutions of the starting material.

4. Incubate the specimens 24 hours at 4°C.

5. Wash in three changes of PBS over 5 minutes. This buffer may be supplemented with 1% Triton X-100 or NP-40 to help with any background problems.

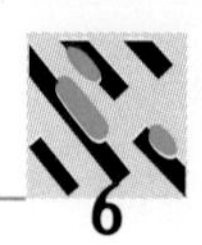


6. Apply the labeled secondary reagent. It is essential to carry out all dilutions in a protein-containing solution such as 1% IgG normal goat/PBS. Useful secondary reagents include anti-immunoglobulin antibodies, protein A, and protein G. In general, we recommend secondary antibodies raised in goat and coupled with horseradish peroxidase. Labeled secondary reagents can be purchased from several suppliers.

   If using a commercial preparation, test dilutions of the secondary antibodies 1/50 to 1/1000. Alkaline phosphatase-labeled reagents should be handled using Tris-buffered saline, not PBS.

7. Incubate with the labeled secondary reagent for 1 hour at 4°C.

8. Wash in three changes of PBS over 5 minutes. This buffer may be supplemented with 1% Triton X-100 or NP-40 to help with any background problems.

9. Dissolve 6 mg of DAB in 9 ml of 0.05 M Tris buffer (pH 7.6).

10. Add 1 ml of a 0.3% wt/vol stock solution of nickel chloride in water (the same amount of cobalt chloride can be used as an alternative).

11. Add 0.1 ml of a 3% solution of hydrogen peroxide in water. Hydrogen peroxide generally is supplied as a 30% solution and should be stored at 4°C, at which temperature it will last about 1 month.

12. If a precipitate appears, filter the solution through Whatman No. 1 filter paper (or equivalent).

13. Apply the solution to the specimen and incubate for 1–20 minutes. Stop the reaction by washing in water. The timing for stopping the reaction can be judged by watching the development of the color under the microscope.

14. **Optional:** When embryos are observed at high magnification, the optical patterns of the cylindrical embryo and the length of the light path through the embryo often cause the specimen to appear opaque. To counter this property, it is common to treat the embryos with different solvents that will change the refractive index of the embryo. This is commonly done by incubating in glycerol or methyl salicylate. For most staining purposes, glycerol works fine.

    Resuspend the embryos in 500 μl of a 50:50 mixture of glycerol:PBS. Incubate for 1 hour at room temperature.

*Methyl salicylate clearing gives a slightly better optical pattern than glycerol, but is more difficult to use. It is volatile, and the smell bothers some workers. In addition, it does not have the viscosity that makes handling the embryos easy. To use, pass the embryos through a graded series of alcohol steps: 5 minutes in 50% ethanol, 5 minutes in 70% ethanol, 5 minutes in 90% ethanol, 2 × 5 minutes in 100% ethanol. Add 500 μl of methyl salicylate. Do not disturb the tube for 10 minutes. The embryos will fall to the bottom. Remove the supernatant and add fresh methyl salicylate. Finish the procedure, substituting methyl salicylate for glycerol.*

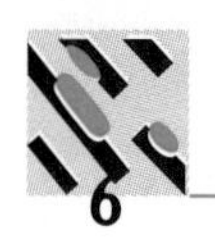



Spin the embryos and resuspend in a 70:30 mixture of glycerol:PBS.

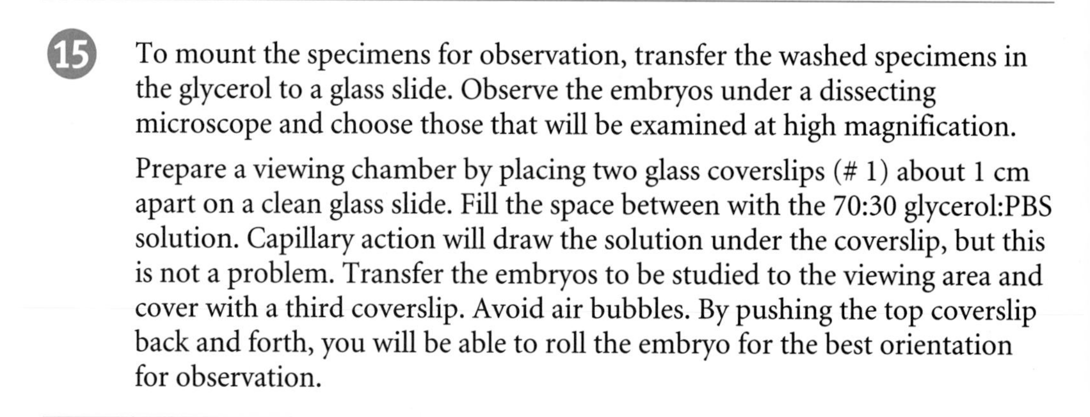

15 To mount the specimens for observation, transfer the washed specimens in the glycerol to a glass slide. Observe the embryos under a dissecting microscope and choose those that will be examined at high magnification.

Prepare a viewing chamber by placing two glass coverslips (# 1) about 1 cm apart on a clean glass slide. Fill the space between with the 70:30 glycerol:PBS solution. Capillary action will draw the solution under the coverslip, but this is not a problem. Transfer the embryos to be studied to the viewing area and cover with a third coverslip. Avoid air bubbles. By pushing the top coverslip back and forth, you will be able to roll the embryo for the best orientation for observation.

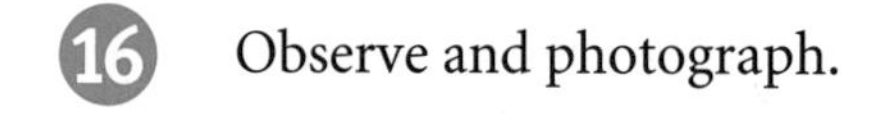

16 Observe and photograph.

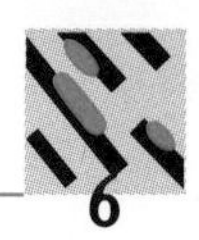


## Antibody addition to Drosophila specimens and detection using fluorochrome-linked reagents

Once the flies are fixed and permeabilized, the antibodies are added. Here, as in many other immunochemical techniques, the antibodies can be labeled directly or they can be detected by using a labeled secondary reagent that binds specifically to the primary antibody. In general, direct labeling of the primary antibody produces cleaner signals with lower background. The major disadvantage of direct detection is the time needed to purify and label each preparation of primary antibody. This makes direct detection much more difficult, and, except in unusual cases, we recommend indirect methods where the secondary detection reagent can be purchased from one of the many commercial sources.

There are two main choices for detection methods. Enzyme-linked reagents are recommended in most cases. They give excellent sensitivity and use a simple light microscope for detection. The previous protocol discusses the use of these approaches. This section covers the use of fluorochrome-linked reagents. This approach should be used when high resolution is needed or two antigens need to be localized simultaneously. Detection using fluorochrome-linked reagents requires access to a confocal microscope.

To counter the background problems commonly found when the preparation of the antigen source has been particularly harsh, as it is during the fixation of flies, workers in this field commonly use several approaches to lower backgrounds. One approach used in fly immunohistochemistry is the use of a preincubation of samples with normal goat serum. Most of the labeled secondary reagents are goat anti-mouse or anti-rabbit immunoglobulin antibodies. Because of this, using nonimmune goat antibodies to block nonspecific interaction sites is an excellent choice to lower background. In addition, lower concentrations of antibodies are commonly used and the incubations are allowed to go overnight. Both of these approaches are good ways to lower backgrounds.

## Controls

Specific staining reactions should always be compared with control reactions. To assess a staining pattern accurately, two antibodies from the same species should be compared. For polyclonal antibodies, the best control is a prebleed from the same animal used to prepare the specific antibodies, but nonimmune serum from the same species is acceptable in most cases. For monoclonal antibodies, the control must be from the same source as the specific antibody, i.e., supernatant versus supernatant, ascites versus ascites, or pure antibody versus pure antibody. If possible, the control antibodies should be of the same class and subclass as the specific antibody. Tissue-culture supernatants from the parental myeloma are never appropriate controls, because they do not contain antibodies. Suitable control hybridoma cell lines are available from the American Type Culture Collection or the European Collection of Animal Cell Cultures. In addition, the secondary reagent should be tested on its own.

### Thinking ahead

The most important preparation for antibody binding and observation is the titering of the primary and secondary antibody preparations. Starting points for the amounts of antibodies to be added are suggested in the technique below, but the single biggest problem in immunostaining is to adjust the input of the primary and secondary antibodies to levels that are sufficient to give strong robust signals, but still below levels that promote nonspecific staining. This is best achieved by doing serial dilutions of each antibody preparation (normally in a protein-containing buffer such as 1% goat IgG in PBS) and doing a test observation. One-in-three dilutions (1 volume into 2 volumes) approximate half-log steps, and this will quickly give a reasonable measure of the desired input. For each preparation of primary antibodies, these titering tests should be repeated. However, once these dilutions have been established for the secondary reagents, they can be used as a standard for that antibody lot.

Finally, whenever possible, flies which carry a deletion of the gene for the antigen under study should be stained. This provides an excellent genetic control for the specificity of the antibody.

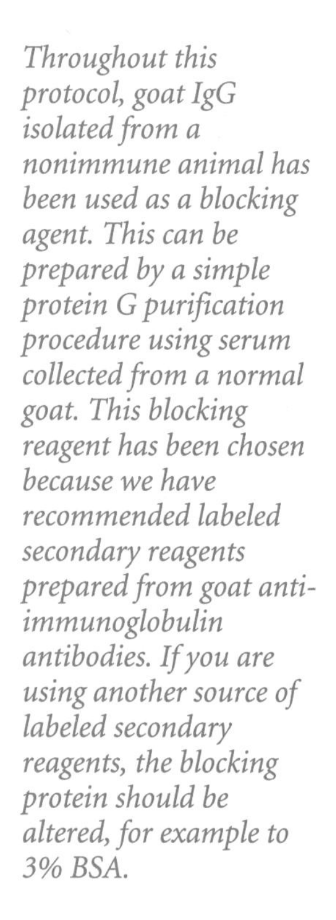
*Throughout this protocol, goat IgG isolated from a nonimmune animal has been used as a blocking agent. This can be prepared by a simple protein G purification procedure using serum collected from a normal goat. This blocking reagent has been chosen because we have recommended labeled secondary reagents prepared from goat anti-immunoglobulin antibodies. If you are using another source of labeled secondary reagents, the blocking protein should be altered, for example to 3% BSA.*

### Needed solutions and reagents

Primary antibody solution
Secondary antibody (most often purchased from a commercial source)
PBS
1% Normal goat IgG in PBS

### Specialized equipment

Confocal microscope

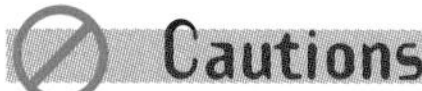

### Cautions

Ethanol, fluorescein, methyl salicylate, see Appendix IV.

1. After the final wash, the specimens are resuspended in 1% normal goat IgG in PBS. Keep the packed volume of embryos or other specimens to less than 50 μl in each 1.5-ml conical tube or 200 μl in a 5-ml snap-top tube. Incubate for 1 hour with rocking.

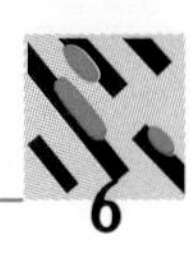

*The use of double-labeling procedures is common in the analysis of antigens in the fly. See p. 142 for these considerations. FITC and Texas Red make a good comparison, but remember the FITC-conjugated antibodies, because of their more intense fluorescent emission, should be used to stain the antigen that is more difficult to detect.*

2. Wash the specimens twice with PBS.

3. Add the first antibody solution. All dilutions must be carried out in protein-containing solutions. For example, use PBS containing 1% goat IgG.

   Monoclonal antibodies are best applied as tissue-culture supernatants (specific antibody concentration of 20–50 μg/ml, use a 1-in-10 dilution as a good starting point). Ascites fluids, purified monoclonal and polyclonal antibodies, and crude polyclonal sera should be tested at a range of dilutions aimed at producing specific antibody concentrations between 0.01 and 1 μg/ml. If the specific antibody concentration of the antibody sample is unknown, prepare and test 1/10, 1/100, 1/1000, and 1/10,000 dilutions of the starting material.

4. Incubate the specimens 24 hours at 4°C.

5. Wash in three changes of PBS over 5 minutes. This buffer may be supplemented with 1% Triton X-100 or NP-40 to help with any background problems.

6. Apply the fluorochrome-labeled secondary reagent. It is essential to carry out all dilutions in a protein-containing solution such as 1% goat IgG in PBS. Useful secondary reagents include anti-immunoglobulin antibodies, protein A, or protein G. In general, we recommend secondary antibodies raised against goat and coupled with horseradish peroxidase. Labeled secondary reagents can be purchased from several suppliers.

   If using a commercial preparation, test dilutions of the secondary antibodies 1/50 to 1/1000. Alkaline phosphatase-labeled reagents should be handled using Tris-buffered saline, not PBS.

7. Incubate with the labeled secondary reagent for a minimum of 1 hour at 4°C.

8. Wash in three changes of PBS over 5 minutes. This buffer may be supplemented with 1% Triton X-100 or NP-40 to help with any background problems.

**Optional:** When embryos are observed at high magnification, the optical patterns of the cylindrical embryo and the length of the light path through the embryo often cause the specimen to appear opaque. To counter this property, it is common to treat the embryos with different solvents that will change the refractive index of the embryo. This is commonly done by incubating in glycerol or methyl salicylate. For most staining purposes, glycerol works fine.

Resuspend the embryos in 500 μl of a 50:50 mixture of glycerol:PBS. Incubate for 1 hour at room temperature.

Spin the embryos and resuspend in a 70:30 mixture of glycerol:PBS.

Methyl salicylate clearing gives a slightly better optical pattern than glycerol, but is more difficult to use. It is volatile, and the smell bothers some workers. In addition, it does not have the viscosity that makes handling the embryos easy. To use, pass the embryos through a graded series of alcohol steps: 5 minutes in 50% ethanol, 5 minutes in 70% ethanol, 5 minutes in 90% ethanol, 2 × 5 minutes in 100% ethanol. Add 500 μl of methyl salicylate. Do not disturb the tube for 10 minutes. The embryos will fall to the bottom. Remove the supernatant and add fresh methyl salicylate. Finish the procedure, substituting methyl salicylate for glycerol.

Observe and record the image using a confocal microscope. For the correct use of these scopes, workers need to consult the instructions for the particular machine they are using. For a general discussion of confocal microscopes, see Spector et al. (1998).

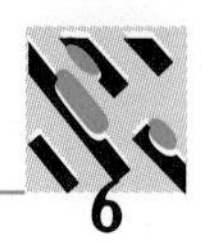


# Protocols for antigen retrieval

Because antigens are so frequently masked by the fixation methods used to prepare tissues for staining, a great deal of research has been devoted to methods for re-exposing the hidden epitopes. These methods are commonly referred to as antigen retrieval.

During the preparation of tissues for staining, antigens are heavily modified by the fixatives. Antigens are frequently modified on free amino groups and, because they are often part of larger cellular structures, they can be hidden by other molecules. In addition, fixation methods are highly denaturing to protein antigens.

The methods for antigen retrieval attempt to counter these changes. They are designed to break local barriers to antibody access and renature protein antigens. The commonly used methods include limited treatment with proteases or heating in the microwave or pressure cooker. All three methods have been used successfully in many cases. However, the correct choice of method will vary from antigen to antigen and from antibody to antibody. Therefore, it is wise to try all three to find an appropriate method.

The mechanism of action of antigen retrieval remains poorly defined but seems to be related to reduction of cross-linking and calcium chelation. The use of heating either in a microwave or pressure cooker in EDTA buffer appears to be the most robust. However, it should be clearly recognized that any of the antigen retrieval methods should be avoided wherever possible because they may introduce artifactual false-positive staining.

Methods for antigen retrieval are specific for each antibody/antigen combination. No attempts to establish quantitative data following these methods should be considered.

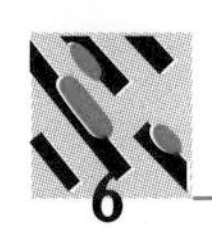



## Unmasking hidden epitopes with proteases

Fixation often masks epitopes. These epitopes can often be reexposed by a gentle incubation with proteases, where these enzymes remove obstructing structures and allow antibody excess. Many proteases work well for this procedure. Very crude preparations of proteases, such as pronase, are often used. However, using a better-characterized protease allows a more controlled reaction and better comparison from one time to the next. In this regard, trypsin works well.

### Needed solutions

PBS
0.1% trypsin, 0.1% calcium chloride,
20 mM Tris (pH 7.8); store at –20°C

---

1. Place the slides or specimens into a rack or other suitable container.

   Slides from paraffin-embedded samples should be dewaxed and rehydrated (steps 7 and 8, p. 164)

2. Incubate the specimens for 10 minutes at room temperature in PBS with occasional agitation.

3. Pour off the PBS and incubate the specimen in a 0.1% trypsin, 0.1% calcium chloride, 20 mM Tris (pH 7.8) solution for 2–20 minutes at room temperature.

   *The length of this incubation and the trypsin concentration determine how much proteolysis will occur. Try various treatment times for each tissue source and antibody combination until suitable conditions are reached.*

4. Stop the digestion by rinsing the specimen under the cold tap for 5 minutes.

**The samples are now ready for antibody addition (p. 166).**

## Unmasking hidden epitopes using the microwave oven

The principle behind using the microwave oven is to use extended periods of heat to break some of the subcellular structures that block antibody access.

### Needed solutions

1.0 mM EDTA (pH 8.0)
PBS

### Specialized equipment

Microwave oven

 **Caution**

Sodium hydroxide, see Appendix IV.

1. Place the slides or specimens into a rack or other suitable container.

   Slides from paraffin-embedded samples should be dewaxed and rehydrated (steps 7 and 8, p. 164).

2. Incubate the specimens for 10 minutes at room temperature in 1.0 mM EDTA (pH 8.0, adjust with sodium hydroxide) with occasional agitation.

   *The traditional buffer for heat recovery of antigens is 10 mM sodium citrate (pH 6.0); however, several researchers have reported recently that the EDTA buffer is superior.*

3. Move the entire container into the microwave oven. Mark the height of the buffer.

4. Microwave the sample at 750 W for three cycles of 5 minutes each. After each cycle, replenish any lost liquid from the slide container by the addition of distilled water to the original marked height of the buffer.

5. Remove the container and allow it to cool to room temperature.

6. Wash the specimens twice with PBS.

**The samples are now ready for antibody addition (p. 166).**

# Unmasking hidden epitopes using the pressure cooker

The principle behind using a pressure cooker is similar to that for using the microwave oven. Extended periods of heat break some of the subcellular structures that block antibody access. Because of the method of handling samples, this approach is appropriate for handling specimens on glass slides. The major advantages of the pressure cooker method are the ability to handle a large number of slides simultaneously, the convenience of using metal racks, and the avoidance of any hot spots in the microwave.

### Needed solutions

1.0 mM EDTA (pH 8.0)
PBS

### Specialized equipment

Pressure cooker

###  Cautions

Sodium hydroxide, see Appendix IV.

1. Place the slides or specimens into a rack or other suitable container.

   Slides from paraffin-embedded samples should be dewaxed and rehydrated (steps 7 and 8, p. 164).

*The traditional buffer for heat recovery of antigens is 10 mM sodium citrate (pH 6.0); however, several researchers have reported recently that the EDTA buffer is superior.*

2. Incubate the specimens for 10 minutes at room temperature in 1.0 mM EDTA (pH 8.0, adjust with sodium hydroxide) with occasional agitation.

3. Fill a stainless steel pressure cooker one-third full of EDTA solution. Heat on a hot plate until the solution boils.

4. Lower the slides into the buffer and then seal the pressure cooker.

5. Allow the pressure to rise to maximum. Leave at maximum for 2 minutes.

6. Remove from heat. Cool the pressure cooker in cold running water.

7. Open and remove slides to PBS. Wash twice with PBS.

**The samples are now ready for antibody addition (p. 166).**

# Frozen tissue sections

Detection limit is approximately 1,000–10,000 molecules/cell if localized.

Detects antigen presence and localization
Qualitative to semi-quantitative
Sensitivity dependent on minimal level and localization of antigen
High local concentration of antigen, so lower-affinity antibody OK

## Cautions

Diaminobenzidine (DAB), DPX, ethanol, hydrogen peroxide, nickel chloride, paraformaldehyde, sodium azide, see Appendix IV.

1. Dissect a small sample, no bigger than approximately 1 $cm^2 \times 0.4$ cm, of undamaged tissue.

2. Place the specimen on one end of a strip of card. Label the card, and submerge the end with the sample in liquid nitrogen. After 60 seconds in the liquid nitrogen, remove the sample and place on dry ice. Trim the card to just larger than the size of the tissue and transfer to a precooled (–70°C), labeled freezing vial.

3. Prior to sectioning, coat clean glass slides with 1% gelatin. Dissolve gelatin in water by heating to 50°C, cool, and add sodium azide to 0.02%. Dip the slides in the solution for 30 seconds, remove, and allow to air-dry.

4. Prepare sections of frozen tissues using a cryostat following the manufacturer's directions. Sections between 5 μm and 10 μm commonly are used. Collect the sections on the coated slides.

5. Allow the sections to air-dry. Dip in freshly prepared 4% paraformaldehyde (see p. 466) for 2 minutes.

6. Wash with several changes of PBS, and place in 1% NP-40, PBS, for 5 minutes. Wash with several changes of PBS.

7. Place slides with the tissue sections in a humidified chamber. Add the first antibody solution. All dilutions must be carried out in protein-containing solutions such as 3% BSA in PBS.

   Monoclonal antibodies are best applied as tissue-culture supernatants (specific antibody concentration of 20–50 μg/ml, use neat). Ascites fluids, purified monoclonal and polyclonal antibodies, and crude polyclonal sera should be tested at a range of dilutions aimed at producing specific antibody concentrations between 0.1 and 10 μg/ml. If the specific antibody concentration of the antibody sample is unknown, prepare and test 1/10, 1/100, 1/1,000, and 1/10,000 dilutions of the starting material.

8. Incubate the slides for a minimum of 60 minutes at room temperature in the humidified chamber. For some reactions, prolonged incubations of up to 24 hours can increase sensitivity.

9. Wash in three changes of PBS over 5 minutes.

10. Apply the horseradish peroxidase-labeled secondary reagent specific for your primary antibody. These reagents can be purchased from several suppliers.

    If the correct amount of secondary reagent is not known, test dilutions of the secondary antibodies 1/50 to 1/1000. Carry out all dilutions in a protein-containing solution such as 3% BSA/PBS.

11. Incubate with the labeled secondary reagent for 30 minutes at room temperature in the humidified chamber.

12. Wash in three changes of PBS over 5 minutes.

13. Prepare the DAB/metal reagent. Dissolve 6 mg of DAB in 9 ml of 0.05 M Tris buffer (pH 7.6). Add 1 ml of a 0.3% wt/vol stock solution of nickel chloride in water (the same amount of cobalt chloride can be used as an alternative). Add 0.1 ml of a 3% solution of hydrogen peroxide in water. If a precipitate appears, filter through Whatman No. 1 filter paper (or equivalent).

14. Apply the solution to the specimen. Observe the sample under a low-power light microscope. When the brown/black precipitate has developed sufficiently, stop the reaction by washing in water. This will normally be between 1 and 20 minutes.

15. Add a few drops of Harris' Hematoxylin to the specimen. Incubate for approximately 5 minutes. The length of time will determine the intensity of the stain.

16. Wash the slide gently in water.

17. Dehydrate the sample by passing through graded alcohols. Incubate twice for 3 minutes each in 75% ethanol, twice for 3 minutes each in 95% ethanol, and twice for 3 minutes each in absolute ethanol. Air-dry.

18. Add a small drop of DPX to the specimen. Carefully place a coverslip (#1) on the drop, avoiding air bubbles. Remove any excess mounting medium with a paper towel.

    DPX will set almost immediately and the samples can be observed and photographed.

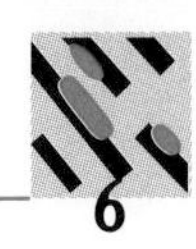


## References


Avrameas S. 1972. Enzyme markers: Their linkage with proteins and use in immunohistochemistry. *Histochem. J.* **4:** 321–330.

Avrameas S. and Uriel J. 1966. Methode de marquage d'antigen et danticorps avec des enzymes et son application en immunodiffusion. *C.R. Acad. Sci. D* **262:** 2543–2545.

Bullock G.R. and Petrusz P. 1982. *Techniques in immunocytochemistry*, vol. 1. Academic Press, Orlando, Florida.

Danscher G. 1981. Localization of gold in biological tissue. A photochemical method for light and electronmicroscopy. *Histochemistry* **71:** 81–88.

Danscher G. and Nörgaard J.O.R. 1983. Light microscopic visualization of colloidal gold on resin-embedded tissue. *J. Histochem. Cytochem.* **31:** 1394–1398.

Heimer G.V. and Taylor C.E.D. 1974. Improved mountant for immunofluorescence preparations. *J. Clin. Pathol.* **27:** 254–256.

Holgate C.S., Jackson P., Cownen P.N., and Bird C.C. 1983. Immunogold-silver staining: New method of immunostaining with enhanced sensitivity. *J. Histochem. Cytochem.* **31:** 938–944.

Iwasaki K., Staunton J., Saifee O., Nonet M.L., and Thomas J. 1997. aex-3 encodes a novel regulator of presynaptic activity in *C. elegans. Neuron* **18:** 613–622.

Kaplan M.H., Coons A.H., and Deane H.W. 1949. Localization of antigen in tissue cells. III. Cellular distribution of pneumococcal polysaccharides types II and III in the mouse. *J. Exp. Med.* **91:** 15

Kilmartin J.V. and Adams A.E.M. 1984. Structural rearrangements of tubulin and actin during the cell cycle of the yeast *Saccharomyces. J. Cell Biol.* **98:** 922–933.

Meek G.A. 1976. *Practical electron microscopy for biologists*, 2nd edition. Wiley-Interscience, Chichester, United Kingdom.

Nakane P.K. and Pierce G.B., Jr. 1967a. Enzyme-labeled antibodies for the light and electron microscopic localization of tissue antigens. *J. Cell Biol.* **33:** 307–318.

———.1967b. Enzyme-labeled antibodies: Preparations and applications for the localization of antigens. *J. Histochem. Cytochem.* **14:** 929–930.

Osborn M. and Weber K. 1982. Immunofluorescence and immunocytochemical procedures with affinity purified antibodies: Tubulin-containing structures. *Methods Cell Biol.* **24:** 97–132.

Polak J.M. and Van Noorden S. 1983. *Immunocytochemistry: Practical applications in pathology and biology.* John Wright & Sons, Bristol, United Kingdom.

Roth J., Bendayan M. and Orci L. 1978. Ultrastructural localization of intracellular antigens by the use of protein A-gold complex. *J. Histochem. Cytochem.* **26:** 1074–1081.

Sheehan D.C. and Hrapchak B.B. 1987. *Theory and practice of histotechnology*, 2nd edition. Battelle Press, Columbus, Ohio.

Spector D.L., Goldman R.D. and Leinwand L.A. 1998. *Cells: A laboratory manual*, vol. 2: *Light microscopy and cell structure.* Cold Spring Harbor Laboratory Press, Cold Spring Harbor, New York.

Sternberger L.A. 1979. *Immunochemistry*, 2nd edition. John Wiley and Sons, New York.

# Immunoprecipitation

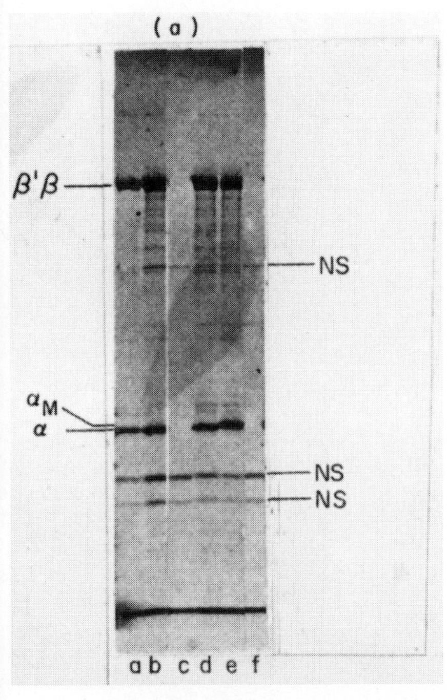


From Horvitz H.R. 1974. Control of bacteriophage T4 of two sequential phosphorylations of the alpha subunit of *Escherichia coli* RNA polymerase. *J. Mol. Biol.* **90:** 727–738. (Reprinted with permission [copyright Academic Press].)

Plate I. Purification of RNA polymerase from crude extracts by antibody precipitation. (a) Autoradiogram of $^{35}$S-label in antibody precipitates analyzed in the presence of sodium dodecyl sulfate on a slab gel. Track a: extract prepared from uninfected cells treated with chloramphenicol and precipitated with antibody to *E. coli* core RNA polymerase, as described in Materials and Methods. Track b: extract prepared from cells pretreated with chloramphenicol and infected with T4 for 10 mn at 30°C; this extract was also precipitated with antibody to RNA polymerase. Track c: same extract as in b precipitated with antibody to protein synthesis factor Tu. Tracks d to f: same as a to c, except cells were not treated with chloramphenicol. This autoradiogram was exposed for 2 days. $\alpha_m$ is T4-modified α. Bands labeled NS are non-specific.

Immunoprecipitations as we know them today rely on a series of technical developments. The figure shown here is one of the first to use slab gels to resolve the immunoprecipitated proteins. The first immunoprecipitations did not include a resolving step such as that used here. They were done by placing an antigen solution in one well of a permeable matrix much like our modern-day agarose. In a nearby well, antiserum was added. As the antibody and antigens diffused into the gel, they began to interact and form large complexes composed of multiple antibodies binding to and bridging between the antigen. At the point in the concentration gradients formed by the diffusing antibodies and antigens where a multimeric lattice formed, a precipitin line was seen as these large protein complexes fell out of solution. In early immunoprecipitations, a variation of this approach was used to create large multimeric interactions in solution that led to these proteins coming out of solution. A later variation used a secondary antibody to generate the lattice with the immune antibody, thus eliminating the need to titrate the primary antibody for each antigen solution. This variation was used in the work shown here. In the mid-1970s, solid-state interactions came to be used. Fixed *S. aureus* with protein A on its surface was used to collect the antibodies and with them the associated antigens. Now this approach has largely been replaced by beads coupled with purified protein A or protein G. Immunoprecipitated proteins can be used for many different tests, all relying on the specificity of the antibody–antigen and the antibody–protein A/G interactions to give a rapid and simple purification.

Immunoprecipitation allows the partial purification of antigens, normally proteins, from complex mixtures of soluble molecules. The antigens can be purified up to 10,000-fold by simple and rapid methods that collect the proteins on inert beads. The technique takes about a day and can be combined with any other method that can utilize immobilized proteins as a starting material. Immunoprecipitations are routinely used to measure the relative molecular weights of protein antigens, check for protein/protein associations, monitor the appearance of posttranslational modifications, determine protein half-lives, and check for intrinsic or associated enzymatic activities.

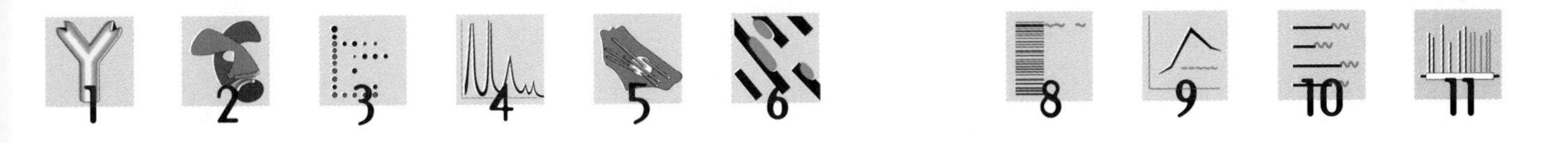




# 7 Immunoprecipitation

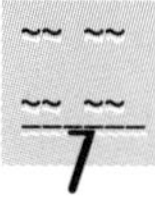


The underlying strategy behind the immunoprecipitation technique is to use the high affinity of antibodies for their antigens as a method to locate and bind target molecules in solution. Once the antibody–antigen complexes are formed in solution, they are collected and purified by using small agarose or polyacrylamide beads with covalently attached protein A or protein G. Both protein A and protein G specifically interact with conserved regions of the antibodies, thus forming an immobilized complex of antibody–antigen bound to beads. Irrelevant molecules in the starting solution are removed by washing the beads. The purified antigens can then be analyzed by any of a number of methods.

Immunoprecipitations are normally one of the first methods used to characterize new protein antigens. When immunoprecipitations are combined with SDS-PAGE, they can be used to determine the relative molecular weight of a protein, look for protein–protein interactions, detect the presence or regulation of posttranslation modifications, or determine the rate of protein degradation. Immunoprecipitated proteins can be used for many different tests and are commonly used to check for intrinsic or associated enzymatic activities or as preparative steps for other assays such as immunoblots or immunizations. This method is one of the most versatile for collecting diverse information about new antigens.

## Major constraints

The success of immunoprecipitations depends on the level of purification and the ease of preparing antigens. These are influenced by two major factors: (1) the abundance of the antigen in the original preparation and (2) the affinity of the antibody for the antigen.

The immunoprecipitation procedure is a very effective purification method used at an analytical scale. Using immunoprecipitations with the proper care and controls, all but the rarest soluble polypeptide can be purified to a sufficient degree that it can be seen as a specific band on an SDS-polyacrylamide gel. Insoluble or highly polymerized antigens may not be able to be studied using immunoprecipitations, because they pellet in the centrifugation steps regardless of whether or not specific antibodies are present. Obviously, abundant soluble proteins are easy to detect and analyze by immunoprecipitation. When rare cellular proteins are studied, the immunoprecipitation procedure must achieve purifications in the order of 100,000- to 1,000,000-fold. Although this level of purification would be difficult using other techniques, when immunoprecipitation is coupled to a technique such as SDS-PAGE such rare polypeptide chains can be identified. Immunoprecipitations themselves can achieve 10,000-fold purifications, and by resolving the resulting proteins on protein gels, a further 10- to 100-fold purification can be achieved, thus allowing the examination of even the rarest of cellular proteins.

The second factor that affects the ease of purification is the affinity of the antibody for the antigen. Comparing the affinities of different monoclonal antibodies provides an excellent example of this problem. Unlike other assays that present the antigen in a highly concentrated local environment, immunoprecipitations rely on the formation of the antibody–antigen complex in solution at relatively low concentrations of the antigen. In practice, this means that quantitative immunoprecipitations normally require antibody affinities of $10^8$ liter $mol^{-1}$ or higher. Affinities of $10^6$ to $10^7$ liter $mol^{-1}$ may allow the antigen to be detected, but it will not be possible to remove the antigen quantitatively from the solution. These observations mean that some monoclonal antibodies that are positive in other tests may not be usable in immunoprecipitations. The use of polyclonal antibodies or pools of monoclonal antibodies may avoid this problem by interacting with multiple epitopes on the antigen. The effect of antibody affinity on immunoprecipitation is discussed in detail in Chapter 2, and the variables for monoclonal versus polyclonal antibodies are discussed in Chapter 3 and below.

## Choosing the correct antibody

Three types of antibody preparations can be used for immunoprecipitations. These are polyclonal antibodies, monoclonal antibodies, and pooled monoclonal antibodies. Their relative advantages and disadvantages are summarized in Table 7.1 and discussed in detail below. Chapter 3 contains a more thorough discussion of the problems of choosing the correct antibody along with a consideration of how to evaluate different antibody sources. The major complicating factors that should influence your choice between available antibodies are the extent of cross-reactions with unrelated antigens, a common problem found with about one-third of monoclonal antibodies, and bad backgrounds, a problem that is more common with polyclonal antibodies. Nonspecific backgrounds can normally be kept to a minimum by titering the amount of antibody to the lowest amount that does not lower the strength of the antigen band (essentially still staying in antibody excess) and by carefully following the preclearing protocols described below.

Table 7.1 *Antibody choice*

| | Polyclonal antibodies | Monoclonal antibodies | Pooled monoclonal antibodies |
|---|---|---|---|
| **Signal strength** | Excellent | Antibody dependent (poor to excellent) | Excellent |
| **Specificity** | Usually good, but some background | Excellent, but some cross-reactions | Excellent by avoiding antibodies with cross-reactions |
| **Good features** | Stable, multivalent interactions | Specificity<br>Unlimited supply | Stable, multivalent interactions<br>Specificity<br>Unlimited supply |
| **Bad features** | Nonrenewable<br>Background | Need high affinity for antigen | Not commonly available |

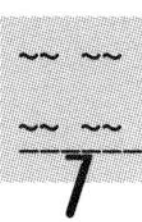



## Immunoprecipitations using polyclonal antibodies

Polyclonal antibodies are the most commonly used reagents for immunoprecipitations. Normally they contain antibodies that bind to multiple sites on the antigen and therefore have a much higher avidity for the antigen (see Chapter 2). Having more than one antibody bound to an antigen also has other important advantages. When the immune complexes are collected on any of the solid-phase matrices, such as protein A beads, the availability of multiple binding sites for the protein A molecules provides a more stable antigen–antibody–protein A complex. Together, multiple antibody–antigen interactions and multiple antibody–protein A interactions provide a multivalent complex that is easy to prepare, stable, and can be treated relatively harshly during the washing procedure.

Although using polyclonal antibodies for immunoprecipitations often produces stable multivalent interactions, their use also yields higher nonspecific backgrounds than the use of other types of antibodies. Multiple interactions that lead to forming large complexes are more apt to trap or bind nonspecific proteins. Because polyclonal antibodies normally are used as whole sera, they contain the entire repertoire of circulating antibodies found in the immunized animal at the time the serum was collected. Therefore, serum may contain antibodies that specifically recognize spurious antigens. Because this type of contamination is specific, it cannot be removed by methods that are designed to lower nonspecific background (e.g., preclearing, adding BSA). In these cases, the easiest method to remove these activities is to switch antibody sources. Other antisera are unlikely to contain identical spurious reactions. In some cases, it may also be possible to block the specific antibodies by preincubating the serum with a solution that contains the contaminating proteins (e.g., an acetone powder from a source that does not express the antigen being studied, p. 437).

Because of contaminating activities and increased nonspecific interactions, immunoprecipitations using polyclonal antibodies normally have higher backgrounds than other antibody preparations. Many of these problems are inherent in this technique, but some of the background can be effectively removed by titrating the amount of antisera needed to immunoprecipitate the antigen. By providing the smallest amount of serum necessary for the quantitative recovery of the antigen, the background can be kept to a minimum. In addition, because of the stability of the complexes, nonspecific background problems may be lessened by more stringent washing.

## Immunoprecipitations using monoclonal antibodies

The biggest advantage of using monoclonal antibodies for immunoprecipitations is the specificity of their interactions. Because monoclonal antibodies bind to only one epitope, they provide an excellent tool to identify a particular structure on an antigen. Given the right antibody, they can be used not only to detect an antigen, but also to distinguish among different forms of the antigen, including conformational changes or posttranslational modifications. In addition, because the immune complexes formed using monoclonal antibodies are not usually multimeric and are smaller than

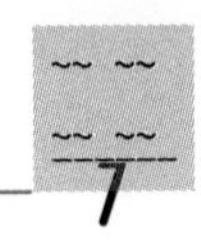

those formed when using polyclonal antibodies, there is less of a problem with nonspecific binding. Therefore, the backgrounds are normally cleaner.

Although using monoclonal antibodies for immunoprecipitations may solve or lessen some of the problems found when using polyclonal antibodies, their use also creates another set of difficulties. The most worrisome problem is affinity. Because the antigen is held only by one antibody–antigen interaction (except when the antigen is multimeric), the affinity of the antibody for the antigen is critically important (see discussions of affinity on p. 28). Monoclonal antibodies with affinities lower than about $10^8$ liter mol$^{-1}$ are difficult to use in immunoprecipitations. Because many screening techniques for hybridoma fusions detect antibodies with affinities as low as $10^6$ liter mol$^{-1}$, not all monoclonal antibodies work well in immunoprecipitations.

A second problem with using monoclonal antibodies is the possibility of detecting spurious cross-reactions with other polypeptides. Because an epitope can be a relatively small protein structure, often composed of only 4 or 5 amino acids, there is a reasonable chance that a similar epitope can be found on another polypeptide. In some cases, the common epitopes form part of an important structural similarity between antigens, and monoclonal antibodies can be used to detect related antigens. Alternatively, the antibodies may detect small structural similarities confined only to the antibody combining site. This is particularly true for antibodies that recognize denaturation-resistant epitopes. Presumably this occurs because these antibodies recognize features found in the primary structure of the polypeptides. Depending on the set of hybridomas, as many as one in three monoclonal antibodies have been shown to display these types of cross-reactions. Because of the frequency of these cross-reactions, the precipitation of an unexpected polypeptide should be treated as a contaminant until proven otherwise.

## Immunoprecipitations using pooled monoclonal antibodies

Using pools of monoclonal antibodies in immunoprecipitation takes advantage of the best properties of both polyclonal and individual monoclonal antibodies. The monoclonal antibodies provide specificity, and the use of multiple antibodies allows the formation of stable multivalent complexes. Consequently, pooled monoclonal antibodies are the best choice of reagents for most immunoprecipitations. Unfortunately, not all antigens have been studied in enough detail to have a set of monoclonal antibodies available for pooling. However, even the use of two antibodies specific for two separate epitopes will greatly increase the avidity for the antigen as well as for protein A or protein G. Therefore, whenever possible, pooled monoclonal antibodies should be used for immunoprecipitations.

# Immunoprecipitation protocols



Each immunoprecipitation has a core set of steps that are discussed in detail below. However, immunoprecipitations are often combined with other methods to make the assays more versatile. For example, immunoprecipitations are often performed on lysates from radiolabeled cells. This allows the identification of proteins from uncharacterized sources and allows investigators to ask about such issues as relative molecular weight, associated molecules, protein modifications, or protein half-lives. When lysates are prepared from unlabeled sources, the immunoprecipitated proteins can easily be quantitated by immunoblotting or checked for enzymatic activities.

The various modifications of the immunoprecipitation method can be used to determine many important characteristics of antigens. Table 7.2 lists these variations and the strategy for determining these characteristics.

## An overview of the basic immunoprecipitation procedure

The actual procedures for immunoprecipitations are quite simple. The method can be divided into three stages: (1) preparation of the antigen solution, (2) preclearing the lysate of nonspecific background, and (3) forming and purifying the immune complexes. The different techniques for each of the three steps are described below beginning on p. 230.

The first step is to prepare the antigen solution. Any solution can be used as a source for performing an immunoprecipitation; however, immunoprecipitation is normally performed on a lysate prepared from a cell or tissue. Lysates can be prepared by any number of methods, but for most purposes some type of mild detergent lysis of cells, such as treating with a nonionic detergent, is the preferred method. This removes the membranes, breaks apart many weak interactions, and releases most antigens from the cell. Importantly, it is mild enough not to destroy the conformation or enzymatic activity of most antigens. If correct conformation or activity of the antigen is not required or if the antigen is more tightly bound, more extreme conditions can be used to prepare the lysate. This can be as violent as boiling in a strong denaturant, which is later diluted or removed prior to immunoprecipitation. Once the cell lysate is prepared, it is ready for the preclearing step.

Because immunoprecipitations are normally used to determine the detailed biochemical characteristics of an antigen, the degree of purification of the final antigen preparation normally needs to be as extensive as possible. Because the interaction between the antibody and antigen behaves essentially according to the inherent properties of the antibody and antigen solutions, the easiest way to improve the signal-to-noise ratio in this technique is to lower the background. This is done by removing any nonspecific binding proteins from the antigen solution by pretreating with a nonspecific antibody that does not bind to the chosen antigen. This method of doing the immunoprecipitation—essentially doing the immunoprecipitation twice, once to lower the background with a nonimmune antibody and once with the antibody under study—is the most effective method for achieving clean immunoprecipitations.

Table 7.2 *Variations on immunoprecipitation procedure*

| Goal | Variations | Recommended approach |
|---|---|---|
| **Relative molecular weight of antigen** | | 1. Radiolabel cells with [$^{35}$S]methionine in methionine-free media<br>2. Immunoprecipitate<br>3. SDS-PAGE and locate by film or imager<br>4. Plot migration versus standards |
| **Quantitation of antigen** | Abundant antigen | 1. Immunoblot |
| | Abundant antigen | 1. Immunoprecipitate<br>2. SDS-PAGE<br>3. Stain by Coomassie blue or silver stain |
| | Rare antigen | 1. Immunoprecipitate unlabeled protein<br>2. SDS-PAGE<br>3. Immunoblot with specific antibody |
| **Rate of degradation of antigen** | | 1. Radiolabel cells with short pulse of [$^{35}$S]methionine in methionine-free media<br>2. Chase with cold methionine<br>3. Immunoprecipitate<br>4. SDS-PAGE and examine by film or imager |
| **Posttranslational modifications** | Any phosphorylation | 1. Radiolabel cells with [*ortho*-$^{32}$P]phosphate in phosphate-free media<br>2. Immunoprecipitate<br>3. SDS-PAGE and locate by film or imager |
| | Tyr-phosphorylation | 1. Immunoprecipitate unlabeled protein<br>2. SDS-PAGE<br>3. Immunoblot with anti-phospho-tyr antibody |
| | N-linked sugar | 1. Radiolabel cells with [$^{3}$H]mannose or [$^{3}$H]galactose in glucose-free media<br>2. Immunoprecipitate<br>3. SDS-PAGE and locate by film or imager |
| | O-linked sugar | 1. Radiolabel cells with [$^{3}$H]mannose or [$^{3}$H]galactose in glucose-free media<br>2. Immunoprecipitate<br>3. SDS-PAGE and locate by film or imager |
| **Associated proteins** | Looking for potential new or studying known associated proteins | 1. Radiolabel cells with [$^{35}$S]methionine<br>2. Immunoprecipitate<br>3. SDS-PAGE and examine by film or imager |
| | Checking on known association | 1. Immunoprecipitate unlabeled protein<br>2. SDS-PAGE<br>3. Immunoblot with antibody for protein partner |
| **Enzymatic activity** | Looking for intrinsic or associated enzyme activity | 1. Immunoprecipitate unlabeled protein<br>2. Wash with reaction buffer<br>3. Add substrate and perform assay |
| **Clear an antigen from a lysate** | Removing a known antigen from solution | 1. Immunoprecipitate unlabeled protein using excess antibody<br>2. Use supernatant from step 1 and repeat immunoprecipitation twice more<br>3. Final supernatant is source for study, but use immunoprecipitates from each step to verify removal (by any method) |

After preclearing, specific antibodies are added to the lysate. Because of the high affinity of antibodies for their respective antigens, the antibody–antigen complexes form rapidly and easily. Then the immune complexes are purified on a solid-phase matrix that has either protein A or protein G linked to an agarose or polyacrylamide bead. Both protein A and protein G have high affinity for the Fc portion of the antibody. After the protein A/G–antibody interaction occurs, the unbound proteins are removed by washing the beads, leaving the purified antibody–antigen complexes bound to the matrix.

After molecules that are not bound to the antigen–antibody–protein A/G beads are removed by washing, the resulting immunoprecipitated proteins are available for further assays. The most common next step is to separate these proteins by SDS-polyacrylamide electrophoresis. This greatly extends the purification by separating the antigen and any remaining associated or contaminating proteins by their relative mobilities in SDS-PAGE. Individual proteins can then be identified by their relative molecular weight and any other specialized property of the antigen. Methods for SDS-PAGE are described on p. 410.

## Lysing cells

Cells and tissues can be lysed by several different techniques. The correct choice of lysis method depends on the types of cells or tissues being studied and the final use of the antigen. Cells without a cell wall can be easily lysed by treating with mild detergents. Cells that have a cell wall, are most often lysed by removing the cell wall by some type of mechanical shearing or enzymatic treatment. If the final preparation of the antigen need not retain its normal three-dimensional shape or biochemical activity, the cells can be lysed by using harsh denaturing conditions and then handled by diluting the denaturants before adding the specific antibody.

Many extraction conditions release proteases in the lysis buffer. If protease digestion becomes a problem during immunoprecipitations, two approaches can be used to lessen its effects. First, care should be taken to keep the samples cold. Temperature has a profound effect on the rate of degradation by most proteases. Second, the lysis buffers can be supplemented with protease inhibitors. The sidebar lists some of the commonly used protease inhibitors. In immunoprecipitations, the two most commonly used inhibitors are aprotinin and phenylmethylsulfonyl fluoride (PMSF); however, a mixture of several of the different protease inhibitors is better, particularly as a starting point for further tests that would identify exactly the right inhibitors to use with your source of antigen.

| *Protease inhibitor* | *Working conc.* |
|---|---|
| *Aprotinin* | *1 μg/ml* |
| *Leupeptin* | *1 μg/ml* |
| *Pepstatin* | *1 μg/ml* |
| *PMSF* | *50 μg/ml* |

***Caution***
*Aprotonin, leupeptin, pepstatin, PMSF, see Appendix IV.*

### *Lysis buffers*

A number of different lysis buffers can be used to release protein antigens from cells, but no one buffer is sufficient for all purposes. In choosing a buffer, there are two important considerations. The antigen must be released efficiently, and it must still be recognizable by the antibody. When beginning the analysis of a new antigen, it is best to test a number of different extraction buffers to identify the most efficient conditions for the release of the antigen. A good strategy is to lyse cells with a relatively strong buffer. If the antigen is released, then begin to alter the composition of the lysis buffer until the mildest conditions to release the antigen are determined (see sidebar p. 231).

Quantitative release should be judged both by testing the amount of antigen in the lysate and by testing the amount of antigen remaining in the cell debris. This can be done most easily by analysis on immunoblots.

In general, the conditions used for lysis should be as gentle as possible to retain the antibody-binding sites and to avoid solubilizing background proteins, but harsh enough to ensure quantitative release of the antigen. For detergents this normally means choosing nonionic detergents over ionic, lower concentrations over higher, and single detergents over mixes.

Probably the two most common extraction buffers for immunoprecipitations are NP-40 and RIPA lysis buffers. They release most soluble cytoplasmic or nuclear proteins without releasing the chromosomal DNA. This strength of release is a good starting point for most studies. It is preferable not to release the DNA if possible, because of the problems that are caused by the viscosity due to the DNA in the resulting solution.

***Build your own lysis buffer***

*Variables that can drastically affect the release of polypeptide antigens include salt concentration, type of detergent, presence of divalent cations, and pH. Salt concentrations between 0 and 1 M, nonionic detergent concentrations between 0.1 and 2%, ionic detergent concentrations between 0.01 and 0.5%, divalent cation concentrations between 0 and 10 mM, EDTA concentrations between 0 and 5 mM, and pH values between 6 and 9 should all be monitored to determine the optimal conditions for extraction. Other possible additions to lysis buffers that may affect some antigens include RNases or DNases. Appendix III contains a short discussion on various detergents that may be chosen.*

## NP-40 lysis

150 mM Sodium chloride
1.0% NP-40
50 mM Tris, pH 8.0

This is probably the most commonly used lysis buffer. It relies on a nonionic detergent, NP-40, as the major solubility agent. In place of NP-40, Triton X-100 can be used with similar results. Useful variations include lowering the detergent concentration, raising the salt concentration, or switching to other detergents such as saponin, digitonin, or CHAPS.

## RIPA lysis

150 mM Sodium chloride
1.0% NP-40
0.5% Sodium deoxycholate
0.1% SDS
50 mM Tris, pH 8.0

This is more denaturing than the NP-40 lysis buffer described above. In addition to the nonionic detergent NP-40, two ionic detergents, sodium deoxycholate and sodium dodecyl sulfate, have been included. This lysis buffer releases most proteins in the cells, but will also break apart many protein–protein interactions.

### Caution

Sodium deoxycholate, SDS, see Appendix IV.

# Lysing tissue-culture cells

LYSING
PRECLEARING, 241
PURIFYING, 244

For cells grown in tissue culture, the most useful method of lysis is treating with detergents. Although many detergents can be used to lyse cells, nonionic ones such as Triton X-100 or NP-40 are most commonly used. Nonionic detergents solubilize the plasma and intracellular membranes, break many weak intermolecular bonds, and solubilize most of the commonly studied protein antigens. These detergents are not effective for the study of large polymeric antigens, but these are difficult to analyze under most conditions. Concentrations between 0.1 and 1% are sufficient for almost all lysis requirements. Nonionic detergent lysis buffers are commonly supplemented with isotonic concentrations of salt and buffered around a neutral pH.

In some situations, somewhat more rigorous extraction conditions may be needed to release the antigen under study or to strip off weakly associated proteins. In these cases, we recommend the use of RIPA lysis buffer. This contains nonionic detergents mixed with ionic detergents and is a considerably more denaturing lysis buffer. This will release all but the insoluble proteins of the cell and will break most weak noncovalent interactions.

*When studying the modifications of proteins by phosphorylation, you should consider including phosphatase inhibitors.*

Unless there are reasons not to use them, we recommend including a mixture of protease inhibitors in the lysis buffer. It is always good to add these in the early stages of investigation of a new antigen. After the protein has been characterized better, a test can be performed to learn whether these inhibitors are needed in all cases. As mentioned above, the most effective method of blocking protease action is to keep all the solutions cold throughout the immunoprecipitation procedure.

## Thinking ahead

Since the immunoprecipitation procedure takes multiple steps and includes several hour incubations, it is helpful to map out the timing of this experiment before starting, noting where overnight pauses can be taken. This will help you decide when you must begin the lysis of cells to fit your schedule.

## Needed solutions

PBS
Lysis buffer (prechilled to 4°C)

1. For monolayer cultures, wash the cells once with room-temperature PBS. Drain well.

   For cells grown in suspension, collect the cells by centrifugation at 400*g* for 10 minutes. Remove the supernatant.

*Lysis buffers stored in a refrigerator are available for use at any time.*

2. For monolayer cultures, place the tissue-culture dish on ice. Add 1.0 ml of lysis buffer (prechilled to 4°C) per 100-mm dish.

*Choice of lysis buffer is discussed on p. 231. For new antigens, RIPA buffer or NP-40 lysis buffer are good first choices.*

For suspension cultures, place the tube containing the washed cell pellet on ice. Resuspend the pellet in 1.0 ml of lysis buffer (prechilled to 4°C) per $10^7$ cells.

3. Incubate the cells on ice for 30 minutes with occasional rocking of the plate for monolayer cultures or gentle mixing for suspension cultures.

4. For monolayer cultures, rock the plate several times to achieve good mixing and then tilt the plate on the bed of ice and allow the buffer to drain to one side. Remove the lysate and transfer to a 1.5-ml conical tube. Some researchers like to scrape the cells from the plate, but this is not required except in unusual cases.

5. For either monolayer or suspension cultures, spin for 10 minutes at 10,000*g* at 4°C. Carefully remove the supernatant to a fresh tube, making sure not to disturb the pellet. Place on ice.

**The supernatant is now ready for preclearing (p. 241).**

## Common problems

The most common problem faced in these settings is the incomplete release of the antigen from the cells. This can be monitored by using immunoblots of the lysate and the remaining cell pellet to check for complete release. Changing the detergent for lysis is the easiest way to improve release. The choice of detergent is discussed in Appendix III.

Cell membranes can also be broken by physical shearing. Common methods include using ultrasound generators, dounce homogenizers, potters, and blenders. These methods are particularly useful when large volumes are being used or when detergents must be avoided. Of these, the gentlest method is dounce homogenization. However, dounce homogenization is efficient only with larger volumes (several milliliters or more). In general, we do not recommend freeze-thaw lysis. For reasons that are not particularly clear, repeated freezing and thawing of lysates leads to excessive proteolytic degradation. Unless your antigen is particularly resistant to proteolytic cleavage or you have previously tested this lysis method, it should not be used as a first choice. In general, detergent lysis is the best method for immunoprecipitations.

# Lysing bacteria by sonication

Several different methods are commonly used for the preparation of bacterial lysates. The most useful method is subjecting the cells to short, intense treatments with ultrasound. This breaks the cell walls of almost all bacteria and also shears the DNA into sizes that will not affect the viscosity of the samples. This method causes some denaturation of the samples but is a reasonable compromise between ease of use, quality of samples, and cost.

## Thinking ahead

Since the immunoprecipitation procedure takes several steps and includes several hour incubations, it is helpful to map out the timing of this experiment before starting, noting where overnight pauses can be taken. This will help you decide when you must begin the lysis of cells to fit into your schedule.

## Needed solutions

PBS
Lysis buffer (prechilled on ice)

## Special equipment

Probe- or cup-type sonicator

##  Caution

DOC, SDS, sodium deoxycholate, see Appendix IV.

1. Collect the cells by centrifugation at 1000*g* for 5 minutes. Remove the supernatant. Resuspend the cells in PBS and spin again. Remove the PBS.

2. Resuspend the bacterial cell pellet in at least 10 cell volumes of ice-cold lysis buffer. RIPA buffer (150 mM NaCl, 1% NP-40, 0.5% sodium deoxycholate, 0.1% SDS, 50 mM Tris, pH 8.0) is usually suitable. Other lysis buffers are discussed on p. 230.

3. Using a probe- or cup-type sonicator (Fig. 7.1), disrupt the bacterial cells with multiple short bursts of maximum intensity (e.g., 10–30 seconds each × 4 repeats). Between each burst, return the cells to an ice bath to keep the temperature from rising.

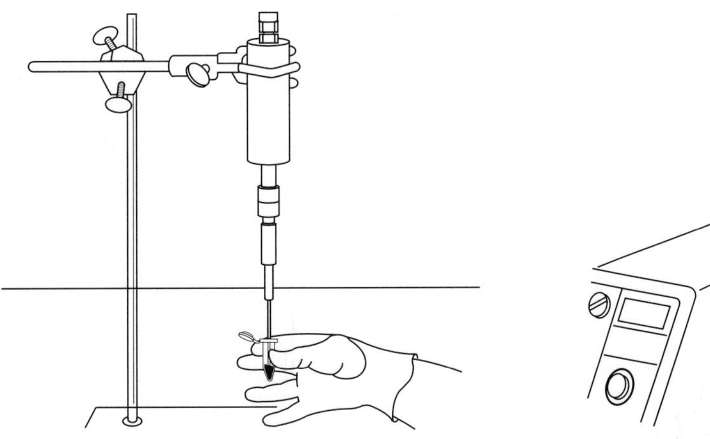

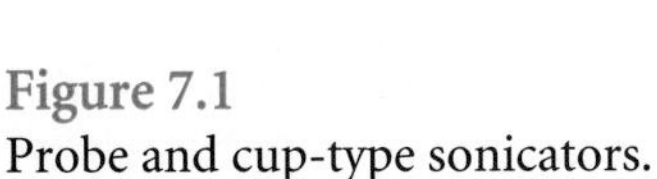

Figure 7.1
Probe and cup-type sonicators.

**4** Spin at 10,000*g* for 10 minutes at 4°C.

**5** Carefully remove the lysate to a fresh tube. Keep on ice.

**6** *Optional:* Spin the supernatant at 100,000*g* for 30 minutes at 4°C to remove aggregated proteins. Carefully remove the supernatant and transfer to a fresh tube. Keep on ice.

**The supernatant is now ready for preclearing (p. 241).**

## Common problems

The most common problem with extracting any bacterial protein is the potential of **denaturing the protein antigens** during lysis. This is particularly true with the sonication procedure. This is a fast and useful method, but it can denature many proteins. If your antigen is not recognized by the antibodies, it is best to try other lysis methods that are more gentle. There are two other methods that we recommend. One is to treat the bacteria with enzymes that will break down the bacterial cell wall (for example, lysozyme treatment of Gram-negative bacteria) and then lyse the cells in detergent-based lysis buffers (p. 230). A second approach is to switch to bacteria that harbor T7 genes, such as lysS. These bacteria constituently make a viral lysozyme that removes the bulk of the cell wall, and the bacteria can be lysed as above by simple detergent treatment.

The other major problem when purifying proteins is the **appearance of proteins in insoluble particles** in the bacteria. This is particularly true when using bacteria to overexpress proteins of interest. In these settings, the proteins are often found in inclusion bodies.

# Lysing yeast cells using glass beads



For yeast, the preferred method of lysis is mechanical shearing by vortexing the cells in the presence of glass beads. In this method, the yeast cell walls are broken by physical shearing caused by crushing the yeast between the rapidly moving glass beads. As one would imagine, this is a powerful lysis method but imparts extensive energy into the lysis procedure and results in considerable denaturation of the samples. For this reason, yeast immunoprecipitations are not as powerful a technique as similar studies in mammalian cells and should not be relied upon for determination of protein properties that require authentic protein structure.

## Thinking ahead

Since the immunoprecipitation procedure takes multiple steps and includes several hour incubations, it is helpful to map out the timing of this experiment before starting, noting where overnight pauses can be taken. This will help you decide when you must begin the lysis of cells to fit into your schedule. Also note that immunoprecipitations of yeast have notoriously high background levels, and that preclearing and use of proteases are both highly recommended.

## Needed solutions

PBS
Lysis buffer (incuding protease inhibitors, prechilled on ice)
Glass beads (500 μm chilled)

## Caution

DOC, hydrochloric acid, see Appendix IV.

1. Collect the cells by centrifugation at 4000*g* for 5 minutes. Remove the supernatant. Resuspend the cells in PBS and spin again. Remove the PBS.

2. Resuspend the yeast cell pellet in a small volume of ice-cold lysis buffer. RIPA buffer (150 mM sodium chloride, 1% NP-40, 0.5% sodium deoxycholate, 0.1% SDS, 50 mM Tris, pH 8.0) is commonly used. Use approximately three cell volumes. In all cases, protease inhibitors should be included (p. 455, 230). Keep on ice.

3. Prepare glass beads (500-μm diameter) by washing twice in 1 N hydrochloric acid and twice in lysis buffer. Store at 4°C in a small volume of lysis buffer.

4. Add a volume of chilled glass beads equal to the total volume of the resuspended yeast cells.

*The extent of lysis can be monitored by observation under the microscope either directly or with the addition of a vital dye.*

5. Vortex vigorously for 30 seconds. Repeat the vortexing step until the bulk of the yeast are lysed.

*Given the problems with background in yeast immunoprecipitations, it will help to spin the supernatant at 100,000g for 30 minutes at 4°C to remove aggregated proteins. Carefully remove the supernatant and transfer to a fresh tube. Keep on ice.*

6 Spin the lysate with the beads at 10,000*g* for 5 minutes at 4°C. Carefully remove the supernatant and transfer to a fresh tube. Keep on ice.

**The supernatant is now ready for preclearing (p. 241).**

## Common problems

The major problem found with this approach is the denaturation of the protein antigens. An alternative that will overcome some of these problems is to treat the yeast with enzymes that degrade the cell wall and produce spheroplasts, which can then be lysed with detergents. This is an effective method, but the high cost of the enzymes makes this approach less appealing for routine high-volume use. However, it is an effective approach for the detailed analysis of a key protein under study.

# Denaturing lysis



For many sources of antigens, one useful method of lysis is treating cells with harsh, denaturing solutions to release most of the protein antigens. The lysates are then diluted or dialyzed to reduce the denaturing conditions to levels that are suitable for the formation of antibody–antigen complexes.

The major consideration in choosing this lysis method is the loss of three-dimensional structural folding during denaturation. This means that all noncovalent protein–protein interactions will be lost and that denaturation-sensitive epitopes will be destroyed. Therefore, this is not an appropriate method for many types of final assays. However, this is a good method for quantitation of the antigen, careful identification of the polypeptide band recognized by the antibody, and display of denaturation-resistant epitopes. As a rule of thumb, an antibody that works well in an immunoblot will work in this type of denaturing lysis.

## Thinking ahead

Since the immunoprecipitation procedure takes multiple steps and includes several hour incubations, it is helpful to map out the timing of this experiment before starting, noting where overnight pauses can be taken. This will help you decide when you must begin the lysis of cells to fit into your schedule.

## Needed solutions

PBS
Denaturing lysis buffer (2% SDS, 50 mM Tris, pH 7.5)
50 mM Tris, pH 7.5, with 2% BSA

## Special equipment

Probe- or cup-type sonicator

## Caution

Hydrochloric acid, potassium thiocyanate, SDS, see Appendix IV.

1. Wash the cells or tissue once in PBS. Transfer the cells by the appropriate method to a test tube. Collect by centrifugation and remove the supernatant.

2. Lyse the cells by adding 10 cell volumes of 2% SDS, 50 mM Tris (pH 7.5). Vortex vigorously.

*For convenience, consider $10^7$ mammalian cells to have a volume of 10 μl.*

3. Place the tube in a boiling water bath for 10 minutes.

4. Shear the DNA by sonication. Either a probe- or cup-type sonicator can be used. Several short bursts at maximum intensity will be sufficient to shear the DNA and reduce viscosity.

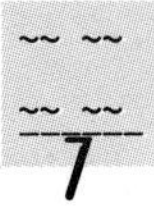

5. Spin at 10,000*g* for 10 minutes. Remove the supernatant and dilute 20-fold in 50 mM Tris, pH 7.5, with 2% BSA.

6. Incubate on ice for 10 minutes. Spin at 10,000*g* for 10 minutes.

7. Carefully remove the supernatant and transfer to a fresh 1.5-ml conical tube. Place on ice.

**The supernatant is now ready for preclearing (p. 241).**

## Common problems

The major problem with this approach is the inability of many antibodies to see the fully denatured protein antigen. This is an inherent property of the antibody and can be changed only by choosing another antibody for use.

There may be cases where removing the denaturant is more problematic. For example, if you are using an antibody that works well on an immunoblot, you can assume that the antibody is recognizing an epitope that either is resistant to denaturation or refolds easily with the removal of SDS. If this type of antibody does not work after denaturing lysis, it is likely that the SDS has not been diluted sufficiently to allow the antibody to recognize the antigen easily. This can be helped by several approaches. First, make sure that BSA is included in the diluent; it acts as a binding sink for excess SDS. Lowering the SDS concentration in the denaturation step should also be tried as a potential remedy. Treatment with 1% SDS is normally sufficient to denature most protein solutions, and concentrations as low as 0.5% may be adequate in some settings. Additionally, you could increase the dilution. This will be limited by how easily you can handle the final volume, by how abundant your antigen is, and by the avidity of your antibody for the antigen. Conveniently, all of these issues will be tested empirically, so the best advice we can give is to try several variations to see what might help. An alternative to the SDS denaturant, such as urea or potassium thiocyanate, may also help. One disadvantage to using SDS, or any detergent for that matter, is that the detergent is difficult to dialyze and has a strong affinity for the protein antigen. Urea concentrations up to 8 M or potassium thiocyanate or guanidine HCl to 4 M will be highly denaturing, and both can be dialyzed effectively.

## Lysis of other cell sources

Almost any source can be used as a starting point for immunoprecipitation. This includes samples from sources as different as whole organisms, frozen tissues blocks, blood samples, column fractions, or environmental samples. If the sample source requires the lysis of cells to release the antigen, it is best to run a series of control experiments to learn the best methods for extraction. In general, the goals should be to release the antigen as completely as possible with as little denaturation as possible, to separate the soluble antigens from the particulate matter, and to either avoid or counteract the problems of releasing long strands of DNA into the solution. Volumes of lysis can be as little as 10-fold over the volume of the packed cells, but we recommend trying to achieve 50- to 100-fold, if possible. Finally, it is best to work on ice or as cold as possible to lower the rate of degradation from released proteases. Unless there are reasons to avoid their use, we recommend including protease inhibitors.

## Preclearing the lysate



Most of the parameters that affect the eventual purity of the final immunoprecipitated proteins depend on the inherent properties of your antibodies and the concentration of the antigen. For example, the abundance of your antigen in the starting solution normally cannot be varied dramatically. Similarly, the qualities of the antibody being used will be fixed. Therefore, the final purity cannot be adjusted by changing these variables. There are some technical tricks that can be used to make the immunoprecipitation step work as efficiently as possible, and we have provided a discussion of these in the section on forming and purifying the immune complexes (p. 244). However, the most useful method for lowering the background and improving the signal-to-noise ratio is to remove proteins in the lysates that bind nonspecifically to the immune complexes or the solid phase prior to the final immunoprecipitation step. This is known as preclearing, and we recommend this as a standard method for all but the very simplest immunoprecipitations.

The recommended method of preclearing is to subject the lysates to a series of steps that mimic the actual immunoprecipitation techniques. An antibody that does not recognize the antigen being studied is added to the lysate and processed as for a normal immunoprecipitation. Here it is hoped that any nonspecific protein that might contaminate the final immunoprecipitation step would be removed by using an irrelevant antibody first. In addition, all of the parameters that might be used to decrease the background, for example, increasing the volume of the reaction, are not used. Essentially, the preclearing step is done in the worst conditions, attempting to remove any contaminating protein.

We recommend using rabbit serum collected from a healthy adult animal that has not been previously immunized. This provides a complex mixture of different antibody types that is not dominated by a particular immune response. We also recommend the use of fixed *Staphylococcus aureus* Cowan I (SAC) as a source of protein A to collect the rabbit antibodies. Protein A beads could be used, but these are considerably more expensive than SAC, and the concentration of protein A on the beads is much lower on the beads than on the surface of the SAC. Therefore, the fixed bacteria provide a much better surface for collecting the rabbit antibodies. Also, the bacteria themselves are inherently more sticky than protein A beads and, hence, are "dirtier," which can be used to your advantage here. If there are reasons to worry about proteins that might bind to agarose or polyacrylamide beads, unmodified beads can be added to the preclearing reactions, or a separate incubation with these matrices can be added.

Preclearing is a step that many investigators choose to skip. After many years of using immunoprecipitations, we strongly believe that this is a poor decision, except in the most unusual situations. There is almost no disadvantage in doing a preclearing, and there are several important advantages, the most important of which is the lowering of nonspecific contaminants. In addition, the preclearing step also adds the advantages found when including serum at an early stage. Serum contains many potent natural protease inhibitors. It also acts as a stabilizing buffer and as a source of proteins that have evolved to act as soluble agents, a property that is not shared with most of the proteins found in a cell lysate.

The only disadvantage of performing a preclearing step is the time that is added to the protocol. In most cases, this is far outweighed by the advantages. The only situation in which we do not recommend preclearing is when the final detection step will be done by immunoblotting. In these cases, the extra steps are truly not necessary.

## Thinking ahead

For convenience, we recommend preparing the *S. aureus* Cowan I (SAC) in advance and storing in 1-ml aliquots of a 10% solution (volume of SAC/volume of buffer) in lysis buffer at –20°C.

## Needed solutions and reagents

Normal rabbit serum 10% solution (volume of SAC pellet/volume of buffer) in lysis buffer

1. To the lysate or antigen solution, add 50 μl of normal rabbit serum per 1.0 ml of sample.

2. Incubate 1 hour on ice.

*If the timing of your immunoprecipitation requires an overnight step to fit the workload into a 2-day procedure, this is the best place to extend an incubation.*

3. While the preclearing step is incubating, wash 100 μl of packed cell volume of fixed *S. aureus* Cowan I (SAC). SAC is available from a number of commercial suppliers. Spin the SAC briefly at 10,000*g* for 30 seconds, remove the supernatant, and resuspend the SAC in lysis buffer by triturating with a pasteur pipet (Fig. 7.2). Spin again at 10,000*g* and remove the wash buffer completely. Set the packed pellet of washed SAC aside on ice.

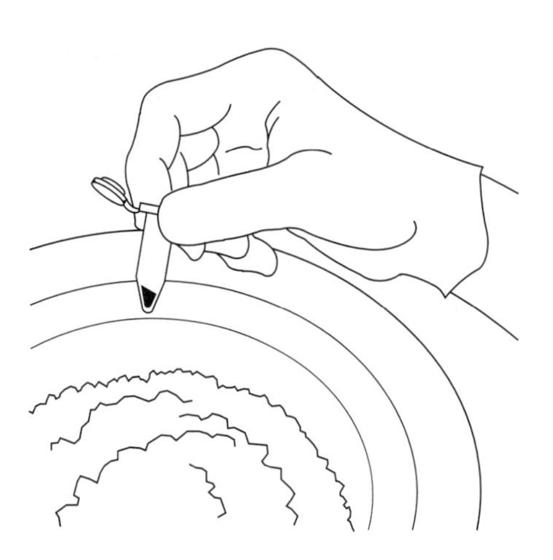

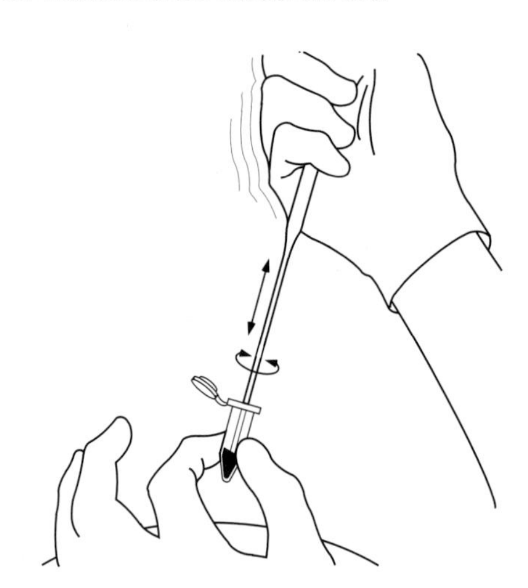

**Figure 7.2**
SAC pellet and resuspending SAC.

 After the 1-hour incubation, use the lysate to resuspend the washed pellet of SAC. Again, this can be done most easily by trituration.

*If backgrounds need to be reduced as much as possible, repeat the SAC step beginning at step 4. Incubate 30 minutes on ice.*

5. Incubate the SAC/lysate slurry for 30 minutes on ice. No mixing is needed because of the high concentration of SAC and large number of protein A molecules on the surface of the fixed SAC.

6. Spin at 10,000*g* for 15 minutes at 4°C. Carefully remove and transfer the supernatant to a fresh tube. Make certain that no SAC is transferred to the fresh tube. Respin if necessary.

**The sample is now ready for antibody addition as described on p. 244.**

## Common problems

Preclearing is a straightforward method that should not generate many problems. However, several precautions can be used to lower any chance of problems. First, it is essential that all of the nonspecific antibody used in the preclearing step be removed quantitatively, or these antibodies will compete for binding in the immunoprecipitation step itself. Any antibody can be used for preclearing, but the best choice is a source whose antibodies bind with high affinity to protein A. For these purposes, we recommend rabbit serum. It is readily available and binds tightly and quantitatively to *S. aureus* protein A. In addition, using SAC will make it easier to collect the rabbit antibodies than when using protein A beads because of the very high concentration of protein A on the surface of the fixed *S. aureus*.

If you are concerned that all of the rabbit preclearing antibody has not been removed, try a simple test with fresh lysis buffer instead of lysate. Begin at step 1 of the preclearing procedure and add 50 μl of normal rabbit serum. Follow the procedure as indicated, but at step 6 transfer the supernatant to a fresh tube and complete the immunoprecipitation as described on p. 244. Run the immunoprecipitated proteins on SDS-PAGE and stain the gel with Coomassie blue. The presence of heavy and light chains in these samples indicates that the rabbit antibodies are not being completely removed from the preclearing step. If this is the problem, increase the concentration of SAC to remove the preclearing antibodies completely.

# Purifying the immune complexes

LYSING, 230

PRECLEARING, 241

PURIFYING

Forming an antibody–antigen complex is the simplest step in an immunoprecipitation. Antibodies are added to the antigen solution, and the antibodies bind to their cognate antigen. Then protein A or protein G beads are added to the solution. This slurry is mixed and the proteins that do not bind to the beads are removed by washing. The variables to be considered are the amount of antibody to be added, the final volume of the immunoprecipitation, and whether to use protein A or protein G.

## Amount of antibody

Although determining how much antigen can be bound by a given amount of antibody is always a useful parameter to learn for any antibody preparation, most investigators do not need to go to extensive lengths to find this out. If you are just trying to characterize your antigen, we recommend the use of 1 μl of serum, 50 μl of tissue-culture supernatant, or 0.5 μl of ascites fluid. For most high-affinity antibodies this will be sufficient to immunoprecipitate a large portion of the available antigen, and the levels of antibody are low enough that you should not experience extensive problems with background or distortion of the gel near the position of the heavy chain.

In all cases where quantitative measurements are needed or when the backgrounds must be kept to a minimum, the amount of antibody to be added should be determined by titration. This amount depends on how much antigen is present, the affinity of the antibody for the antigen, and the volume in which the immunoprecipitation takes place. The correct amount of antibody to be used can be determined by titrating the volume of antibody versus a constant amount of antigen. A general starting titration range is between 0.05 μl and 5 μl of a polyclonal serum, 1 μl and 100 μl of a hybridoma tissue culture supernatant, or 0.01 μl and 1 μl of an ascites fluid. At the midpoint of these three suggested ranges, the amount of heavy chain will be approximately 1 μg. This is sufficient that the heavy chain can be detected easily by Coomassie blue staining of an SDS-PAGE. The presence of a stained band is used for troubleshooting because it indicates that efficient binding of the antibody to the protein A or protein G beads has occurred.

Another advantage of titrating the amount of antibody is that this often helps to lower the nonspecific background.

## Volume of the immunoprecipitation

Several competing factors need to be considered when choosing the final volume of the immunoprecipitation. The final volume determines the rate at which the binding equilibrium between the antibody and antigen is reached. Small volumes reach this equilibrium more quickly than larger volumes. Although one might assume that as small a volume as possible is the preferred approach, smaller volumes also promote the affinity of nonspecific interactions. So using larger volumes can be an effective method of keeping the backgrounds down. Also, it is important to get good mixing after the addition of the protein A or protein G beads. Larger volumes promote the ease of keeping the beads in a good mix with the antigen/antibody solution. To balance these variables, we recommend using a final volume of approximately 0.5 to 0.75 ml in a 1.5-ml conical tube. In general, most of the antibodies that have been selected for use in immunoprecipitations have a relatively high affinity for the antigen, making the volume of the reaction less important. In addition, for most investigators, the background problems are more worrisome than making certain that 100% of the antigen is captured. Increases in the final volume can be made by the addition of lysis buffer. If desired, this diluent can be made with 1% bovine serum albumin to help reduce any nonspecific protein binding.

In settings where the background is not a problem or when trying to remove all of the antigen from a solution, keeping the volumes as small as possible will drive the antigen/antibody interaction toward completion.

Finally, there may be cases where the types of antibodies you are using should be considered. When using a polyclonal antibody, the volume of the reaction is seldom a concern. In fact, the avidity is normally high enough to allow efficient binding and, eventually, removal of the antigen from solution even with dilute samples. With monoclonal antibodies of high affinity, similar approaches are possible. However, with low-affinity monoclonal antibodies, using high concentrations of the antibody in low volumes will help drive the reaction toward completion.

## Protein A versus protein G

All of the methods for purifying immune complexes rely on secondary reagents that bind to the antibody. The antibody is removed from the solution by binding to the secondary reagent, and the antigen remains associated with the antibody throughout the purification. The earliest versions of this method used anti-immunoglobulin antibodies to form a large complex of antibody–anti-immunoglobulin antibodies. This multicomponent complex of molecules is known as a lattice. When a lattice is suitably large, it can be removed from solution by centrifugation. This procedure is still one of the best at yielding clean immunoprecipitations. However, the ability to form large enough complexes to be collected by centrifugation is critically dependent on the molar ratio of anti-immunoglobulin antibodies to primary antibodies. For quantitative removal of the immune complexes, the ratio must be determined empirically for each primary antibody that is used. To some degree, the size of the lattice also depends on the amount and type of antigen. A large quantity of a multimeric antigen changes the potential size of any lattice work compared with a rare, monomeric antigen. A monoclonal antibody gives a different set of problems to forming the lattice.

As a solution to these problems, Kessler (1975) suggested the use of protein A-bearing *S. aureus* Cowan 1 (SAC) as a solid phase to collect the antibody–antigen complexes. Protein A forms a portion of the cell wall of these bacteria. The cell-wall proteins are fixed by treating with formaldehyde, the bacteria are killed by heat treatment, and the resulting particles form an excellent solid-phase matrix to bind to the antibodies. The protein A binds to the Fc domain of the antibody, thus, its attachment to the antibody does not affect the interaction with the antigen.

In recent years, the use of SAC has been replaced by the widely available recombinant protein A and protein G. They are available covalently coupled to a number of different bead matrixes. Use of this solid phase also lowers some of the background problems encountered with SAC. The choice of either protein A or protein G beads is based on the affinity of the antibodies for protein A or protein G.

## Controls

The correct controls for immunoprecipitation reactions should include nonimmune antibodies that are as close to the specific antibody as possible. For example, polyclonal serum should be compared to other polyclonal serum from the same species. The best control is a prebleed from the same animal used for immunization. For monoclonal antibodies, the control must be from the same source as the specific antibody; i.e., supernatant versus supernatant, ascites versus ascites, or pure antibody versus pure antibody. If possible, the control antibodies should be of the same class and subclass as the specific antibody. Tissue-culture supernatants from the parental myeloma are never appropriate controls because they do not contain antibodies. Suitable control hybridoma cell lines are available from the American Type Culture Collection and the European Collection of Animal Cell Cultures.

*For most purposes, we recommend adding approximately the equivalent of 1–2 μg of antibodies. This will provide an excess of antibody for rare or moderate-abundance proteins and enough heavy and light chains that these bands can be found by Coomassie blue staining if any troubleshooting is needed. These volumes are given as a standard starting point, and the amount of protein A or protein G beads has been adjusted to remove the amount of antibodies commonly found in these volumes. If your source of antigen is unusual, your antigen is abundant, or you need to remove your antigen quantitatively, the amount of antibody to be added should be determined by titration prior to the final experiment.*

### Thinking ahead

The protein A or protein G slurries can be prepared prior to use and stored at 4°C with the addition of sodium azide.

### Needed solutions

Lysis buffer
Source of antibodies
Protein A or protein G beads (10% vol/vol in lysis buffer with 0.02% sodium azide stored at 4°C)
Laemmli sample buffer without DTT (2% SDS, 10% glycerol, 60 mM Tris, pH 6.8, and 0.02% bromophenol blue)
1 M DTT (stored at –20°C)

### Special equipment

Rocking platform, aspiration source (most often a line to a vacuum flask hooked to a house vacuum source)

### Caution

DTT, lithium chloride, potassium thiocyanate, sodium azide, SDS, see Appendix IV.

1. Aliquot samples of the lysate into the appropriate number of 1.5-ml tubes. Add lysis buffer to bring the final volume to approximately 0.5 ml. For good starting volumes, add serum (1 μl), hybridoma tissue-culture supernatant (50 μl), or ascites fluid (0.5 μl) to a sample of lysate. For a titration, compare serum at 0.5–5 μl, hybridoma tissue-culture supernatant at 10–100 μl, and ascites at 0.1–1.0 μl.

2. Incubate on ice for 1 hour. High-affinity reactions will be substantially complete considerably sooner than 1 hour; however, the 1-hour incubation time provides a reasonable compromise for most antibodies.

*Overnight reactions, although suggested in some protocols, are seldom any advantage, and will increase the background. We do not recommend their use here, unless there are unusual circumstances.*

3. Add 100 μl of protein A or protein G bead suspension (10% vol/vol in lysis buffer) to the antibody–antigen reaction. Incubate 1 hour at 4°C with rocking (Fig. 7.3).

**Polyclonal antibodies**

| | Protein A | Protein G |
|---|---|---|
| Cow | | ✓ |
| Dog | ✓ | |
| Donkey | | ✓ |
| Goat | | ✓ |
| Guinea pig | ✓ | |
| Horse | | ✓ |
| Human | ✓ | |
| Mouse | | ✓ |
| Pig | ✓ | |
| Rabbit | ✓ | |
| Rat | | ✓ |

**Monoclonal antibodies**

| Species | Isotype | Protein A | Protein G |
|---|---|---|---|
| Mouse | $IgG_1$ | | ✓ |
| | $IgG_{2a}$ | ✓ | |
| | $IgG_{2b}$ | ✓ | |
| | $IgG_3$ | ✓ | |
| Rat | All | | ✓ |
| Human | All | ✓ | |

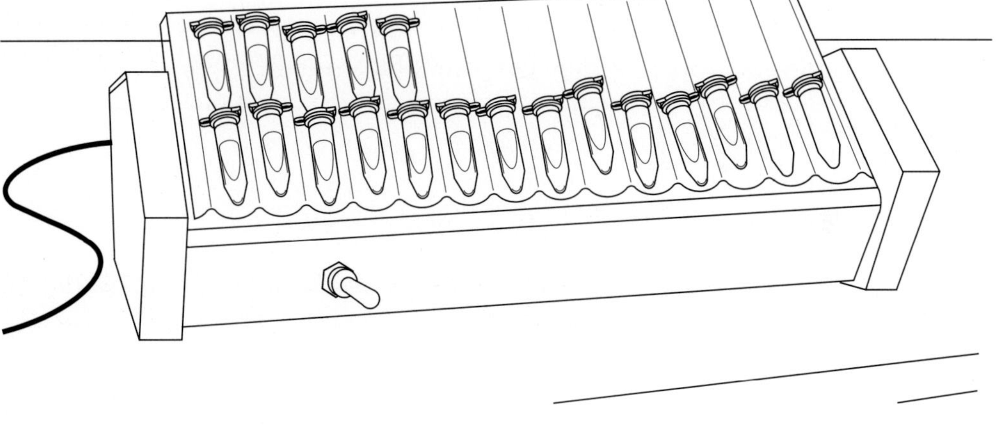

Figure 7.3
Rocking tubes.

*Removing the wash buffer as completely as possible at the end of each step will lower the background. We recommend the use of a 23-gauge needle or a micropipettor tip at the end of the vacuum aspirator line to slow the liquid flow and allow more precise handling of the beads. If the tip is small, it can be inserted directly into the beads to remove the remaining wash buffer. Any beads that adhere to the needle can be removed by gently flicking it on the lip or side of the tube.*

Collect the beads by centrifugation at 10,000*g* for 15 seconds at 4°C. Wash the immune complexes three times with lysis buffer. The lysate and wash buffers are easily removed by aspiration (Fig. 7.4).

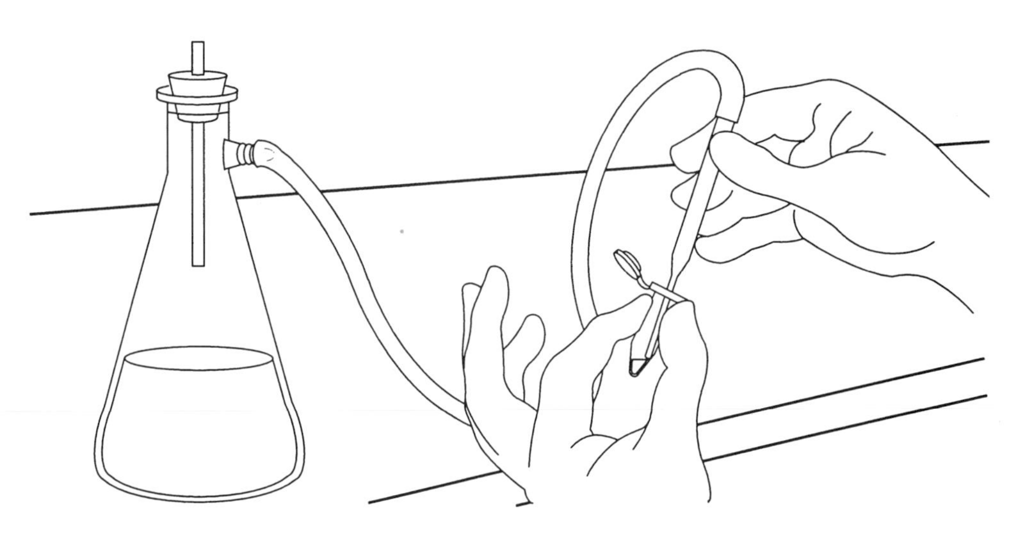

Figure 7.4
Aspirating immune complex.

Remove the final wash as completely as possible, and use the immune complexes for the appropriate assay.

For SDS-PAGE, add 50 μl of Laemmli sample buffer (2% SDS, 10% glycerol, 100 mM DTT, 60 mM Tris, pH 6.8, and 0.01% bromophenol blue). Heat to 85°C for 10 minutes. Spin, remove supernatant, and load supernatant onto gel (p. 410). Samples can be stored at –20°C if the gel will be run later.

## Common problems

Probably the most frequently asked question about immunoprecipitations concerns methods for lowering the number and type of background proteins that contaminate the washed immune complexes. Background problems come from many different sources and can be either specific or nonspecific. Antigens that are recognized directly by spurious antibodies in the antibody preparation give rise to specific background bands. There are only two methods for dealing with these problems. First, the contaminating antibodies can be removed by purifying the antigen-specific antibodies on an antigen affinity column (p. 77). Second, the activities can be blocked by adding a saturating amount of the cold proteins that are bound by the contaminating antibodies (p. 437).

Nonspecific background proteins result from a number of sources. They can form noncovalent bonds with the immune complexes or protein A/G beads. They can bind to particulate matter in the preparation. Some contaminating proteins aggregate or polymerize to a large enough size that they are removed by centrifugation. Proteins can be trapped within the latticework of the antigen–antibody–protein A/G complex. The contaminating proteins can bind to the plasticware that is used to centrifuge the immune complexes.

Below are some suggestions for dealing with nonspecific background problems:

- Add saturating amounts of competitor proteins. BSA, gelatin, acetone powders (p. 437), or 5% nonfat dry milk are commonly used. Store SAC or protein A beads in buffers containing 2% BSA.
- Spin the lysate at 100,000*g* for 30 minutes prior to the addition of the antibody to remove aggregated proteins.
- Try a different antibody.
- Centrifuge the antibody at 100,000*g* for 30 minutes and titrate.
- Use more stringent washes. Try 1.0 M NaCl, 0.5 M lithium chloride, 1 M potassium thiocyanate, 0.2% SDS, or 1% Tween 20. Also, alternating wash buffers from high salt to low salt or different detergents may help. Try washing with distilled water for one wash.
- Increase the number of washes. Leave the solid phase in the wash buffers for 10 minutes at each wash.
- If using radioactivity detection, lower the number of cpm of the radiolabel to the minimum needed for antigen detection.
- Make certain the lysates are not frozen before use.
- If specific proteins remain, remember that your antigen may consist of more than one polypeptide chain.

With unusual antibodies or when the volumes needed for the antigen solution are particularly large, it may not be possible to bind the immune complexes efficiently to the protein A or protein G beads. In these settings it may be helpful to include anti-immunoglobulin antibodies half-way through the immunoprecipitation incubation. When using anti-immunoglobulin antibodies, it is important to titrate the amount of the anti-immunoglobulin antibody that is needed to bind all of the primary antibody. This should be determined for each batch of antisera.

# Variations on the immunoprecipitation procedures

The basic method of immunoprecipitation can be applied to any goal that relies on the specific collection or removal of an antigen from a solution. These variations take advantage of the high affinity of the antibody for the antigen and can be applied to any purpose that needs the purification of analytic amounts of the antigen. For large-scale purification of antigens, Chapter 9 covers the major approaches for immunoaffinity purification.

Immunoprecipitations are commonly used to determine the relative molecular weight, half-life, associated molecules, and posttranslational modifications of protein antigens. When combined with immunoblotting, immunoprecipitations can be used to determine an accurate quantitation of the antigen as well as association with other known proteins. Immunoprecipitated proteins can be checked for intrinsic or associated enzymatic activities or as sources for these enzymatic activities to use on other molecules under study.

Another application of immunoprecipitation is to remove an antigen from a lysate. Although the methods above refer to techniques that have capturing the antigen as a goal, in many cases immunoprecipitations can be used to clear an antigen from solution. This is helpful when trying to learn what portion of an activity in a lysate is due to a particular antigen.

Because all of these methods demand slightly different approaches in the preparation of the lysate, the parameters of the immunoprecipitation, or the use of the collected antigen, each of these variations is discussed individually below. The methods are sufficiently different that we cannot provide detailed protocols; however, we have tried to provide sufficient information so that once you are familiar with the basic immunoprecipitation technique, you will be able to apply these modifications easily.

Table 7.2 (p. 229) lists the various outcomes that you may wish to achieve and suggests what steps may be employed to reach these goals.

## Determining the relative molecular weight of a protein antigen

*The relative molecular weight is often used as a temporary mechanism of identification, because many proteins take their relative molecular weight as their first name—often given as the abbreviation "p," for protein, followed by their molecular weight. One excellent example of this is the tumor suppressor protein p53. p53 was named and studied in great detail using this abbreviation, even before any biological significance was placed on its function. Thus, the relative molecular weight provides a good signature for any polypeptide.*

One of the key identifying properties of any protein is its relative molecular weight. This is the most commonly used characteristic of a protein antigen, and this allows the rapid comparison of proteins, often before their sequence, biochemical activities, or biological function is known.

The relative molecular weight of an antigen is determined by the migration of the polypeptide chain through SDS-polyacrylamide gels (Fig. 7.5). The relative migration of a polypeptide in an SDS-polyacrylamide gel is dependent on a number of variables, including the size of the polypeptide, the flexibility of its alpha carbon backbone, and its ability to bind to SDS. The primary determinant of migration in SDS-polyacrylamide gels is the charge of the protein–SDS complex that is formed when polypeptides are solubilized in SDS solutions. The dodecyl chain of SDS binds to most peptide sequences, and the number of molecules that can bind is roughly determined by the size of the polypeptide. Thus, the number of SDS molecules bound is an approximation of the length of the polypeptide chain. To achieve separation of the SDS–polypeptide complexes, the molecules are placed in a polyacrylamide matrix and charge is ap-

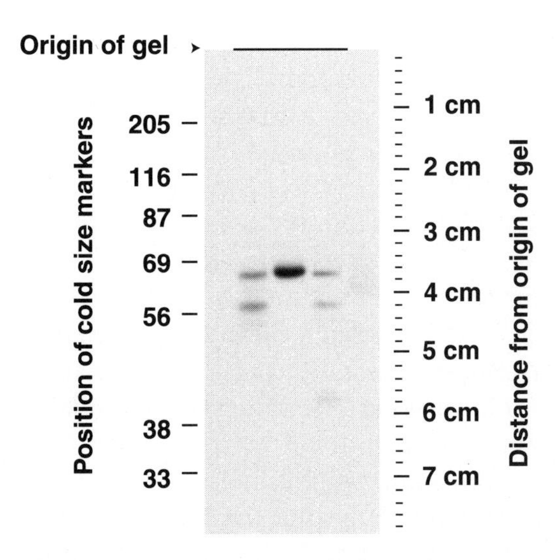


Figure 7.5
Example of molecular weight in gel.

plied. The SDS–polypeptide complexes are negatively charged and migrate to the positive electrode. Their rate of migration is also controlled by the sieving of the polyacrylamide matrix, with higher concentrations slowing larger complexes. With the proper choice of polyacrylamide concentration, a polypeptide can be separated from molecules that approach 1% differences in size. This level of resolution allows comparison of the relative migration of your polypeptide with other, previously characterized, polypeptides. From these comparisons it is possible to assign a relative molecular weight value.

In reality, this value is only a comparison of migration rates and not a true assessment of molecular mass. Values achieved for relative molecular weight should be considered only as a useful characteristic of the polypeptide and only a rough estimate of molecular size. Two properties of proteins are known to affect their relative molecular weights significantly. Highly acidic polypeptides migrate abnormally slowly in SDS-polyacrylamide gels. This is due to the inability of the dodecyl group to bind well to these regions and the concomitant decrease in migration rate. Another property of polypeptides that affects their rate of migration is the number of proline residues in the chain. Because proline residues are fixed in the rotation around the phi angle, they restrict the flexibility of the polypeptide chain. This makes the sieving process of migrating through the polyacrylamide gel slower and gives a corresponding higher relative molecular weight. In both these cases, when polypeptides are high in acidic or proline residues, their migration will be slower than expected. Nevertheless, even when the relative molecular weight is not an accurate predictor of molecular size, the migration rate is still consistent for a particular polypeptide chain and therefore becomes an important identifier for the polypeptide.

## *Technical approaches for determining the relative molecular weight of a protein*

The most common method for determining the relative molecular weight of a protein is to label the protein by growing cells in a radioactive amino acid precursor, most frequently [$^{35}$S]methionine. The cells are then lysed and the protein of interest is immunoprecipitated as described above. The final immune complexes are dissolved in SDS sample buffer and resolved on SDS-polyacrylamide gels (p. 410). If the weight of the protein antigen is completely unknown, you may need to run several different gel concentrations to find one that allows good separation from closely sized proteins. On these same gels, you will need to run a negative control which uses an antibody that does not recognize your antigen so you will be able to distinguish any background bands from your antigen. In addition, you will need to run a series of molecular-weight standards of known relative molecular weights to compare to the migration of the new protein antigen. These are available from many companies and come both as radiolabeled or cold versions. The radiolabeled standards are easiest to use and compare to the new antigen, as both the standards and the samples will be detected on the same exposure of film or on the phosphorimager output. If you wish to use cold markers (they are considerably cheaper than radioactive markers), stain the gel with Coomassie Blue and then expose to film or phosphorimager. The relative molecular weights of these markers will be provided by the manufacturer or check the list on p. 438. Next measure the migration of the markers and your protein from the top of the wells. Plot the migration versus the relative molecular weight of all the proteins on semi-log paper. The migration of the markers should form a straight line when displayed in this fashion (Fig. 7.6). Find the relative molecular weight of the new antigen.

To be particularly careful about relative molecular weight, we recommend using several different acrylamide and bisacrylamide concentrations and then checking the migration at each concentration. Most antigens migrate differently under various gel concentrations, and this is helpful in getting a more accurate molecular weight. It also may be good background information for later experiments, when you are trying to separate your antigen from other similarly sized proteins.

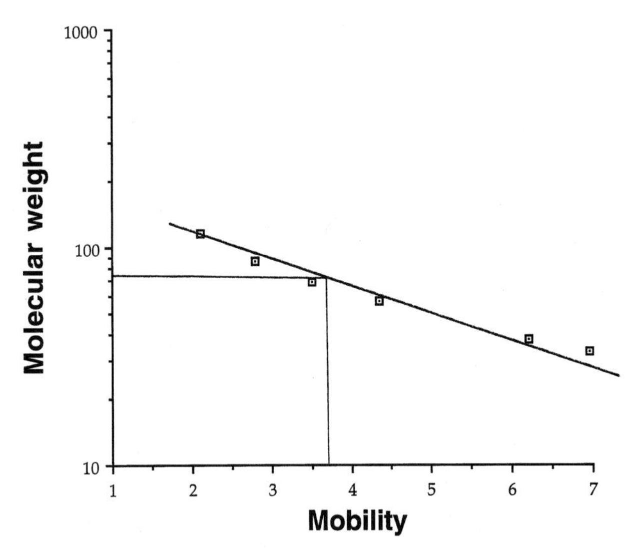


Figure 7.6
Calculation of molecular weight.

## Steady-state levels of proteins

Once the protein of interest can be reliably identified as a band on a polyacrylamide gel, it is possible to determine the total amount of this antigen in any solution. The most important aspect of these comparisons is that all of the antigen can be recognized by the antibodies. Antibodies of lower affinity or ones that recognize only a subset of the total amount of protein will not be useful in determining the steady-state levels of a protein.

### *Technical approaches to determine the steady-state levels of a protein antigen*

There are three variations for determining steady-state levels. When the protein levels are high, the antigen can be most easily quantitated by direct immunoblotting. Samples of the total lysate are resolved on a SDS-polyacrylamide gel and transferred to a membrane. The levels of the antigen are determined by binding with an antibody. Here, some standards of antigen will be needed for comparison. This could be a purified sample of the protein, in which the several concentrations of known amounts can be compared in adjacent lanes of the SDS-polyacrylamide gel, or a standard from a reliable but unpurified source could be used as a relative comparison. For example, you might compare the antigen level in an unknown sample with a lysate from a well-characterized cell line that is commonly used in your lab. This will not give you the absolute number of molecules but will provide a unit of comparison to determine the relative amount of any protein.

The second method also is appropriate only for relatively high levels of the antigen. In this method, the immunoprecipitated proteins are separated on SDS-polyacrylamide gels and stained with Coomassie Blue or silver stain (pp. 425–428). When compared to protein markers of known concentrations, the approximate steady-state level of the protein can be determined (Fig. 7.7). Because different proteins are stained to

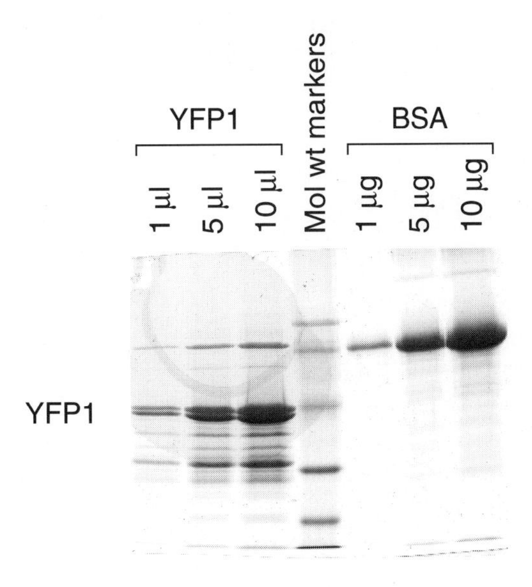


Figure 7.7
Determining protein levels by Coomassie Blue staining.

different extents, these comparisons can be used only to gain an approximation of protein levels. It is also essential that all of the protein be removed from the lysate under study. This can be tested by saving the supernatant from the first centrifugation step after the addition of the protein A or protein G beads. Test this supernatant for the presence of any remaining antigen.

A third method for determining the steady-state levels of proteins is to analyze immunoprecipitated proteins on immunoblots. The techniques for immunoblots are described in Chapter 8, but the strategy is straightforward. Proteins are removed from a test solution by immunoprecipitation. The immune complexes are resolved by SDS-PAGE and immunoblotted with an antibody specific for the antigen. This approach has two major advantages. One is the avoidance of any radioactivity. The second is that rare and/or dilute antigens can be studied by this approach. The immunoprecipitation step works to concentrate the antigen and allows almost any type or source of antigen to be studied. This provides a reliable and versatile method to study varied antigens in almost unlimited settings. The major disadvantage is that the immunoprecipitation must go to near completion to allow an accurate determination of the protein level. This means that only high-avidity reagents can be used in these comparisons. Again, the method could be used to determine a relative measure of an antigen when the results are compared to a stable and well-characterized source. Alternatively, if a purified source of the antigen is available, a comparison can be made to a titration of known amounts of the protein run in parallel lanes of the SDS-PAGE. This would lead to a good estimate of the actual concentration of the antigen in the starting solution.

## Determining the half-life of a protein antigen

By combining other techniques with immunoprecipitation, the rate of degradation of a protein antigen can be determined (Fig. 7.8). Two methods are in common use. In the first method, known as a pulse-chase, a radioactive amino acid is added to the

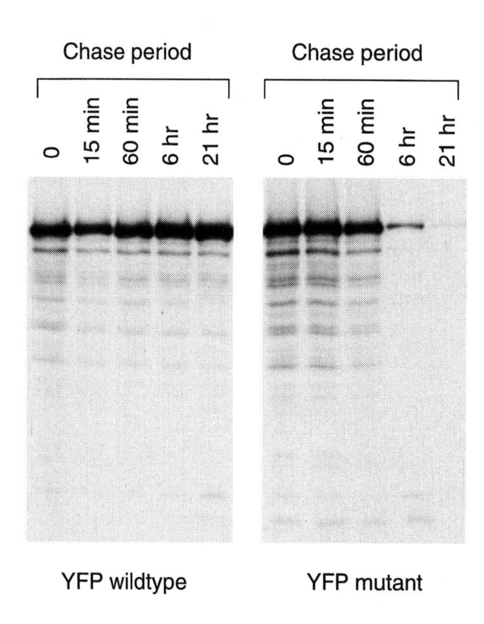


Figure 7.8
Half-life determination.

medium for a short time. After this "pulse" in which the amino acid is incorporated into the protein during synthesis, the radioactive amino acid is removed from the medium and replaced by saturating amounts of unlabeled amino acid. At various times after the medium change, this "chase" is monitored by immunoprecipitations of your antigen. The rate of loss of radioactivity is a measure of the rate of decay of the labeled antigen. In the second method, following radiolabeling of your antigen, a drug is added to block further protein synthesis. Periodic immunoprecipitations, following the addition of the drug, can monitor the rate of protein turnover for your antigen.

Of these methods, the drug treatment is a considerably easier method, but it makes more assumptions that cannot be directly validated. For example, if the continued presence of a second protein is required to establish the correct half-life of a protein, blocking protein synthesis could also eliminate this regulatory factor. Therefore, we recommend that half-life measurements made by blocking protein synthesis be used as a rapid method for preliminary studies only. Formal reporting of half-life times should be confirmed by the pulse-chase method.

### *Technical considerations for pulse-chase determination of half-lives*

*Some workers supplement the complete media with a 10-fold excess of unlabeled amino acid. For most media the concentration of methionine is approximately 15 mg/liter, so if you are using methionine the final concentration of unlabeled methionine should be 150 mg/liter.*

First, the amount of label needed to detect a specific band in a relatively short labeling period and after a reasonable exposure time should be determined. The incorporation of [$^{35}$S]methionine is linear up to at least 10 mCi per $5 \times 10^6$ cells. Short detection times are needed to have a good chance to detect the band in several time points during the chase. Although any length of time could theoretically be used for the pulse, most workers try to keep the labeling time below 1 hour, with 2 hours being the longest time commonly used. Longer labeling times stress the cells, because they will be missing a key component in the growth media. Another reason to avoid long pulse times is that the length of the pulse and chase times plus the immunoprecipitation steps leads to an excessively long day. Once suitable and reliable conditions for labeling the antigen have been determined, the pulse-chase experiment can begin.

Several plates of cells are radiolabeled for the appropriate pulse time, usually with [$^{35}$S]methionine, and the radioactive precursor is removed. The cells are washed with fresh medium, and then incubated with fresh complete medium. In general for short pulses, for example under 1 hour, cells should be labeled in medium without serum. For longer pulses or with cells that require the continued presence of serum, use dialyzed and filter-sterilized serum. At different time points after the pulse, one of the plates is harvested and lysed. The proteins from each chase time point are immunoprecipitated. After collecting all time points and completing all immunoprecipitations, the immune complexes are resolved by SDS-polyacrylamide gel electrophoresis. The amount of radioactivity in the protein band is determined either by densitometric tracing, counting excised bands, or use of a phosphorimager. The rate of decay should be plotted versus time. With careful manipulation of the length of the chases, three points that fall on a straight line can be found. These data points can be used to determine the half-life of the protein. It is essential that three points on a straight decay line can be established, because early in the chase period there will be a balance between continued incorporation of radioactive methionine remaining in the cell and decay. Only after incorporation has finished will a standard rate of decay be found.

*Intracellular methionine pools are relatively small, so achieving an effective pulse of incorporation is relatively straightforward. However, pulses with other amino acids may need to be preceded by a short "starvation" incubation in media with no precursor. This time should not be longer than the pulse time.*

**Caution**

Radioactive substances, see Appendix IV.

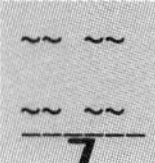


### *Technical considerations for drug block determination of half-lives*

Many labs have begun to report the determination of protein half-lives by using protein synthesis inhibitors to initiate the chase period. Commonly this is done using cycloheximide at concentrations of 1–10 μg/ml added from concentrated stocks. Protein levels are then determined by simple immunoblots at different times post treatment with the protein synthesis inhibitor. This methodology is appropriate only when preliminary tests show that pulse-chase results are correlated with those from the drug blocks. There are many examples now reported in the literature in which protein turnover is dramatically different in the presence of protein synthesis inhibitors. Therefore, the preferred technique is the pulse-chase methodology described above. However, there may be cases when many different conditions need to be tested for altering protein half-life or when use of radioactive precursors is inappropriate.

## Checking for posttranslational modifications

A number of proteins are modified after their synthesis, commonly by the addition of sugars, phosphates, or sulfates. These additions are used for many purposes including to mark proteins for particular intracellular or extracellular transport systems, to help ensure a specific protein-folding option, or as regulatory events that change a key feature of the target substrate. By growing cells in the presence of a radioactive precursor specific for a modifying group, immunoprecipitations can be used to identify proteins that undergo posttranslational modifications.

There are several hundred different potential posttranslational modifications, but many modifications are not commonly studied using specific radioactive precursors. This is because the correct precursors are not commercially available, the precursors cannot be taken up by cells, or the intracellular pools are too large to achieve high enough specific activities to identify the group. However, a number of modifications can be studied in this manner. Several of these are summarized below.

### *Phosphorylation by radiolabeling*

Phosphorylation of proteins is one of the most common methods of regulating protein function. Phosphorylation is used to turn enzymes off and on, to mark proteins for transport, to stimulate interaction with other molecules, and to designate protein scheduled for proteolytic degradation. Phosphorylation of proteins is catalyzed by the transfer of the gamma-phosphate of ATP to a target site by a class of enzymes known as protein kinases. Phosphorylated proteins can be detected by growing cells in the presence of radiolabeled orthophosphate. Commonly this will be $^{32}$P, a beta-particle emitter, but $^{33}$P, a low-energy beta-emitter, is becoming more frequently used. It is more expensive than $^{32}$P, but the half-life of $^{33}$P makes it more useful in some settings. The phosphate is readily taken up by the cells and is converted to labeled ATP primarily through standard nucleotide synthesis pathways. Labeling cells with radioactive ATP is not possible, because ATP is not transported across the cell membrane.

Protein phosphorylation is detected by lysing the labeled cell population and immunoprecipitating the antigens using standard techniques. The labeled proteins are located after SDS-PAGE either by using film autoradiography (intensifying screens at –70°C give the most sensitive film detection) or by detection using a phosphorimager.

Phosphate labeling is performed in phosphate-free media, which can be purchased from several different commercial suppliers. The highest specific activity $^{32}P$ that can be obtained is normally used. This is because the intracellular pools of phosphate are relatively large, and this decreases the percentage of proteins that contain the labeled phosphate moiety. Fortunately, the detection of $^{32}P$ is efficient, so high specific activity of the final phosphorylated proteins is not required. Labeling for most proteins is linear in mammalian cells only for about 1–2 hours and levels of incorporated phosphate rise only until about 4 hours. Labeling times beyond 4 hours should be avoided unless the medium is supplemented with 10% complete medium with phosphate. Commonly, researchers label with 100 μCi/100-mm dish to 1 mCi/100-mm dish. The choice of amount of label is based on the abundance of the protein, the number of phosphorylated residues, and the turnover rate of these sites. Since this is often not known prior to the first phosphate labeling, the levels are commonly determined empirically. For initial tests, we recommend using 500 μCi/100-mm dish.

*A good starting point to examine phosphorylations of proteins would be to transfer a 100-mm dish of cells into 2 ml of phosphate-free medium for 15 minutes at normal growth conditions, then add 500 mCi of $^{32}P$-orthophosphate. Incubate for 1 hour. Then wash cells twice with ice-cold PBS and process for a normal immunoprecipitation.*

One disadvantage of using $^{32}P$ as a radionuclide for labeling proteins is that it causes DNA damage. This occurs in two manners. First, as expected, the $^{32}P$ is incorporated into the DNA backbone, and its decay breaks the resident chain and the local decay also likely breaks the opposite strand, yielding a double strand break. In addition and more frequently, as all of the $^{32}P$ decays, it exposes the cells to a local and very intense treatment of ionizing radiation. Both of these treatments lead to the induction of the normal DNA damage response in the cell. If the levels of $^{32}P$ are sufficiently high, cell cycle arrest will occur. Therefore, shorter labeling times and lower levels of radiolabel are preferable.

### *Tyrosine phosphorylation by immunoprecipitation/immunoblot*

Phosphorylation of proteins on tyrosine residues can be tested by using antibodies raised against the phosphotyrosyl moiety. This can be most easily tested by immunoprecipitating the antigen under study directly from unlabeled cells. The immunoprecipitated proteins can be separated by SDS-PAGE and transferred to nitrocellulose using standard immunoblotting methods (see Chapter 8). Develop the blot with antibodies specific for phosphotyrosines.

### *Glycosylation*

Having specific antibodies that will immunoprecipitate your antigen is a major advantage in studying protein glycosylation. Glycosylation is normally first noticed when proteins migrate unusually on SDS-polyacrylamide gels. Immunoprecipitated proteins that are glycosylated run considerably larger in molecular weight than expected, perhaps as much as 30–50% larger than their predicted mass, and they will generate quite broad bands. Glycosylation is used for many purposes in cells, but it is primarily employed to mark proteins for particular stages of protein trafficking, to alter the structure of a protein to change its activity, or to provide extracellular binding domains that function in intercellular signaling and tissue development.

Glycoslyation occurs in two general forms based on the type of linkage that is made to the polypeptide chain. N-linked glycosylation links a sugar, almost exclusively *N*-acetylglucosamine, to asparagine through its amino group. O-linked glycosylation links a wide range of sugars to serine or threonine reacting with the hydroxyl. Proteins are seldom modified by single sugars. What makes glycosylation difficult to study is the wide range of different sugars that appear in the glycan, the different orders in which sugar subunits are added to the growing sugar backbone, and the variations in the extent and complexity of the branching.

There are two general strategies to study protein glycosylation. These are (1) to label cells with radioactive monosaccharides and allow these sugars to be processed and added to the sugar backbone or (2) to treat purified polypeptides with specific chemical or enzymatic cleavage agents to remove all or portions of the sugars. Both approaches are helped by the availability of specific antibodies. Following growth in labeled sugars, proteins can be precipitated and examined for the presence of the radioactivity after separation on SDS-polyacrylamide gels. Proteins that are marked by labeling with[$^{35}$S]methionine or another amino acid that gets incorporated into the polypeptide chain can be immunoprecipitated and then left untreated or treated with chemical or enzymatic cleavage agents. These proteins can then be resolved on SDS-polyacrylamide gels and checked for changes in mobility. Both approaches have some difficulties. Radiolabeling is done by growing cells in the presence of [$^{3}$H]galactose or [$^{3}$H]mannose. Labeling times should be kept to the absolute minimum incubation—seldom longer than 1 hour—because sugars are quickly shunted into many different biosynthetic pathways and their labels will quickly appear in other macromolecules in addition to just sugar-containing compounds. Cleavage is equally problematic because there are no single methods that will hit all glycosylations or all N-linkages or all O-linkages. Therefore, a large number of potential agents have been discovered and are used frequently. Enzymatic cleavage of N-linked sugars is now done with peptide-*N*-glycosidase F, which will cleave most of the commonly studied N-linked gylcans. Other useful enzymes include endoglycosidase H and endoglycosidase F. Chemical cleavage is more complicated technically but is believed by many workers to be more reliable once the method is set up and working in the lab. The most useful reagent to use for chemical cleavage is anhydrous trifluoromethanesulfonic acid.

For more detailed discussions of these problems, the reader is referred to Varki (1994) for radiolabeling approaches and one of the recent manuals on cell biology (e.g, *Cells: A Laboratory Manual* by Spector, Goldman, and Leinwand is an excellent compendium of methods) for appropriate conditions for enzymatic or chemical cleavage.

### *Prenylation*

It has been suggested that between 0.1% and 0.5% of all cellular proteins are modified by the addition of an isoprenoid. The known isoprenoids used for protein modification are farnesyl and geranylgeranyl. These hydrophobic moieties are used for such processes as anchoring proteins in lipid membranes. The modifications are found exclusively at carboxy-terminal cysteine residues, linked through a thioester.

Detecting prenylation can be done by metabolic labeling with a precursor of the isoprenoids, [$^{3}$H]mevalonate. Four variations on the labeling method can be considered. Early experiments relied on relatively low levels of incorporation and were performed by adding high levels of [$^{3}$H]mevalonate to the media (up to 500 μCi/ml were used). A variation that helps boost incorporation is to block the endogenous synthesis of mevalonate. In cells, mevalonate is synthesized from conversion of HMG CoA by HMG CoA reductase. In metabolic labeling experiments, HMG CoA reductase can be inhibited to slow this synthesis reaction and increase the incorporation of [$^{3}$H]mevalonate into the precursors of farnesyl and geranylgeranyl groups. This now can be done by using a drug specific for the HMG CoA reductase, mevinolin (available from Merck, Rahway, New Jersey). A third variation is to increase the rate of transport for

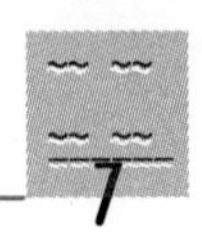

mevalonate. A transporter for mevalonate has recently been cloned (Kim et al. 1992), and this can be transfected into cells you wish to test. Finally, there are a few cell lines that have been selected for high levels of transport. Your gene of interest can be transfected into these cells and studied for prenylation there.

In additon, there are chemical detection methods that allow the identification of farnesyl and geranylgeranyl groups. For more details on these modifications, readers are referred to Spector et al. (1998).

### *Sulfation*

Many extracellular proteins are modified by the addition of sulfate. Some of the best characterized are the glycosaminoglycans, such as the heparin sulfate proteoglycans, and the granins. Sulfation can be detected easily by growing cells in small volumes of sulfate-free medium ($MgCl_2$ replacing $MgSO_4$) in the presence of [$^{35}$S]sulfate. If serum needs to be included, use dialyzed and refiltered sterilized samples to remove the sulfate in the medium. Final concentration of the radiolabeled sulfate should be approximately 0.5 μCi/ml. Labeling times should be kept relatively shorter than those used for peptide chain elongation. Times as short as 5 minutes are used to label proteins still in the secretory pathway itself, whereas labeling incubations of 30–60 minutes are commonly used for secreted proteins and extracellular matrix proteins.

Secreted proteins can be studied by immunoprecipitating directly from the media. Intracellular proteins are released from cells after washing the cells and treatment with lysis buffers. Immunoprecipitations are performed using standard methods and sulfate-labeled proteins are detected on SDS-polyacrylamide gels by film autoradiography or phosphorimaging.

## Protein-protein interactions

When lysates are prepared under gentle conditions, specific antibodies immunoprecipitate not only the antigen under study, but also any other macromolecules that are bound to it. Immunoprecipitations are often the most useful method for studying these types of interactions, and thereby allow workers the possibility of studying heteropolymeric complexes.

Immunoprecipitations are still considered the gold standard for arguments of protein–protein interactions (Fig. 7.9). Because immunoprecipitations have many points at which specific and nonspecific contaminants can be detected, extreme care must be used before any band is classified as an associated protein. Good minimal evidence for association should meet several criteria. First, all antibodies that are used must be shown to be specific, that is, to recognize only one of the proteins in question. Second, the association needs to be demonstrated by more than one method. Useful combinations include:

1. Perform a second immunoprecipitation with an antibody specific for the potential binding partner. If the association can be demonstrated from both partners, this forms a strong argument for in vivo binding.
2. Use more than one independent antibody against the protein antigen. If two or more antibodies that can be shown to recognize independent epitopes can precipitate the potential interacting partner, this is reasonably good evidence for binding. Problems could be caused by unexpected cross-reactions between the antibodies,

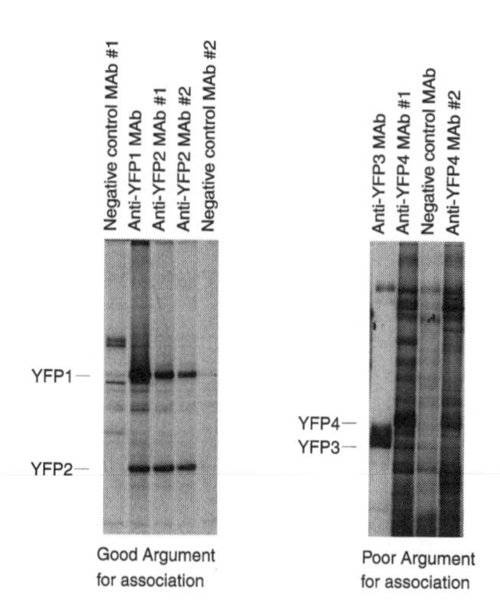


Figure 7.9
Protein–protein interactions.

or by the two antigens having multiple epitopes in common, as seen with protein families or with spliced variants of the same gene.

3. Less convincing but still helpful are coprecipitation and copurification of the two proteins following one or more standard purification steps, such as gel filtration or velocity gradient sedimentation. This method is most easily interpreted when the proteins are mostly pure. Copurification from crude samples should only be used to support association claims.

Excellent evidence for association would be to include multiple examples from the above list. All claims should contain clear evidence of antibody specificity for only one member of the protein complex.

Other methods also provide helpful approaches to study protein–protein interactions. In vitro binding, binding following transfection of two expression constructs, or two hybrid interactions are useful first steps to look for interactions or good methods to map interaction domains, but they are prone to overinterpretation and should not be considered sufficient evidence to claim an in vivo interaction. Even clear evidence generated by immunoprecipitation from lysates needs a careful interpretation because proteins may bind after lysis of the cells and never touch each other in vivo.

In many cases, the choice of buffers or detergents used in the lysis step will determine whether a multimeric complex remains intact. The properties of various detergents are discussed in the Appendix (pp. 469–471). Try various combinations to test for weaker interactions.

## *Technical approaches for identifying or studying protein–protein interactions*

There are two useful methods using immunoprecipitations to identify and study protein–protein interactions. Immunoprecipitation of radiolabeled proteins is an effective method to look for new interacting proteins. Because most proteins are labeled with an amino acid such as [$^{35}$S]methionine, an immunoprecipitation with a specific antibody may detect the specific antigen and any other interacting protein. In this method, cells are grown in a radioactive amino acid precursor, and immunoprecipitation is performed as usual. The immunoprecipitated proteins are resolved by SDS-PAGE. By examining the gels for bands (in addition to the antigen) that are specific for immune lanes but not present in the control lanes, one can look for potential associated proteins.

The second approach uses immunoblotting to study known proteins. Immunoprecipitations are performed from unlabeled sources. The immunoprecipitated proteins are resolved on SDS-PAGE and transferred to membranes, as described in Chapter 8. The blot is then developed with an antibody against a known protein. This method is very sensitive, because the immunoprecipitation step represents a powerful concentration step. Consequently, investigators must be careful that the experiments include controls for the total amount of each protein. Comparing this to the amount in the complex gives a good indication of the percentage of the protein that is associated. This can be done by running samples of lysates that have not been precipitated or by immunoprecipitating and immunoblotting with the same antibodies. Researchers should show that associations detected in this manner represent a reasonable proportion of the total protein present in the solution. It is a good practice to examine closely and be skeptical of complexes that represent less than about 5% of the total protein.

Several controls should be included when using either the radiolabeled or immunoblotting approaches. As mentioned above, the antibodies for these experiments must be well characterized to show that they are specific only for their cognate antigens. Appropriate controls should always include a negative antibody that does not recognize any of the proteins in the potential interactions.

## Checking for intrinsic or associated enzymatic activities

Because immunoprecipitated proteins can be prepared in relatively mild conditions, the final protein complexes often retain many of their biochemical properties. For example, immunoprecipitated kinases often retain their ability to recognize and phosphorylate their natural substrates. This allows the use of a variation of the immunoprecipitation method to examine not only the intrinsic enzymatic activities of any antigen, but also the activities of any proteins that are associated with the antigen under study.

### *Technical approaches to studying enzymatic activities*

Immunoprecipitated proteins or protein complexes often retain their enzymatic activities. Following the third wash, the immune complexes bound to the beads are washed one additional time in the reaction buffer. This last reaction buffer wash normally does not contain the intended substrate and should also omit any ATP or other energy source. This will remove most contaminating detergents of other agents, such as EDTA, that might block or slow enzymatic activities. The immune complexes and beads can then be resuspended in reaction buffer and aliquoted for the desired number of reactions.

Several points should be kept in mind while designing these experiments. First, remember that the enzyme kinetics will be altered dramatically in this setup. The enzymes are still bound to the beads, so they will not be able to diffuse through the solution and hence the reaction will follow essentially second-order kinetics. Second, the beads are dense and will drop to the bottom of your tube quite quickly. This may mean you will need to rock closed tubes during the reaction period. Alternatively and more easily, you can occasionally resuspend the beads by flipping the bottom of all the tubes during the reaction period.

To stop the reaction, several approaches can be used. The correct choice depends on the next step. If you will be detecting the transfer of a radioactive moiety to a protein substrate, such as the transfer of the [$^{32}$P]gamma phosphate of ATP to a protein in a protein kinase reaction, you can stop the reaction by the addition of Laemmli sample buffer. In other cases, heating the reactions will kill enzymatic activity. Other choices might include adding EDTA to chelate divalent cations (EGTA for $Ca^{++}$) or freezing the samples.

One other advantage of this approach that is not often used, but investigators should keep in mind, is that the enzymes in this setting are most often still bound to the beads. This is equivalent to a small-scale immunoaffinity purification. This will allow the simple separation of the enzyme from the substrates by centrifugation and removal of the supernatant.

## Clearing a lysate of an antigen

When immunoprecipitations are performed in conditions that lead to complete or near-complete removal of the antigen, they allow a rapid and effective method to clear an antigen and all molecules bound to it from a lysate. With the availability of the correct antibody, this allows an investigator to learn the effects of losing an antigen from a solution. Uses for this approach include removing an antigen and determining what proportion of an associated protein is bound to antigen versus what remains, and learning how the activities of a lysate, when depleted of an antigen, are changed.

This is a useful approach for analytical-scale projects. When large solutions are being studied, clearing is more easily done by using the methods described in Chapter 9.

### *Technical approaches to clearing a lysate of an antigen*

Preclearing a lysate of an antigen is normally done by performing the immunoprecipitation in antibody excess and often is accomplished by performing the immunoprecipitation several times in succession with the same lysate (Fig. 7.10).

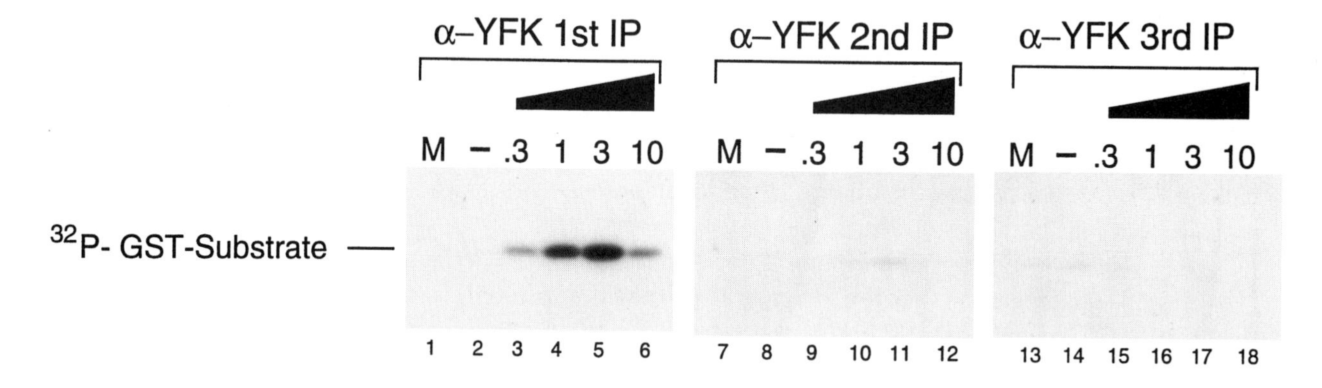


**Figure 7.10**
Preclearing lysate of antigen.

## References

Horvitz H.R. 1974. Control by bacteriophage T4 of two sequential phosphorylations of the alpha subunit of *Escherichia coli* RNA polymerase. *J. Mol. Biol.* **90:** 727–738.

Kessler S.W. 1975. Rapid isolation of antigens from cells with a staphylococcal protein A-antibody adsorbent: Parameters of the interaction of antibody-antigen complexes with protein A. *J. Immunol.* **115:** 1617–1623.

Kim E., Goldstein J. and Brown M. 1992. cDNA cloning of MEV, a mutant protein that facilitates cellular uptake of mevalonate, and identification of the point mutation responsible for its gain of function. *J. Biol. Chem.* **267:** 23113–23121.

Spector D.L., Goldman R., and Leinwand L. 1998. *Cells: A laboratory manual.* Cold Spring Harbor Laboratory Press, Cold Spring Harbor, New York.

Varki A. 1994. Metabolic radiolabeling of glycoconjugates. *Methods Enzymol.* **230:** 16–32.

# Immunoprecipitation


## Summary

Determines antigen presence, quantity, size, turnover, modifications, associations
Multiple steps over 1/2 to 1 day
Semi-quantitative to quantitative
Sensitivity dependent on relative quantity of antigen and affinity of antibody
Needs high affinity/avidity antibody


1. Add 50 μl of normal rabbit serum per 1.0 ml of antigen solution.

2. Incubate 1 hour on ice.

3. During this incubation, wash fixed *S. aureus* Cowan I (SAC) once in lysis buffer. Use 100 μl of packed SAC per 50 μl of normal rabbit serum. It is easiest to spin SAC briefly at 10,000*g* for 30 seconds and resuspend the pelleted SAC by triturating with a pasteur pipet. Spin again at 10,000*g* and remove the wash buffer. Set the packed pellet of washed SAC aside on ice.

4. After the 1-hour incubation, use the lysate to resuspend the washed pellet of SAC.

5. Incubate 30 minutes on ice.

6. Spin at 10,000*g* for 15 minutes at 4°C. Carefully remove and save the supernatant.

7. Divide the supernatant and aliquot into the appropriate number of 1.5-ml conical tubes. To individual tubes, add the immune or control serum (1 μl), hybridoma tissue-culture supernatant (50 μl), or ascites fluid (1 μl). Other volumes will be appropriate in specific settings as determined by titration of antibody volume versus a constant antigen amount.

8. Incubate on ice for 1 hour.

9. To the antibody–antigen reaction, add protein A or protein G beads depending on the type of antibody used (see Table, below). Add 100 ml of a 10% vol/vol slurry made in lysis buffer (final bead volume will be 10 ml). Close the caps securely. Incubate 1 hour at 4°C with rocking.

10. Collect the beads by centrifugation at 10,000*g* for 15 seconds at 4°C. Wash the immune complexes three times with lysis buffer. The lysate and wash buffers are easily removed by aspiration through a 23-gauge needle.

11. Remove the final wash as completely as possible.

12. Use the immune complexes for the appropriate assay, often SDS-polyacrylamide electrophoresis.

| Antibody source | Protein A | Protein G |
|---|---|---|
| Monoclonal antibodies | | |
| mouse $IgG_1$ | | √ |
| Mouse $IgG_{2a}$, $IgG_{2b}$, $IgG_3$ | √ | |
| rat | | √ |
| Polyclonal antibodies | | |
| human | √ | |
| rabbit | √ | |
| mouse | | √ |
| rat | | √ |
| horse | √ | |
| goat | | √ |
| donkey | √ | |
| pig | √ | |
| guinea pig | √ | |
| dog | √ | |
| cow | √ | |

# Immunoblotting

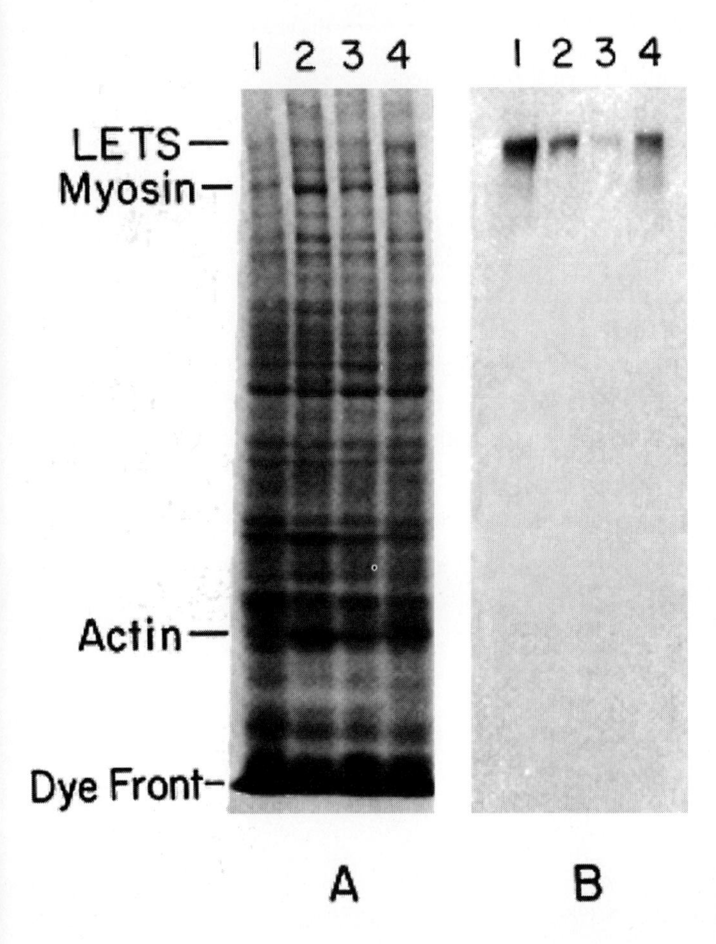


From Burridge K. 1976. Changes in cellular glycoproteins after transformation: Identification of specific glycoproteins and antigen in sodium dodecyl sulfate gels. *Proc. Natl. Acad. Sci.* 73: 4457–4461. (Reprinted with permission).

Fig. 6. Identification of the LETS protein gel band by direct "staining" of a $NaDodSO_4$ gel with antibody against the LETS protein. A 7.5% $NaDodSO_4$ slab gel was used to fractionate parallel samples of whole cells: Py3T3 *(1)*, 3T3 *(2)*, SV3T3 *(3)*, Sv101 *(4)*.... For economy of antiserum, small gel slots were used (3 mm compared with 6 mm) and 25 μg of protein was put in each one. Parallel slices were stained for protein (A) or with antibody against LETS protein (B), followed by the second iodinated antibody as described in the *text.*

Immunoblots are a relatively recent technical development. This figure from Burridge's 1976 paper is the first example of combining the resolving power and ease of use provided by SDS-polyacrylamide slab gels with antigen localization after the gel. In this approach, the antigens were detected directly in the gel by soaking the gel with labeled antibody and then washing out unbound antibody. Later methods captured the antigens by covalently binding them onto modified paper as they diffused from the gel. This approach gave an image of the separated proteins on a convenient paper surface. Then noncovalent binding to nitrocellulose filter paper was used and the proteins were collected not by diffusion but by electoelution. The recent application of chemiluminescense to the detection step greatly extended the sensitivity and has made immunoblotting one of the most widely used immunochemical techniques.

Immunoblotting provides a reliable method to check any sample for the presence of a protein antigen. The assay identifies the protein on the basis of both its interaction with a specific antibody and its relative molecular weight. Immunoblotting can be used to determine other characteristics of your antigen, such as the relative abundance of the antigen or association with other well-characterized antigens. It also is a useful method to characterize new antibody preparations. Immunoblotting involves multiple simple steps that take about a day to complete. The method is robust, relatively simple, and quite sensitive.

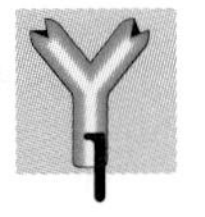
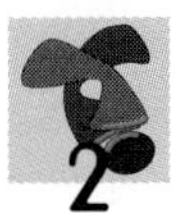
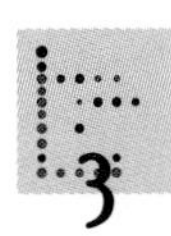
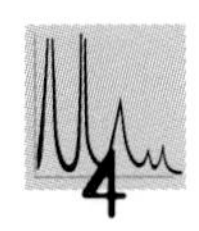
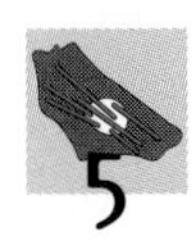
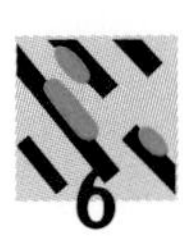
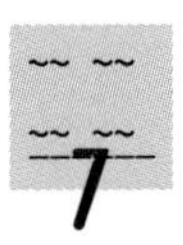
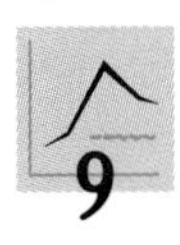
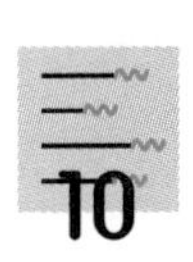
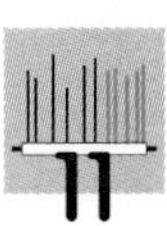



# 8 Immunoblotting

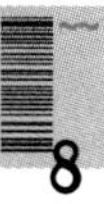



Immunoblotting combines the resolution of gel electrophoresis with the specificity of immunochemical detection. The strategy behind the immunoblotting technique is to separate protein antigens by gel electrophoresis and then transfer the proteins out of the gel onto a membrane support, thus making a replica of the separated proteins. The location of the antigen is then determined by using specific antibodies.

Immunoblotting can be used to determine a number of important characteristics of protein antigens. Essentially any experimental question that requires one to know the presence and quantity of an antigen or the relative molecular weight of the polypeptide chain can be answered by immunoblotting. Immunoblotting is particularly useful when dealing with antigens that are insoluble in detergent lysates, difficult to label, or easily degraded, and thus less amenable to analysis by immunoprecipitation. When immunoblotting is combined with immunoprecipitation, it can be used to allow very sensitive detection of minor antigens and to study specific interactions between antigens. Immunoblotting also can be used to determine whether tyrosine phosphorylation has occurred on a protein and can determine how well an antigen is extracted. It is a particularly powerful technique for assaying the presence, quantity, and specificity of antibodies from different samples. In addition, it can be used to purify small samples of specific antibodies from polyclonal sera. Because the antigen is not labeled, only the steady-state level can be determined, and detailed analyses of a protein's biochemical properties, modifications, or half-life are not possible except where specialized antibodies are available. These are properties that are more amenable to study using immunoprecipitations (see Chapter 7).

## Major constraints

The major factor that determines the success of an immunoblotting procedure is the nature of the epitopes recognized by the antibodies. Most high-resolution gel electrophoresis techniques involve denaturation of the antigen sample, so only antibodies that recognize denaturation-resistant epitopes will bind. Most polyclonal sera contain at least some antibodies of this type, and so are likely to work in immunoblotting procedures. However, many monoclonal antibodies do not react with denatured antigens, because they recognize epitopes dependent on the correct three-dimensional folding of the protein.

The second major factor that affects the difficulty of immunoblotting is the abundance of the antigen in the starting protein solution. Average molecular weight proteins (about 50 kD, for example) will need to be present at about 1 in $10^6$ to be detected without difficulty. With current technology, proteins levels down to 0.1 ng can be detected. Rarer proteins need to be partially purified prior to gel electrophoresis, and we recommend immunoprecipitation as an easy method to prepare samples and extend the range of immunoblotting. Both the calculations of detection limits and the use of immunoprecipitations with immunoblots are discussed below.

Immunoblotting does not require particularly high-affinity antibodies. For example, some antibodies that bind poorly to antigens in solution are satisfactory for use in immunoblotting. This is due to the high local concentration of antigens on the membrane. The high local concentration provides a better chance for the antibody to bind through both Fab arms, thus greatly raising the avidity of the interaction (see Chapter 2 for a more detailed discussion). The antigen density also favors the retention of low-affinity antibodies on the membrane by increasing the frequency with which antibodies leaving the membrane rebind to adjacent sites.

## Choosing the correct antibody

The two major worries in choosing the correct antibody are whether the antibodies will recognize the denatured proteins on the membrane after the gel electrophoresis and transfer processes and whether there are cross-reacting bands (Table 8.1).

### Recognition of denatured proteins

*If all of the available antibodies recognize only native epitopes, you should consider raising the antibodies with the appropriate characteristics by immunizing animals with samples of denatured protein.*

The most important property that an antibody must have to work successfully in an immunoblot is the ability to recognize denaturation-resistant epitopes. The epitopes that are displayed on the membrane will almost exclusively be those that are formed by linear stretches of amino acids or amino acid modifications. These are the types of epitopes that remain intact following gel electrophoresis and transfer to the membrane support. The simplest method to check a set of antibodies for this property is to do a simple test run of the immunoblotting procedure using a protein source that is known to contain your antigen.

### Extra bands

Another potential problem to be considered in choosing the correct antibody preparation for immunoblotting is the presence of antibodies binding to other proteins on the blot. The best antibodies for immunoblotting recognize only the antigen under study, but this is not always the case. Extra bands on the blots arise from two sources. They may be background bands caused by spurious antibodies in your preparation or they may be cross-reactions to polypeptides that have epitopes which are structurally related to your antigen.

Whole sera contain a wide range of antibodies that comprise the entire repertoire of antibody response present in the animal at the time of serum harvest. This may include any autoantibodies against cellular components and antibodies against microorganisms that have infected the host animal, either at the time of collection or at any recent time, that have left circulating antibodies, or other antigens that are contaminating your immunizing preparation. These antibodies bind to the cognate, or any closely related, antigens on your blot, generating additional bands and potentially obscuring the bands of interest. Because this type of contamination is specific, it is unlikely to be removed by methods that are designed to lower nonspecific backgrounds (e.g., more extensive blocking of the membrane or more vigorous washing).

Table 8.1 *Antibody choice*

| | Polyclonal antibodies | Monoclonal antibodies | Pooled monoclonal antibodies |
|---|---|---|---|
| Signal strength | Usually good | Antibody dependent (zero to excellent) | Excellent |
| Specificity | Good, but some background | Excellent, but some cross-reactions | Excellent |
| Good features | Most recognize denatured antigen | Specificity<br>Unlimited supply | Signal strength<br>Specificity<br>Unlimited supply |
| Bad features | Nonrenewable<br>Background<br>Need to titer | Many do not recognize denatured antigen | Availability |

The second type of unexpected or additional bands arise from cross-reactions. Because an epitope is a relatively small protein structure that can be composed of only four or five amino acids, there is a chance that a similar epitope can be found on another polypeptide. In some cases, the common epitopes form part of an important structural similarity between antigens, and in these cases, monoclonal antibodies can be used to detect related antigens. Alternatively, the antibodies may detect small structural similarities confined only to the antibody combining site. Here the cross-reaction is less interesting, but problematic because it does not allow the precise identification and characterization of your desired antigen. Because these bands arise from the same antibodies that will be important in recognizing your antigen, they cannot be removed by any mechanism that will interfere with the antibody–antigen interaction.

If you have an independent method to confirm the identity of your antigen and if any other band is in a region of the gel that does not interfere with the interpretation of the work, it may not be necessary to worry about other bands. However, in most cases, extra bands pose serious problems in interpretation. The multiple bands on a blot can be characterized by several methods:

### *Negative control antibodies*

Comparing the pattern of bands seen with a carefully matched set of antibodies will allow you to determine whether the additional bands are due to a common spurious antibody in the serum or in the detection reagent. For polyclonal sera, the best control serum is a sample taken from the same animal prior to immunization. Less desired but still acceptable is a serum from the same species. For monoclonal antibodies, the correct control is another antibody from the same isotype as your antibody.

### *Antigen blocking*

If you add saturating amounts of a preparation of your antigen (for example, purified from bacterial or baculoviral overexpression) to your antibody prior to adding to the

*A band can be confirmed as your antigen by several methods. A required first step is to show that your band has the correct size as your antigen. A purified preparation or well-characterized sample that gives an easily identified band is a good first characterization. A second step is to show that the band under study and your control preparation are both recognized by your antibody. Size and immune recognition provide a strong, although still not definitive, argument for identification. This should be followed by at least one other method to confirm the identity of your antigen. These methods might include: (1) use of multiple antibodies recognizing different epitopes or regions of the antigen; (2) if looking at an exogenously produced antigen, use of a tagged version that can be located with an independent antibody; (3) if looking at an exogenously produced antigen, use of truncated (either amino-terminal or carboxy-terminal) versions that can show a change in electrophoretic mobility of the antigen; or (4) comparison of partial proteolysis products.*

blot for developing, you will be able to see which bands arise from the specific antibodies. This will indicate either that these bands are your antigen or that they share an epitope with your antigen.

### Nonspecific blocking

In these cases, the easiest solution to removing these spurious activities is to block the specific antibodies by preincubating the serum with a preparation that contains the contaminating protein (e.g., an acetone powder from a cell that does not express the antigen being studied, p. 437).

### Change antibodies

If the extra bands on the blot make interpreting your results confusing, the easy solution is to use another preparation of antibodies.

### Use multiple antibodies

If there are confusing bands on your blot, it may be possible to identify the correct band by using more than one antibody specific for your antigen. For example, if you have two antibodies that are raised to independent epitopes or regions of your antigen and they both recognize the same band, this forms a strong argument to concentrate your characterization studies on this band.

### Immunoprecipitate first

Since extra bands arise from the mixture of proteins loaded on the gel, it may be possible to simplify your pattern of bands by purifying the antigen prior to running the gel. This can be done by many methods, but one of the most convenient is to immunoprecipitate the antigen prior to running the gel. This eliminates the nonspecific background bands. It does require, however, that you have a good antibody available for immunoprecipitation, and it is best if this is a different antibody from your detection reagent and preferably an antibody that recognizes different epitopes than your immunoblotting antibody recognizes.

### Titrate

Often spurious bands on a blot can be lessened by using your antibody at much lower concentrations. More often than not, the immune antibodies are the highest concentrations in serum, and thus titrating can lower the levels of the contaminating antibodies to levels that will not interfere with your analysis.

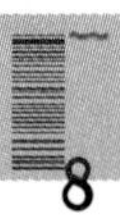



## Immunoblotting with polyclonal or monoclonal antibodies

Immunoblots can be done with either polyclonal or monoclonal antibodies. Both have specific advantages and disadvantages. Although not as frequently used, pools of well-chosen monoclonal antibodies have the advantages provided by monoclonal and polyclonal antibodies with few of their disadvantages. Whenever possible, we recommend the use of pooled monoclonal antibodies for immunoblotting.

### *Immunoblots using polyclonal antibodies*

Polyclonal antibodies probably are the most widely used type of antibody preparation for immunoblotting. Most sera contain antibodies that will bind to a number of denaturation-resistant epitopes on the antigen. This results in multiple antibody molecules binding to a given polypeptide and generates a relatively stronger signal than a monoclonal antibody. Because polyclonal sera most normally contain high concentrations of specific antibodies, they can often be diluted extensively. Therefore, dilution can be used to reduce nonspecific background problems without reducing sensitivity.

Because polyclonal antibodies normally are used as whole sera, they also contain the entire repertoire of circulating antibodies found in the immunized animal at the time the serum was collected. Therefore, the serum may contain high-titered antibodies that specifically recognize spurious antigens. Strategies to minimize the problems of spurious antibodies that bind to proteins other than your antigen are discussed above (p. 271).

### *Immunoblots using monoclonal antibodies*

The major advantage of using monoclonal antibodies for immunoblotting is the specificity of their interactions. Because monoclonal antibodies bind to only one epitope, they provide an elegant tool for identifying a particular region of the antigen. Monoclonal antibodies that function well in immunoblotting usually interact with epitopes that are defined by short stretches of the protein's primary sequence. As such, they can be used to examine the presence and origin of quite small regions of the antigen, and this can be useful in studies of polypeptide processing or in mapping other processes that rely on small protein domains.

The principal difficulty in using monoclonal antibodies in immunoblotting is that many do not recognize epitopes that are destroyed by the denaturing reagents used in the preparation of the sample. However, some monoclonal antibodies work well and can give extremely clean and sensitive results.

A second problem with using monoclonal antibodies in immunoblotting is the possibility of detecting cross-reactions with other polypeptides. Depending on the set of hybridomas, as many as one in three monoclonal antibodies will display these types of cross-reactions. Unless there are other reasons to suggest that extensive and physiologically significant similarities accompany a cross-reaction (such as multiple sites in common), an unexpected band on an immunoblot should be treated as a spurious cross-reaction until proven otherwise.

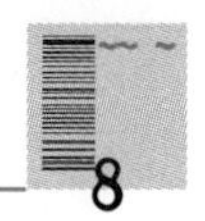


### *Immunoblots using pooled monoclonal antibodies*

Using pools of monoclonal antibodies in immunoblotting takes advantage of the best properties of both polyclonal and individual monoclonal antibodies, combining specificity and sensitivity. Obviously, the pool must be composed of monoclonal antibodies that react with distinct denaturation-resistant epitopes and that do not show spurious cross-reactions. An increasing number of antigens have been studied in enough detail to have such sets of antibodies available, and, whenever possible, a well-chosen pool of monoclonal antibodies should be used for immunoblotting.

## Detection limits

For chemiluminescent detection systems and most antibody preparations, the detection will be relatively routine down to levels that approach 2 femtomoles. For a 50,000-kD protein, this is approximately 0.1 ng, and levels higher than this will be relatively easy to detect. For standard SDS-polyacrylamide gels, the capacity of a lane is approximately 150 μg (or 15 μg for a minigel) (see p. 283). Distortion is seen if larger amounts are used. Therefore, an average protein antigen of 50 kD must be present at 0.1 ng/150 μg of sample (or 1 part in 1,500,000). When analyzing total proteins from mammalian cells, this limit represents approximately 1,000 molecules of a 50,000-kD protein per mammalian cell. To detect proteins present at lower levels, partial purification of the antigen is required. This may be done conveniently by cell fractionation, chromatography, or immunoprecipitation.

Unless the molecular weight of your antigen is similar to that of an abundant protein in the cell, for example actin, the capacity of the transfer membrane will not be limiting.

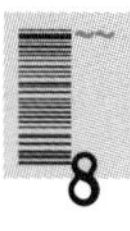



# Immunoblotting protocols

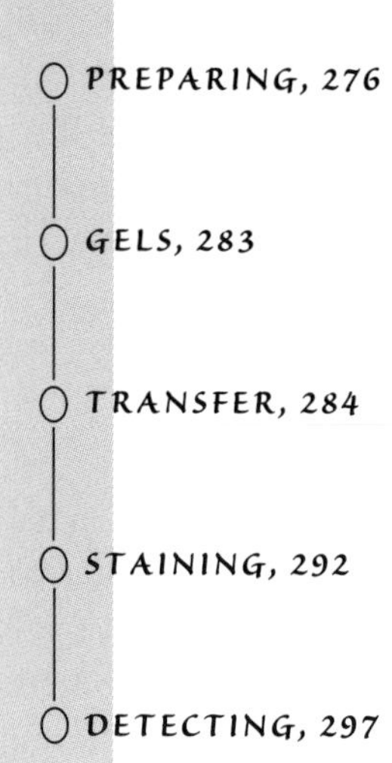


The immunoblotting method has evolved from early stages where antibodies were used to "stain" proteins directly within polyacrylamide gels (Burridge 1976; Showe et al. 1976) to more versatile approaches using replica techniques, where the separated polypeptides are transferred to nitrocellulose membranes, chemically activated paper, or nylon sheets (for review, see Gershoni and Palade 1983; Towbin and Gordon 1984; Beisiegel 1986). Although there are a number of variations on this basic theme, the most common and easiest method involves electrophoretic transfer to nitrocellulose sheets (Towbin et al. 1979; Burnette 1981), and this is the method we recommend for most applications.

## Overview of the basic immunoblotting procedure

The immunoblotting procedure can be divided into five steps:

1. Preparation of the antigen sample
2. Resolution of the sample by gel electrophoresis
3. Transfer of the separated polypeptides to a membrane support
4. Staining the blot for total protein (optional)
5. Antigen detection

A solution of proteins, often an extract of cells or tissues, is prepared in a gel electrophoresis sample buffer. The proteins are separated by gel electrophoresis, and the resolved proteins are transferred to a membrane that binds all proteins nonspecifically. Transfer usually is achieved by placing the membrane in direct contact with the gel and then placing this sandwich in an electric field to drive the proteins from the gel onto the membrane. In some cases, the blot can now be stained to detect the position of transferred proteins. Then remaining binding sites on the membrane are blocked to eliminate any further reaction with the membrane. Finally, the location of specific antigens is determined, usually using an unlabeled primary antibody followed by a labeled secondary antibody.

## Sample preparation

Almost any protein sample can be used as a source for immunoblotting. The protein sample is mixed with standard sample buffer, separated by gel electrophoresis, and then processed for the immunoblot. Samples that are commonly used include purified or partially purified preparations, crude cell lysates, or immunoprecipitated samples.

One of the strengths of the immunoblotting technique is that it permits the analysis of proteins from sources that cannot be studied using other immunochemical techniques. For example, samples that cannot be labeled or are insoluble in gentle extraction buffers often can be analyzed by immunoblotting. This includes crude samples from tissues, organs, or whole organisms.

Three variations of the most commonly used sample sources—protein solutions, cell lysates, and immunoprecipitated protein—are discussed below; however, any sources of protein could be adapted to this approach.

# Preparing protein solutions for immunoblotting

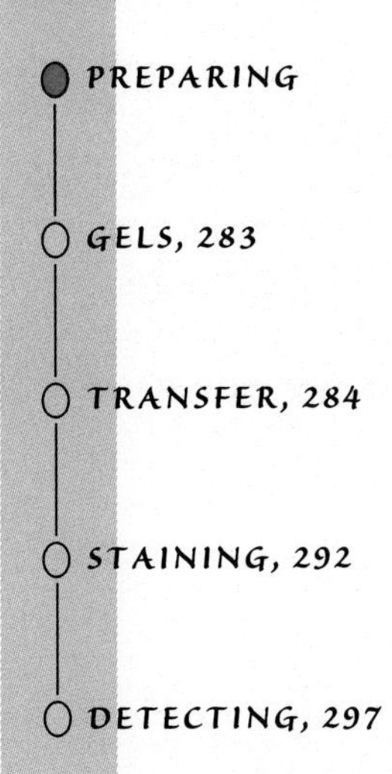


*Be sure to consider how to normalize protein samples if multiple samples will be compared. For example, if you are comparing antigen levels in different cells, then standardize to cell number or total protein level. If you are examining various preparations of purified proteins, it would normally be convenient to normalize for total protein content. However, for column fractions you may need to compare to the total volume of each fraction. The total amount of protein in the sample can be determined by many of the commonly used protein concentration methods. Protein quantitation will be easier without the addition of bromophenol blue. This can be left out of the sample buffer with no detrimental effects.*

Most protein solutions can be mixed with sample buffer and analyzed directly using immunoblots. The approach described here can be used on detergent lysates of cells, samples from column eluates, and most other sources of antigens.

To analyze a protein sample directly, two criteria must be met: (1) The protein sample must be in a solution that is compatible with the gel electrophoresis system. For Tris/glycine SDS-polyacrylamide gels, the pH of the protein solution should be approximately neutral, salt concentrations should be below approximately 200 mM unless a large dilution into the sample buffer will be used, but most other buffer components will not affect the running of the gel. Standard methods for exchanging buffers are appropriate. Normally this can be accomplished easily by dialysis or a small gel filtration column used as a desalting column. (2) The concentration of proteins in the sample must not exceed the loading capacity for the particular gel system. Representative values for both of these variables are given in the gel electrophoresis discussion below (p. 283), but a good rule of thumb is to not run more than 150 μg of total protein per lane (or 5 μg per lane for a minigel).

## Controls

Two sets of controls should be included in an immunoblot that starts from protein solutions. These controls should include both a positive sample that is known to contain your antigen and test samples that can be developed with a negative control antibody. The positive control could be any source that contains a known or standard amount of your antigen. This might be from a bacterial or baculovirus overexpression system or might come from a well-characterized cell line. It will provide a test to show that the immunoblot has worked successfully, it will give a precise comparison of relative molecular weight of the antigen, and, if the amount of the antigen in the positive control is known, it will provide a rough estimate of the amount of antigen in the test solution. Samples that are developed with a nonimmune antibody will give you some reading of the background in your sample.

### Thinking ahead

Prepare a water bath at 70°C.

### Needed solutions

Laemmli sample buffer without DTT (2% SDS, 10% glycerol, 60 mM Tris, pH 6.8, and 0.01% bromophenol blue)
1 M DTT (stored at –20°C)

*The samples can be used immediately or frozen. At –20°C samples are stable for months.*

## Cautions

DTT, SDS, see Appendix IV.

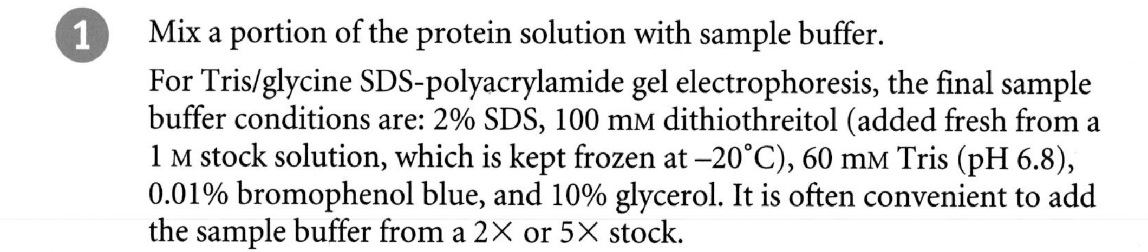

1. Mix a portion of the protein solution with sample buffer.

   For Tris/glycine SDS-polyacrylamide gel electrophoresis, the final sample buffer conditions are: 2% SDS, 100 mM dithiothreitol (added fresh from a 1 M stock solution, which is kept frozen at –20°C), 60 mM Tris (pH 6.8), 0.01% bromophenol blue, and 10% glycerol. It is often convenient to add the sample buffer from a 2× or 5× stock.

2. Heat the sample to at least 70°C for 5 minutes.

**The samples are now ready for electrophoresis (p. 283).**

# Preparing cell lysates for immunoblotting



*When comparing the levels of antigens from multiple samples of cells, be certain to consider how they will be normalized. For example, will the comparison make most sense when corrected for the total amount of protein in the sample or when corrected for cell number? Protein concentration can be done by many of the commonly used protein quantitation methods. Protein quantitation is often easier without the addition of bromophenol blue, which can be left out of the sample buffer with no detrimental effects.*

It is often important to compare the total amount of an antigen from many different sources or to learn if a particular source has the antigen under study. In this procedure, cells, tissues, or other sources are disrupted directly in an electrophoresis sample buffer. After the chromosomal DNA is sheared to lower viscosity, the samples are processed and run as usual for the particular gel system. In the example given here, the samples are prepared for electrophoresis in a standard Tris/glycine SDS-polyacrylamide gel.

Some samples need to be treated to shear the chromosomal DNA to reduce viscosity. This can be done most conveniently with a sonicator; either an immersible tip or cuphorn is suitable.

## Controls

Two sets of controls should be included in an immunoblot that starts from cell lysates. These controls should include both a positive sample that is known to contain your antigen and test cell lysates that can be developed with a negative control antibody. The positive control could be any source that contains a known or standard amount of your antigen. This might be from a bacterial or baculovirus overexpression system or might come from a well-characterized cell line. It will provide a test to show that the immunoblot has worked successfully, it will give a precise comparison of relative molecular weight of the antigen, and, if the amount of the antigen in the positive control is known, it will provide a rough estimate of the amount of antigen in the test solution.

Cell lysates that are developed with a nonimmune antibody will give you some reading of the background in your sample. If available, a useful third control to include would be a cell lysate that does not contain your antigen, for example from a genetic null.

### Thinking ahead

Prepare a water bath at 70°C.

### Needed solutions

Laemmli sample buffer without DTT (20% SDS, 10% glycerol, 60 mM Tris, pH 6.8, and 0.1% bromophenol blue)
1 M DTT (stored at –20°C)

### Special equipment

Sonicator, if using yeast or bacteria

## Cautions

DTT, SDS, see Appendix IV.

*The samples can be used immediately or frozen. At –20°C samples are stable for months.*

1. Measure the volume of sample to be lysed. For tissue-culture cells, $10^9$ cells ≈1 ml ≈1 gram.

   For tissues or organs, weighing the sample will be sufficient, 1 gram ≈1 ml. For bacterial or yeast cells, spin the samples and estimate the volume just by comparison with known volumes in similarly sized tubes.

2. Add 10 volumes of sample buffer. Mix vigorously.

   For Tris/glycine SDS-polyacrylamide gel electrophoresis, the 1× sample buffer is: 2% SDS, 100 mM dithiothreitol (added fresh from a 1 M stock solution, which is kept frozen at –20°C), 60 mM Tris (pH 6.8), 0.01% bromophenol blue, and 10% glycerol.

3. For yeast or bacteria, lyse the cells by sonication. Resuspend the cells in sample buffer and sonicate at full intensity for four bursts of 15–30 seconds each. Between each sonication step, transfer the samples to ice for 15 seconds.

4. Heat the sample to at least 70°C for 5 minutes.

5. Centrifuge at 10,000*g* for 10 minutes to remove the supernatant. Remove the supernatant to a fresh tube.

**The samples are now ready for electrophoresis (p. 283).**

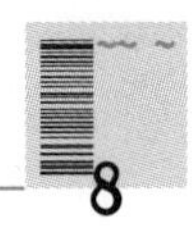


# Using immunoprecipitated proteins for immunoblotting

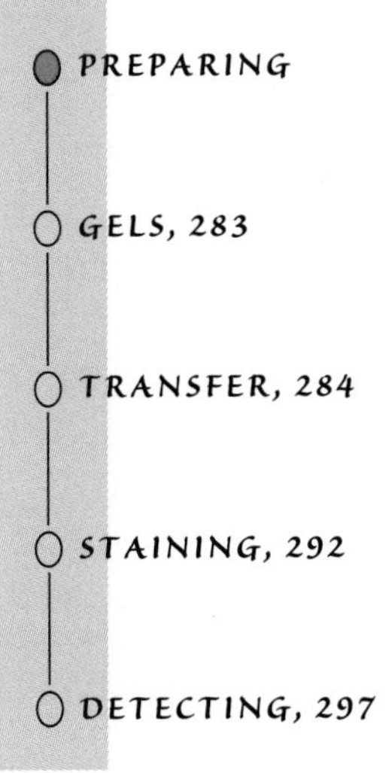


In most cases, crude samples may be run directly on a gel without further purification. However, there are two situations where immunoprecipitated proteins can be a useful preparative step prior to immunoblotting. The first is to examine very rare proteins. Because the total amount of protein that can be resolved adequately on a gel is limited, it is often impossible to load sufficient levels of proteins to detect very rare antigens. In these cases, the protein of interest can be purified and concentrated by standard immunoprecipitation techniques. In this way, immunoprecipitation with an antibody with the same specificity as the immunoblotting antibody greatly extends the range of detection of the immunoblotting technique. A second use of this approach is to check for protein–protein interactions. Here the immunoprecipitating antibody will be specific for one protein of a complex and the immunoblotting antibody will be specific for a second member of the complex. This approach is only useful when the complex is sufficiently well characterized to know which antibodies to use, but it does provide a useful method to study protein–protein interactions.

## Controls

Controls for an immunoblot that starts from immunoprecipitated proteins should include samples precipitated with the immune antibodies under study and nonimmune antibody. This comparison will identifiy bands specifically recognized by the immune antibody and will identify any background bands (for example, from the heavy chain) that show up in a nonspecific manner. In addition, you should include a positive sample that is known to contain your antigen. This positive control could be from any source that contains a known or standard amount of your antigen. This might be from a bacterial or baculovirus overexpression system or might come from a well-characterized cell line. This sample need not be immunoprecipitated but should be run on an adjacent lane. It will provide a test to show that the immunoblot has worked successfully, it will give a precise comparison of relative molecular weight of the antigen, and, if the amount of the antigen in the positive control is known, it will provide a rough estimate of the amount of antigen in the test solution.

### Thinking ahead

Prepare a water bath at 70°C.

### Needed solutions

Laemmli sample buffer without DTT (2% SDS, 10% glycerol, 60 mM Tris, pH 6.8, and 0.01% bromophenol blue)
1 M DTT (stored at –20°C)

## Cautions

DTT, SDS, see Appendix IV.

1. Add sample buffer to the washed protein A or G beads with the bound antibodies and antigens. Use sufficient sample buffer to make at least a 2-to-1 ratio of sample buffer to bead volume. Ratios of about 5 to 1 are better, but there is seldom any need to exceed 10 to 1.

   For Tris/glycine SDS-polyacrylamide gel electrophoresis, the final sample buffer conditions are: 2% SDS, 100 mM dithiothreitol (added fresh from a 1 M stock solution, which is kept frozen at –20°C), 60 mM Tris (pH 6.8), 0.01% bromophenol blue, and 10% glycerol.

*The samples can be used immediately or frozen. At –20°C, samples are stable for months.*

2. Heat the sample to at least 70°C for 5 minutes. Except in unusual situations, it is not necessary to remove the beads prior to loading the gel.

**The samples are now ready for electrophoresis (p. 283).**

## Common problems

One problem to keep in mind when immunoprecipitated proteins are used for immunoblots is that the antibodies from the immunoprecipitation will appear on the blot. Depending on the source of the antibody, they may be detected by the secondary reagent. Often the sizes of the heavy and light chains of the antibodies do not cause any problem of identification of the antigen. However, if the antigen under study is around 50 or 25 kD (the approximate size of heavy- and light-chain polypeptides), there are two solutions. In the first, the immunoprecipitating antibodies can be covalently coupled to the protein A or protein G beads (p. 321). Alternatively, the detection can be done using a direct detection technique.

# Gel electrophoresis

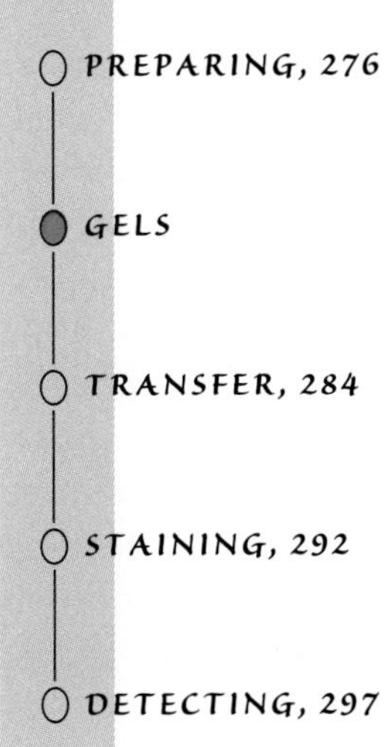


Although Tris/glycine SDS-polyacrylamide gels (p. 403) are the most common method for separating proteins for immunoblotting, any gel separation technique can be used. Other techniques for high-resolution separation of proteins that have been used successfully for immunoblotting include isoelectric focusing, isoelectric focusing followed by SDS-polyacrylamide gels, SDS-polyacrylamide gels using buffers other than Tris/glycine, urea-polyacrylamide gels, and native low-salt polyacrylamide gels. Nonetheless, by far the most widely used system is the standard Tris/glycine discontinuous gel system.

Two decisions concerning the conditions for electrophoresis need to be made prior to immunoblotting: first, the total amount of protein that can be loaded on a gel without distortion and, second, the physical dimensions and acrylamide concentration of the separating gel. If an extract from whole cells will be used, the total amount of protein should not exceed approximately 30 $\mu g/mm^2$ of loading surface (about 150 μg for a 5-mm × 1-mm slot or 15 μg for a 2-mm × 0.025-mm slot). For individual bands, loading more than 0.3 $\mu g/mm^2$ will lead to distortion (or 1.5 μg/5-mm × 1-mm slot); however, because immunoblots are so sensitive, this upper limit for individual proteins will seldom be used.

Since all blotting techniques require a successful transfer of proteins from the gel, some consideration as to the kind of gel to be used is helpful. Crudely, the lower the percentage of the acrylamide and cross-linker, the easier the transfer will be. Therefore, running the softest gel that yields the desired resolution is best. For efficient transfer of high-molecular-weight proteins, the concentration of the acrylamide should be lowered to a level where the protein of interest migrates at least one-third of the distance from the top of the separating gel to the bottom within the time it takes the dye front to reach the bottom. In general, proteins that run slower than this are difficult to elute.

Transfer is faster and more complete from thinner gels, although ultra-thin gels may cause handling problems. In most cases, a 0.4-mm thickness represents the lower practical limit for handling gels. Remember that during transfer, all the proteins in the width of a band become concentrated at the membrane surface, so running larger samples on thicker gels will increase sensitivity. Transfers from gels over 2 mm in width are inefficient, however.

*If needed, run prestained or radioactive markers on the gel to serve as internal markers for transfer and molecular-weight determinations.*

Given these variables, we recommend that you make the selection of the gel thickness and size based on the desired final results. If you are looking for maximum resolution of the proteins, longer gels are better than shorter ones. If needed, you can even run some of the markers off the bottom of the gel to let higher-molecular-weight proteins migrate further through the gel. If you are looking for maximum sensitivity, use gels up to 1.5 mm in thickness and load the maximum amount of protein per lane that does not give distortion. If speed is the most important variable, we recommend using mini-gels (about 3 inch × 1.5 inch and about 0.5 mm in thickness).

**After the gels are run, proteins are transferred by the methods on p. 284.**

# Transfer of proteins from gels to membranes

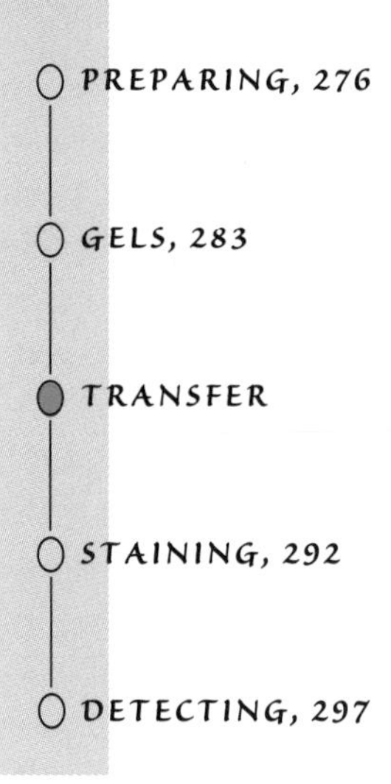


Transfer of proteins from the gel onto a membrane for detection of the antigens can be achieved in several ways. The earliest methods used simple diffusion (Renart et al. 1979; Bowen et al. 1980). Later, vacuum-assisted solvent flow (Peferoen et al. 1982) and electrophoretic elution (Towbin et al. 1979; Bittner et al. 1980; Reiser and Wardale 1981; Kyhse-Andersen 1984) were introduced. Electrophoretic elution or electroblotting has become the standard method. Its principal advantage lies in the speed and completeness of transfer. Electrophoretic elution can be achieved either by complete immersion of a gel-membrane sandwich in a buffer (wet transfer) or by placing the gel-membrane sandwich between absorbent paper soaked in transfer buffer (semi-dry transfer). For the wet transfer, the sandwich is placed in a buffer tank with platinum wire electrodes. For the semi-dry transfer, the gel-membrane sandwich is placed between plate electrodes. Apparatuses for both types of transfers are available commercially. Both work well, and different labs favor each method.

Nitrocellulose, activated paper, and activated nylon have all been used successfully to bind the transferred proteins (Renart et al. 1979; Towbin et al. 1979; Gershoni and Palade 1982). Nitrocellulose is the most commonly used, and it or more recently developed derivatives are highly recommended. However, nitrocellulose does have certain disadvantages. The proteins are not covalently bound, and nitrocellulose can be brittle, especially when dry. With appropriate care, however, it will fit most applications.

## Other membrane supports

Several other membrane supports can be used for immunoblotting. Nitrocellulose is the most commonly used and is the best choice for most settings. The other two membrane supports that are used in some settings are positively charged nylon and chemically activated paper. Of these, positively charged nylon is more commonly used.

Nylon itself can bind only a small amount of protein and is not suitable for most applications. However, it has excellent mechanical strength and does not change size during washing or drying. Positively charged nylon (PVDF; Immobilon) allows the binding of proteins to the membranes and can be used in a similar fashion to nitrocellulose. Because of the high number of protein-binding sites in the activated nylon, the backgrounds are normally considerably worse, but careful blocking will eliminate many of these problems. One of the most common uses of PVDF membranes is in the preparation of polypeptides for protein chemistry methods. Proteins bound to PVDF are common starting points for proteolysis and sequencing methods.

Another membrane that is used occasionally is diazotized paper. Activated paper can be purchased commercially and covalently binds proteins. It has good mechanical strength, but unfortunately, the coupling method is incompatible with many gel electrophoresis systems. The linkage is through primary amines,

so systems that use gel buffers without free amino groups must be used with this paper (for alternative electrophoresis buffers, see Jovin et al. 1970). Also, the paper is expensive and the reactive groups have a limited half-life once the paper is activated. Consult commercial suppliers' instructions for using this paper.

## Cutting blots after transfer

There are a number of reasons to cut the blot after transfer into smaller pieces for independent processing. Individual lanes can be run with identical samples and may be separated from each other to allow different antibodies to be used to probe samples run side by side. Membranes can be cut horizontally so that antigens of different sizes can be detected in the same samples. Occasionally there may be different types of markers in some specific lanes that need to be processed separately.

To find the lanes simply and accurately, you should include sufficient amounts of proteins (either they may be from your samples or you can add nonspecific proteins that you know will not interfere with your detection) and stain the blot with Ponceau S after running. This will identify the location of major proteins and allow you to easily cut one lane from another.

In some cases, you may wish to use higher-molecular-weight regions of the blot to probe for one antigen and use another region for a different molecular weight protein. To locate different regions of the blot that correspond to a particular range of molecular weights, you should include proteins of known molecular weight in marker lanes. Then you can orient the blot and cut out the appropriate region.

To find special lanes, you might try just spiking one lane with a known protein and then locating it by Ponceau S staining.

The advantage of Ponceau S staining is that it is simple, cheap, and reversible. During the blocking step, the staining disappears and will not interfere with any subsequent detection methods.

An alternative approach is to spike your samples with any of the prestained molecular-weight markers available commercially. Although these markers are more expensive than the Ponceau S approaches, they provide good guides for cutting the blot after transfer. For those with money to burn, there are even markers with different colors that brighten the look of your running gel and the transfer. The colors don't add anything but cost to your experiment, but they are pretty while they are running.

In some cases, it may be important just to cut side lanes and process them to determine the location of your antigen. Store the main portion of the wet blot in plastic wrap. After detection, reassemble the blot and use the stained side strips to cut the desired portion of the blot.

Finally, several companies offer an apparatus that allows multiple different antibodies to be compared on the same blot without cutting the blot into individual strips. This is done by clamping a Plexiglas template on both sides of the blot and providing narrow channels where antibody samples can be applied. This is an effective method to analyze up to 50 antibody samples simultaneously.

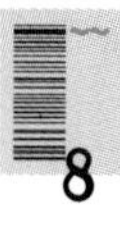



# Semi-dry electrophoretic transfer*

PREPARING, 276
GELS, 283
TRANSFER
STAINING, 292
DETECTING, 297

Transfer of proteins from a gel to nitrocellulose using a semi-dry method is achieved by placing the gel next to a piece of nitrocellulose filter and placing this sandwich directly between two plate electrodes. The plates can be made of graphite, which is relatively cheap but will need to be exchanged after approximately 100 uses, or platinum, which is much more expensive but will be good for the life of the blotter. The proteins then are eluted by electrophoresing them from the gel onto the filter, much in the same way that migration through the gel is achieved, but now perpendicular to the plane of the gel. This method gives even and rapid transfer and does not require a large power source. In the original description, different buffers were described for the anode and cathode, but a simple buffer system using diluted Tris/glycine SDS-polyacrylamide gel running buffer is much easier. Good contact between the electrodes, gel, and filter is maintained by using several sheets of prewetted glass fiber filter paper on both the cathode and anode sides.

## Needed solutions or reagents

Distilled or deionized water
Transfer buffer (0.04% SDS, 20% methanol in 48 mM Tris, 39 M glycine)
Absorbent paper (Whatman 3 MM or equivalent)
Nitrocellulose paper
Coomassie blue stain (p. 425–426)

## Special equipment

Semi-dry transfer apparatus (some manufacturers label these as dry transfer)

## Caution

SDS, methanol, see Appendix IV.

1. Rinse electrode plates of the semi-dry apparatus with distilled water.

2. Cut the gel to the desired size for transfer. This will normally involve removing the stacking gel and the lanes of the gel that have not been used. Mark the gel to establish orientation of the number one lane (normally clipping the bottom left-hand corner is sufficient). Put the gel in transfer buffer while preparing the filters (see step 5 for transfer buffer).

3. Cut six sheets of absorbent paper (Whatman 3 MM or equivalent) and one sheet of nitrocellulose to the size of the gel.

   Wear gloves and use virgin nitrocellulose sheets. The types of bonds that hold proteins to nitrocellulose are not known; however, the binding is blocked by oils or other proteins.

*Make sure the paper is cut to the correct size. If the paper overlaps the edge of the gel, the current will short-circuit the transfer and bypass the gel, preventing efficient transfer. An alternate approach is to make a Parafilm mask to serve as a collar around the gel and separate the plates.*

*Kyhse-Andersen (1984).

4. Soak the nitrocellulose membrane in distilled water. Nitrocellulose should always be wetted by carefully laying it on the surface of the water. Allow the nitrocellulose to wet by capillary action from the bottom (several minutes), and then submerge the sheet in the water for 2 minutes. Place the nitrocellulose in transfer buffer.

5. Wet the absorbent paper by soaking in transfer buffer. The transfer buffer is:

| | Concentration | for 1000 ml |
|---|---|---|
| Tris base | 48 mM | 5.8 g |
| Glycine | 39 mM | 2.9 g |
| SDS | 0.04% (vol/vol) | 0.37 g |
| Methanol | 20% | 200 ml |
| Distilled water | | Make up to 1000 ml |

6. Assemble the gel, nitrocellulose, and paper on the bottom plate of your apparatus. Check to see whether your bottom plate is cathode or anode (Fig. 8.1).

–bottom plate anode
–three layers absorbent paper soaked in transfer buffer
–one nitrocellulose membrane soaked in transfer buffer
–polyacrylamide gel slightly wetted in transfer buffer
–three layers absorbent paper soaked in transfer buffer
–cathode

or

–bottom plate cathode
–three layers absorbent paper soaked in transfer buffer
–polyacrylamide gel slightly wetted in transfer buffer
–one nitrocellulose membrane soaked in transfer buffer
–three layers absorbent paper soaked in transfer buffer
–anode

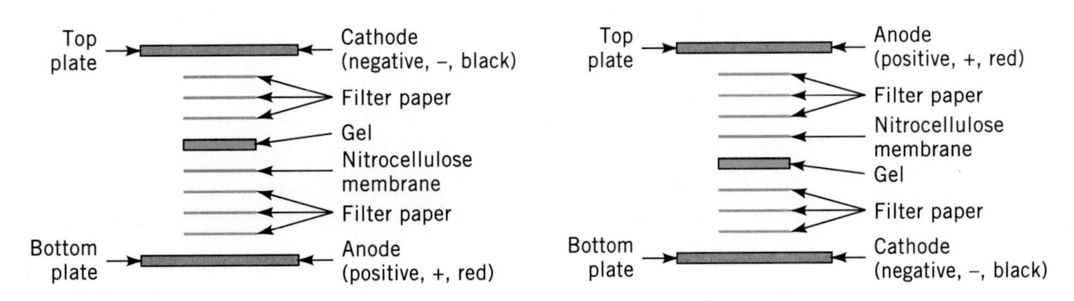


Figure 8.1
Two potential gel assemblies for bottom anode or cathode.

7. Check carefully for air bubbles and gently remove them either by using a gloved hand or by rolling a clean pipet over the sandwich. Dry any buffer that may surround the gel-paper sandwich. Many apparatuses have a gasket that surrounds the gel-paper sandwich to lessen the chance of allowing a short circuit of the transfer.

8. Carefully place the upper electrode on top of the stack. Connect the electrodes (positive or red lead to the anode) and commence transfer. Run for 45 minutes to 1.5 hours with a current of 0.8 $mA/cm^2$ of gel. Avoid extending the running time, because this can cause drying out.

9. Disconnect the power source after transfer. Carefully disassemble the apparatus. Mark the membrane to follow the orientation (usually by snipping off lower left-hand corner, the number one lane). Rinse the electrodes with distilled water after use.

10. The polyacrylamide gel can now be stained with Coomassie Blue (pp. 425–426) or silver stain (pp. 427–428) to verify transfer.

**Process the nitrocellulose sheet for staining (p. 292) or blocking (p. 296) as appropriate.**

## Common problems

To make transfer effective, a good electrical contact must be maintained between the electrodes and through the filter/gel/nitrocellulose/filter sandwich. The electrical current must be even over the entire surface of the electrodes. This means the electrodes must be kept clean and free of any nonconductive substance. In addition, any direct connection between the two electrodes, such as a misplaced glass fiber filter, will provide a low resistance path for the current and will short-circuit and effectively block the transfer. Any bubbles in the filters/gel/nitrocellulose/filter sandwich will block transfer at that site.

The other common problem is the difficulty of transfer of large-molecular-weight proteins. This is an inherent problem with transfer. If the protein runs slowly through the separating gel, it follows that the transfer out of the gel will also be slow. If this is a problem, we recommend lowering the concentration of the separating gel. If more than one polypeptide of different sizes need to be studied and the same gel concentration will not work for both, try running two separate gels with different acrylamide concentrations.

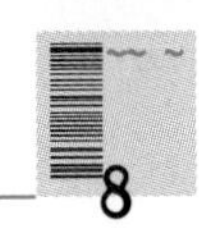

# Submerged electrophoretic transfer*

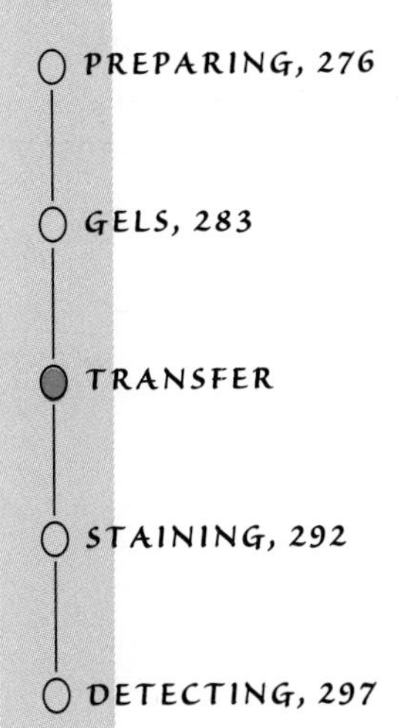


Transfer of proteins from a gel to nitrocellulose using the submerged method is achieved by placing the gel next to a piece of nitrocellulose filter, submerging this sandwich in a large volume of transfer buffer in a transfer tank, and running current from one side of the transfer tank to another. The proteins then are eluted by electrophoresing them from the gel onto the filter, much in the same way that migration through the gel is achieved, but now perpendicular to the plane of the gel. If carefully assembled, this is an effective method to transfer many proteins to a membrane. It demands a slightly longer time to set up than the semi-dry transfer and uses more buffer, but it is less finicky.

For submerged transfers, no one set of transfer conditions offers complete and even transfer of proteins with good retention on the membrane. We recommend the use of one of two buffers based on the size of the protein to transfer. Different transfer times will need to be determined by empirical examination. The times below should be used as a starting guide for transfer.

## Needed solutions and reagents

Nitrocellulose paper
Absorbent filter paper (Whatman 3 MM or equivalent)
Distilled water
Transfer buffer 1 (proteins 20,000–400,000 kD; 0.1% wt/vol SDS, 20% methanol in 50 mM Tris base, 380 mM glycine [not pH-ed])

*or*
Transfer buffer 2 (proteins < 80,000 kD; 20% methanol, 25 mM Tris base, 190 mM glycine [not pH-ed])
Coomassie Blue stain (p. 425)

## Special equipment

Submerged transfer apparatus

## Caution

Methanol, SDS, see Appendix IV.

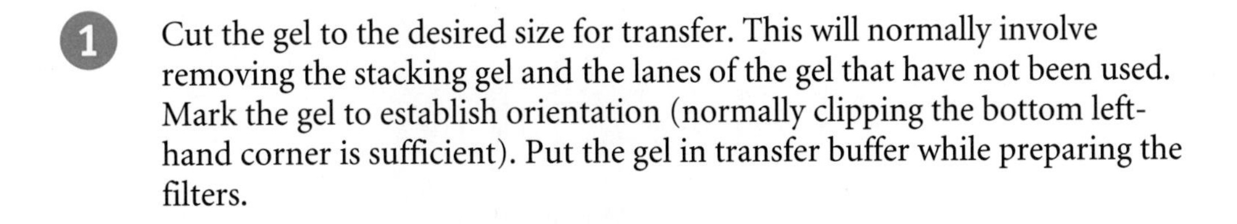

**1** Cut the gel to the desired size for transfer. This will normally involve removing the stacking gel and the lanes of the gel that have not been used. Mark the gel to establish orientation (normally clipping the bottom left-hand corner is sufficient). Put the gel in transfer buffer while preparing the filters.

**2** Cut one sheet of nitrocellulose paper and four sheets of absorbent filter paper (Whatman 3 MM or equivalent) to the size of the gel.

Wear gloves and use virgin nitrocellulose sheets. The types of bonds that hold proteins to nitrocellulose are not known. However, the binding is blocked by oils or other proteins.

*Towbin et al. (1979).

**3** Soak the nitrocellulose membrane in distilled water. Nitrocellulose should always be wetted by carefully laying it on the surface of water. Allow the nitrocellulose to wet by capillary action from the bottom (several minutes), then submerge the sheet for 2 minutes. Move the membrane to soak in transfer buffer for 5 minutes. Wet the absorbent paper by soaking in transfer buffer.

Transfer buffer 1 (proteins 20,000–400,000 kD):

| | Concentration | for 1000 ml |
|---|---|---|
| Tris | 48 mM | 5.8 g |
| Glycine | 390 mM | 29.3 g |
| SDS | 0.1% (wt/vol) | 1.0 g |
| Methanol | 20% | 200 ml |
| Distilled water | | Make up to 1000 ml |

Transfer buffer 2 (proteins < 80,000 kD):

| | Concentration | for 1000 ml |
|---|---|---|
| Tris | 25 mM | 3.0 g |
| Glycine | 190 mM | 14.5 g |
| Methanol | 20% | 200 ml |
| Distilled water | | Make up to 1000 ml |

**4** Immerse gel, membrane, filter papers, and support pads in transfer buffer to ensure that they are thoroughly soaked. Be careful to exclude air bubbles from the support pads.

**5** Assemble the transfer sandwich as shown below (Fig. 8.2). Keep all the components wet and make sure that good contact is made between the gel and filter.

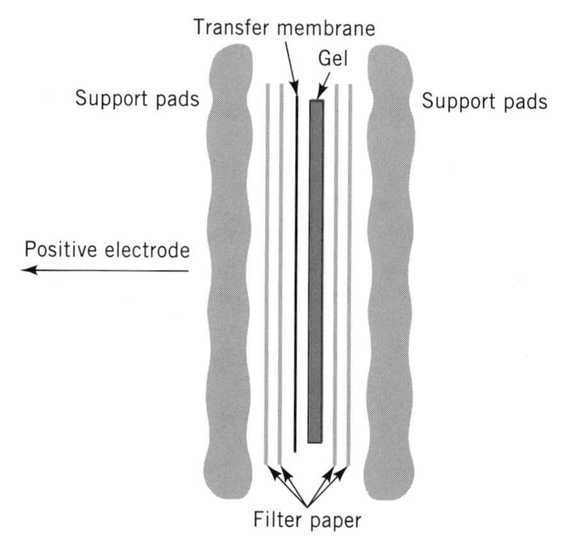


Figure 8.2
Transfer sandwich.

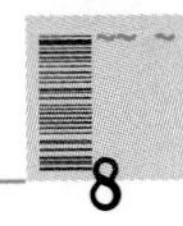



6. Place the complete sandwich in the transfer tank with the membrane closest to the positive electrode (anode, red electrode).

7. Transfer for 4–18 hours. Thicker gels and higher-molecular-weight proteins require longer transfers. The following conditions have been optimized to permit transfer and retention of a very wide range of molecular weight proteins.

   For proteins over 100,000 kD on a 15 × 15 × 0.1-cm gel, transfer at 28 volts for 1 hour, then at 84 volts for 14–16 hours.

   For proteins under 100,000 kD on a 15 × 15 × 0.1-cm gel, transfer at 63 volts for 4–16 hours.

   In all transfers, the temperature will rise substantially during the run. It is essential to use a cooling coil or to run the transfer in a cold room to avoid the generation of gas bubbles in the sandwich.

8. After transfer, disconnect the power supply. Disassemble the sandwich and mark the nitrocellulose membrane by clipping one corner (normally the bottom left-hand corner, the number one lane).

9. The polyacrylamide gel can now be stained with Coomassie Blue (pp. 425–426) or silver stain (pp. 427–428) to verify transfer.

**Process the nitrocellulose sheet for staining (p. 292) or blocking (p. 296) as appropriate.**

## Common problems

The only major problem that will be encountered with this method is the lack of transfer because of bubbles in the transfer sandwich. If this is a problem, try assembling the sandwich in a shallow tray filled with transfer buffer. This will allow you to make sure no bubbles are present by basically assembling the transfer unit under water.

The other common problem is the difficulty of transfer of large-molecular-weight proteins. This is an inherent problem with transfer. If the protein runs slowly through the separating gel, it follows that the transfer out of the gel will also be slow. If this is a problem, we recommend lowering the concentration of the separating gel. If more than one polypeptide of different sizes need to be studied and the same gel concentration will not work for both, try running two separate gels with different acrylamide concentrations.

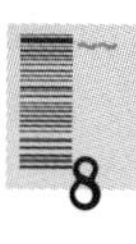



## Staining the blot for total protein (optional)



Prior to probing blots for the presence of an antigen, the total composition of the proteins transferred to nitrocellulose can be determined by staining the membrane. Staining for proteins can be used to determine the position of molecular-weight markers and to ensure that efficient transfer has occurred. This method also gives a remarkably good picture of the complexity of the transferred proteins. The conventional procedures used for staining polyacrylamide gels are unsuitable for staining immunoblots. Both Coomassie Blue and silver staining methods give high backgrounds due to nonspecific dye adsorption, and when using nitrocellulose, these methods damage and distort the membrane. A number of suitable staining methods have now been developed that give a sensitive and high-quality stain of nitrocellulose replicas.

There are any number of useful methods for staining the blot prior to blocking the remaining protein-binding sites on the blot (Table 8.2). Both the India ink and the Ponceau S methods below work well and are extremely easy. The India ink method is considerably more sensitive and is generally more useful when low amounts of proteins are being transferred, such as when immunoprecipitated or purified protein preparations are being studied. When unpurified protein preparations are being used, both methods are suitable.

Table 8.2 *Stains used for immunoblots*

| Stain | Advantages | Disadvantages |
|---|---|---|
| Ponceau S | Cheap<br>Compatible with all antigen detection methods | Insensitive<br>Not permanent |
| India ink | Cheap<br>Sensitive<br>Compatible with radiolabel detection | For enzyme detection block in Tween, detect, then stain<br>Incompatible with enzymatic detection methods, both chemiluminescence and chromogenic substrate |

## Staining the blot with Ponceau S

PREPARING, 276

GELS, 283

TRANSFER, 284

STAINING

DETECTING, 297

Ponceau S is applied in an acidic aqueous solution. Staining is rapid but not permanent; the red stain will wash away in subsequent processing. Because the binding is reversible, the stain is compatible with all antigen visualization techniques. Therefore, Ponceau S can be used routinely to verify transfer and to locate molecular-weight markers or other internal controls (Fig. 8.3). However, the stain is not very sensitive and is rather difficult to record photographically. The stain can be used effectively by marking the position of molecular-weight markers and lane positions with pencil or indelible pen.

### Needed solutions

2% Ponceau S (3-hydroxy-4-[2-sulfo-4-(sulfo-phenylazo]-2,7-naphthalene disulfonic acid) in 30% trichloroacetic acid

30% Sulfosalicylic acid

PBS

### Caution

Sulfosalicylic acid, trichloroacetic acid, see Appendix IV.

*The stock solution is stable at room temperature for over 1 year.*

*If using PVDF membranes (Immobilon), adjust the final working solution of the Ponceau S stain to 1% acetic acid.*

1. Prior to staining, prepare a concentrated stock of Ponceau S. The concentrated solution is 2% Ponceau S (3-hydroxy-4-[2-sulfo-4-(sulfo-phenylazo)phenylazo]-2,7-naphthalene disulfonic acid) in 30% trichloroacetic acid, 30% sulfosalicylic acid. The concentrated dye solution is diluted 1 in 10 with water to prepare the working solution.

2. Wash the nitrocellulose sheet once in Ponceau S solution.

3. Add freshly diluted Ponceau S and incubate for 5–10 minutes at room temperature with agitation.

4. Transfer the nitrocellulose sheet to PBS and rinse for 1–2 minutes with several changes of PBS.

5. Mark position of transfer and molecular-weight markers as required.

**The nitrocellulose sheet is now ready for blocking and addition of the antibody (p. 296).**

## Common problems

There are seldom any problems with this approach except that it is not particularly sensitive. If more contrast or sensitivity is needed, try the India ink staining method.

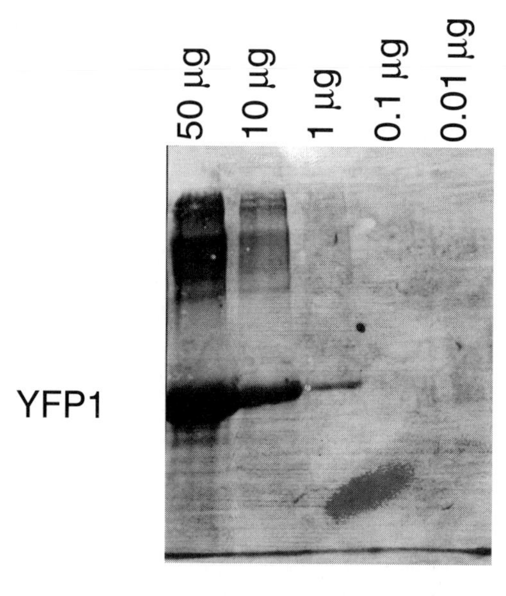


Figure 8.3
Ponceau S.

## Staining the blot with India ink*



If you are not using chemiluminescence, this method of staining blots is highly recommended. It is cheap, reliable, sensitive, and yields a permanent record and therefore is very useful when staining with a radioactive antibody. Importantly, it does not interfere with subsequent binding of antibody to the antigen (Glenney 1986). It is also an excellent choice when staining a duplicate blot. Because of a lack of contrast between the colored reaction product and the interference with chemiluminescence, India ink is not compatible with enzyme-based chromogenic detection methods.

The staining depends on the preferential adherence of the colloidal carbon particles in India ink to the immobilized protein on the filter. It is essential that the correct India ink be used. Pelikan Fount India drawing ink (Original Recipe, Black) or equivalent is suitable (Fig. 8.3).

### Needed solutions

0.03% Tween 20/PBS

India ink suspension (0.1% India ink in 0.3% Tween 20/PBS)

PBS

1. Wash blot in 0.3% Tween 20/PBS, with two changes of 100 ml at 5 minutes each.

2. Place blot in ink solution (100 μl of ink in 100 ml of 0.3% Tween 20/PBS).

3. Incubate at room temperature for 15 minutes to 18 hours. Longer incubations will increase sensitivity.

4. Destain by washing the blot in multiple changes of PBS.

**The nitrocellulose sheet is now ready for blocking and addition of the antibody (p. 296).**

### Common problems

India ink cannot be used with chemiluminescence; in this case, Ponceau S should be used instead. If you are using an enzymatic detection method that relies on the precipitation of chromogenic products, the black color of the India ink may make photography of the gel difficult. If this unusual setting is being used, try another detection method or switch to Ponceau S. One other solution to this problem is to delay staining the blot until after the detection step has been completed. This works well provided that a non-protein-containing blocking buffer, such as Tween, is used.

*Hancock and Tsang (1983).

# Antigen detection

PREPARING, 276
GELS, 283
TRANSFER, 284
STAINING, 292
DETECTING

Antigen detection depends primarily on the availability of effective reagents, most particularly good antibodies that will detect the denatured and immobilized antigens on the membrane.

The process for detection is straightforward. Before the blot can be processed for antigen detection, it is essential to block the membrane to prevent nonspecific adsorption of the immunological reagents. Blocking can be achieved by incubating the blot with a range of protein or detergent solutions. The antigen is then located by binding antibodies to the proteins immobilized on the membrane. The antigen is detected by labeling the antibodies with conveniently identified tags. The antibodies can be labeled themselves and, thus, can detect the location of the antigen directly, or more commonly, the antibodies can be used unlabeled and located by labeled secondary reagents. Common labeling methods include coupled enzymes, normally horseradish peroxidase or occasionally alkaline phosphatase.

### *Blocking nonspecific protein-binding sites on the membrane*

Table 8.3 summarizes the commonly used blocking solutions and their advantages and disadvantages. Although all of these solutions work satisfactorily in some circumstances, a careful choice is necessary to ensure compatibility with the detection reagent. For example, using whole serum to block is inappropriate if protein A is used as a detection reagent. The compatibility of the blocking reagent with the detection system can be tested by taking a fresh piece of membrane, blocking it, and then treating with the detection system.

Table 8.3 *Blocking solutions*

| Blocking buffer | Composition[a] | Advantages | Disadvantages |
|---|---|---|---|
| 5% Nonfat dry milk | 5% wt/vol nonfat dry milk in PBS | Cheap<br>Clean background | Deteriorates rapidly<br>Disguises some antigens<br>Incompatible with avidin/streptavidin technique |
| 5% Nonfat dry milk/Tween | 5% wt/vol nonfat dry milk<br>0.2% Tween 20<br>in PBS | Cheap<br>Clean background | Deteriorates rapidly<br>Disguises some antigens |
| Tween | 0.2% Tween 20<br>in PBS | Allows staining after antigen detection | May get some residual background |
| BSA | 3% BSA (Cohn fraction V)<br>PBS | Cheap<br>Good signal strength | Relatively expensive |

[a] If blocking buffers are not made fresh each time, include 0.01% Merthiolate as a preservative. Sodium azide should be avoided, as this blocks horseradish peroxidase enzyme activity.

Two blocking solutions that are compatible with nearly all detection systems are nonfat dry milk (Johnson et al. 1984) and BSA (Towbin et al. 1979). If protein-blocking solutions cause problems with excessive background or interfere with the detection system, blocking in Tween 20 should be tried (Batteiger et al. 1982).

### *Direct versus indirect detection methods*

Direct detection is the term to describe methods in which the primary antibody is purified and labeled. Binding of this reagent to the blot generally leads to lower backgrounds and allows multiple different antibodies with different specificities or origins to be studied on the same blot. However, direct detection is considerably more work, relies on homemade reagents, and has lower sensitivity than indirect methods.

Indirect detection is achieved by using unlabeled primary antibodies, followed by labeled secondary antibodies that bind to epitopes on the primary antibodies. This immune complex allows a single source—often commercial—to be used to detect all of the primary antibodies from a single species and has a much higher sensitivity because of the number of secondary antibodies that can bind.

It is our recommendation that except when the specificity of direct detection is needed, immunoblots should be analyzed using indirect methods. For most purposes, we suggest that the primary antibody be detected using commercial anti-immunoglobulin antibodies coupled with horseradish peroxidase. This allows the use of a small number of detection reagents, each specific for a different species of primary antibody. Thus, one lab can effectively use a relatively small number of common reagents for mouse, rat, rabbit, or other primary antibodies. The secondary reagents can be titered and used with confidence in many immunoblotting protocols.

### *Detection methods*

There are any number of potential methods to detect the location of the antibodies bound to the immobilized proteins on a blot. Over the last several years, the method of chemiluminescence (CL) has become the most commonly used approach. This method works by chemical oxidation of a cyclic diacylhydrazide, creating an unstable intermediate that decays with the emission of light. This light emission can be captured on standard X-ray film to yield an excellent record that is easy to display.

The chemiluminescent method is more sensitive than previously used chromogenic or radioactive detection methods. The extra increase in sensitivity is widely disputed but appears to be about 20-fold more sensitive than chromogenic methods and probably severalfold more sensitive than radioactive detection methods.

The key to this method is the use of horseradish peroxidase-coupled secondary reagent. Horseradish peroxidase can be covalently coupled to an anti-immunoglobulin antibody, protein A, protein G, or other reagents that will bind specifically to the primary antibody. In the presence of hydrogen peroxide, the peroxidase catalyzes the oxidation of luminol, which in turn releases light.

### *Increasing the sensitivity*

Several methods commonly are used to increase the sensitivity of immunoblots. The first relies on the purification and concentration of the antigen by immunoprecipitation prior to electrophoresis. This is discussed on p. 281. This method can be used to concentrate a very dilute antigen and separate it from most of the contaminating proteins prior to running the gel and doing the immunoblot, allowing very minor antigens to be studied.

Other approaches to increasing the sensitivity of detection are designed to intensify the strength of the signal itself. This can be done by using better and more intensive fluors or by localizing more enzyme at the band. A number of companies continue to introduce new and better chemiluminescent detection systems, and workers should constantly be on the lookout for better and more sensitive reagents.

The signal can also be intensified by using a triple-layer detection system, i.e., primary, secondary, and tertiary antibodies are all complexed to the antigen. This increases the number of potential labeled antibodies that can be bound. For example, if five secondary antibodies can bind to the primary antibody and five tertiary antibodies can bind to each secondary antibody, a 25-fold increase in the signal over a labeled primary antibody can be achieved.

*A band can be confirmed as your antigen by several methods: (1) By comparing to a purified preparation that gives a single band run in an adjacent lane, (2) by use of multiple antibodies recognizing different epitopes or regions of the antigen, (3) by use of a tagged version of the antigen that can be located with an independent antibody, or (4) by use of truncated (either amino- or carboxy-terminal) versions that can show a change in electrophoretic mobility of the antigen.*

## Thinking ahead

In planning for antigen detection, the major issues to consider are the best concentrations of primary and secondary antibodies to use. In the steps below, we have suggested amounts of the primary antibody to use as a starting point; however, the concentration of specific antibodies in every antibody source will be different. Therefore, a titration of antibody will be helpful to achieve the best signal-to-noise ratio. Similar preliminary steps for secondary reagents will also help. Here, however, once the correct concentration is found, it can be used for each blot developed with the same lot of secondary antibodies.

## Needed solutions and reagents

PBS
3% BSA/PBS
Blocking solutions (see Table 8.3)
Primary antibody solution
Labeled secondary reagent (most often horseradish peroxidase-labeled anti-immunoglobulin antibodies)
Solutions for chemiluminescence (most often purchased or prepared as described on p. 461)
X-ray film

## Caution

DOC, hydrogen peroxide, SDS, see Appendix IV.

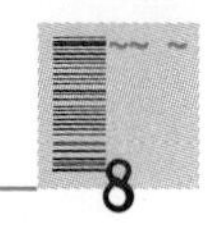

1. Rinse the filter several times with PBS.

2. Add one of the blocking solutions (see Table 8.3).

   Different antigens or applications may require different blocking buffers. For example, both BSA (fraction V) and milk contain both phosphotyrosine and biotin. This confuses the interpretation of tests with antibodies specific for anti-phosphotyrosine antibodies and gives problems with the use of avidin/streptavidin detection. Alkaline phosphate is inhibited by some preparations of milk. If no signal or a high background is detected, check different blocking buffers.

*If using small strips of the blot, each strip can be put into its own test tube. Five-ml tubes with sealable tops work well for this. Use 0.5 ml for a 15 × 0.5-cm strip.*

3. Incubate at room temperature with agitation. Incubations between 20 minutes and 2 hours are appropriate.

4. Remove the blot from the blocking solution and wash twice for 5 minutes each in PBS.

5. Add the primary antibody solution. Use 10 ml per 15 × 15-cm blot. All dilutions should be done in protein-containing solutions such as 3% BSA/PBS. Incubations can be performed in shallow trays.

   Use tissue-culture supernatants either undiluted or diluted up to 1 in 10. This yields an antibody concentration between 1 and 50 μg/ml. For polyclonal sera, ascites fluid, or purified antibodies, the final antibody concentration should also be approximately in this range. A dilution of 10 μl in 10 ml will normally be sufficient. If the concentration of an antibody solution is unknown, try several dilutions to determine the correct range.

6. Incubate the blot with antibody for at least 1 hour at room temperature with agitation (Fig. 8.4). Some workers have reported increased sensitivity by using overnight (12–18 hours) incubation.

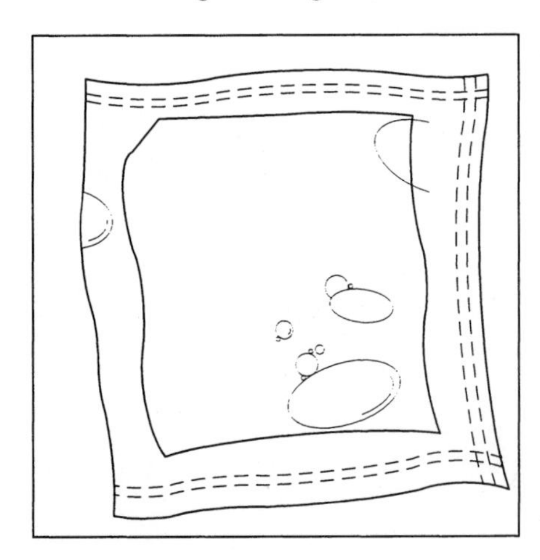

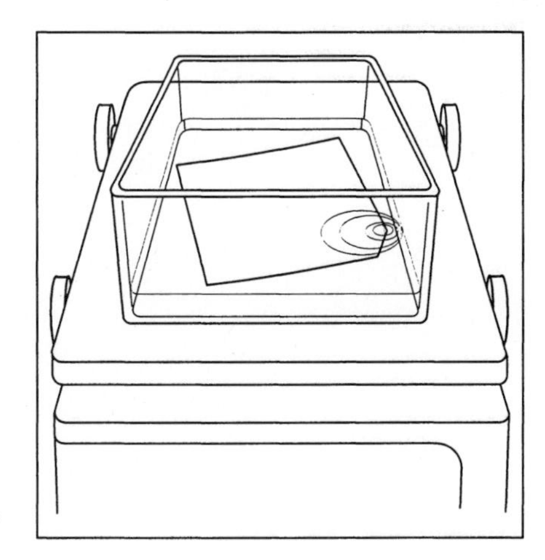

**Figure 8.4**
Blot in sealed bag (*left*); blot in containers (*right*).

7. Wash the blot with four changes of PBS for 5 minutes each.

8. The blot is now ready for the addition of the labeled secondary reagent. Incubation can be done in a shallow tray when probing a full blot. All dilutions should be done in protein-containing buffers such as 3% BSA/PBS.

   In general, commercial enzyme-labeled secondary conjugates should be used at concentrations of 5–0.5 μg/ml (usually a dilution of 1/200 to 1/2000 of commercial stocks). Reagents labeled with horseradish peroxidase should be diluted in blocking buffer without sodium azide. Enzyme-labeled protein A, anti-immunoglobulin antibodies, avidin, and streptavidin are all available commercially.

9. Incubate for 1 hour at room temperature with agitation.

10. Wash the blot with four changes of PBS for 5 minutes each.

11. Immediately prior to use prepare fresh chemiluminescence reagent. Prepare only as much reagent as needed, because the reagent has a very short shelf life.

    Most workers currently use commercial solutions for chemiluminescence. In this case, mix the two solutions in a 1:1 ratio. One solution contains hydrogen peroxide, and the other contains the luminol and may contain a chemical enhancer. If you are not using commercial reagents, useful substitutes for the two solutions are found on p. 461.

12. Incubate with the blot for 1 minute.

13. Drain the blot and remove excess chemiluminescence reagent by blotting the edge or corner of the filter with a paper towel. Place the blot in plastic wrap to ensure a dry surface for film exposure.

14. Expose the blot to film in the darkroom for 1 minute. Develop the film and determine the correct exposure time for your antigen (Fig. 8.5). Exposure times may be as short as a few seconds to several hours.

## Common problems

The major problems encountered while using immunoblots are unexpected bands or bad backgrounds. Methods to identify the origin of unexpected bands are discussed above on p. 271, and strategies to counter band backgrounds are found in the box on p. 301.

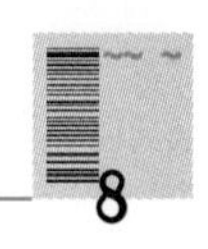

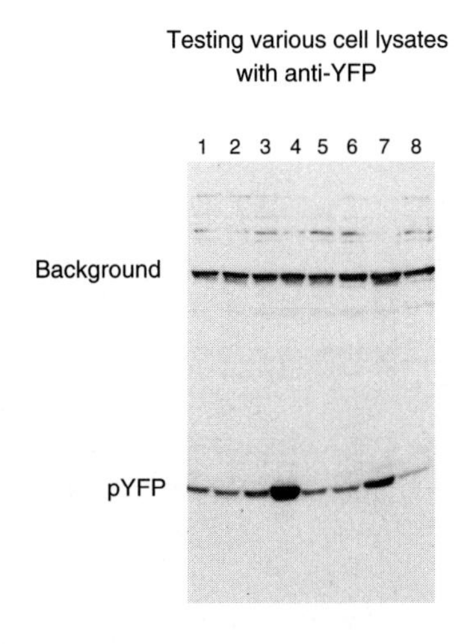


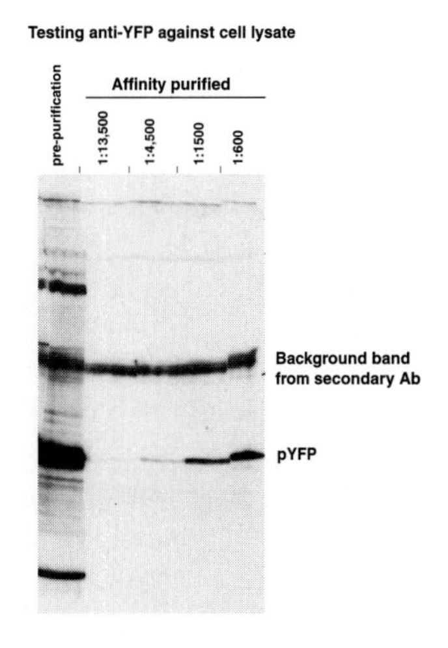


Figure 8.5
Full blot (*left*) vs. strips (*right*).

## Troubleshooting—Bad backgrounds

The most frequently encountered problem in immunoblots is the presence of a high background consisting either of extra, discrete bands or of a general diffuse signal covering the entire membrane.

Specific background bands are generated either by contaminating antibodies present in polyclonal sera or by specific cross-reactions when your antigen and another in the sample share an epitope recognized by your antibody. The latter problem is especially prevalent with monoclonal antibodies. Nonspecific diffuse backgrounds result either from insufficient blocking of the membrane or from a specific reaction of the detecting reagent with a component of the blocking buffer.

***Diffuse backgrounds***

- If using an indirect technique, first determine whether the secondary reagent is contributing to the background. Omit the primary antibody and observe the background generated by the secondary reagent alone. If the background is generated by the secondary reagent: (1) reduce the time of incubation with the secondary reagent; (2) try adsorbing the secondary reagent with high concentrations of protein. Adding 3% BSA to the secondary reagent would be a first good attempt. If the background persists, try a sample of the starting antigen preparation (an acetone powder may be suitable); (3) use an alternative secondary reagent.
- Use a different blocking buffer.
- Try 5% nonfat dry milk/Tween, if presently using anything else.
- Titrate the concentration of the primary and/or secondary antibodies and look for a lower concentration that will give an acceptably strong signal.
- Reduce the incubation time of the primary and secondary antibodies.
- Wash the filter at each step in RIPA buffer (1% NP-40, 0.5% DOC, 0.1% SDS, 150 mM sodium chloride, 50 mM Tris, pH 8.0).

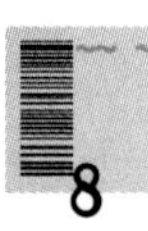


- Add 1% NP-40 or 0.3% Tween and 3% BSA to the primary and secondary antibodies.
- Increase the duration of each washing step.

*Specific background bands*

- If using an indirect technique, first determine whether the secondary detecting reagent is contributing to the background. Omit the primary antibody and observe the background generated by the secondary reagent alone. If the background bands are generated by the secondary reagent, first use an alternative label. Second, try adsorbing the secondary reagent with a sample of the starting antigen preparation. An acetone powder may be suitable.
- If using a monoclonal antibody, use another monoclonal antibody if available. But please note, the continued presence of the same band may suggest an amino acid homology between your antigen and the other band.
- If using a polyclonal serum as a source of primary antibodies, try adsorbing the serum with a protein preparation that does not contain the antigen of interest.

# Variations in the detection methods

There are many different methods for detecting antibodies bound to the blot, and although the horseradish peroxidase/chemiluminescence detection has become a useful standard for the field, the approach will not solve all problems or fit all situations. The two major problems for which chemiluminescence is not well suited are when accurate quantitation is needed or when the level of detection must be limited because of strong signals.

## Detection method variation 1: Accurate quantitation

The horseradish peroxidase/chemiluminescence method described above provides an output that can be used to compare relative film darkening. These comparisons can be used to estimate the relative levels of proteins from any source that is amenable to immunoblotting techniques. The comparisons can be made to another sample as a reference point or to known amounts of purified standards. However, because the final measure will be film darkening, it is difficult to establish accurate quantitation. Like all film-darkening comparisons, the level of darkening is only linear in a short range of exposure, and accurate comparisons are possible only through densitometer readings.

A more robust method of comparison is to use a radioactive detection method that can be accurately determined. For this, we recommend the use of $^{125}$I-labeled secondary reagents. $^{125}$I-labeled reagents can be purchased coupled to anti-immunoglobulin antibodies, protein A, protein G, and other reagents that can specifically bind to primary antibodies immobilized on the blot. They are easy to quantitate by excising labeled bands from the membrane and counting them directly or by quantitating on a phosphorimager.

## Detection method variation 2: Controlled development

One annoying aspect of horseradish peroxidase/chemiluminescence is that the light emission cannot be controlled easily. Other methods of detection do not have this problem. For example, enzyme-linked reagents can be used to act on chromogenic substrates that will change color and precipitate at the site of the enzyme, generating a result that can be monitored just by visual inspection. This allows the worker to stop the reaction at exactly the point in the development of the signal to allow maximum signal-to-noise ratios for whichever antigen is being studied.

For visual development of blots, we recommend alkaline phosphatase-labeled antibodies with the bromochloroindolyl phosphate/nitro blue tetrazolium substrate (BCIP/NBT). The BCIP/NBT substrate generates an intense black-purple precipitate at the site of enzyme binding. The substrate solution is stable in the absence of enzyme. The reaction proceeds at a steady rate, thus allowing accurate control of the development of the reaction. This allows the relative sensitivity to be controlled by the length of incubation. The BCIP/NBT substrate characteristically produces sharp bands with very little background coloring of the membrane. Coupled reagents should be pur-

*NBT: Dissolve 0.5 g of NBT in 10 ml of 70% dimethylformamide.*

*BCIP: Dissolve 0.5 g of BCIP (disodium salt) in 10 ml of 100% dimethylformamide.*

***Alkaline phosphatase buffer:** 100 mM sodium chloride, 5 mM magnesium chloride, 100 mM Tris (pH 9.5).*

chased with eukaryotic alkaline phosphatase, because this enzyme is readily inactivated with EDTA. The bacterial enzyme is difficult to stop, causing overdevelopment and leading to high background.

The three required stock solutions are described in the sidebar.

## Caution

BCIP, NBT, see Appendix IV.

1. Just prior to developing the blot, prepare fresh substrate solution. Add 66 μl of NBT stock to 10 ml of alkaline phosphatase buffer. Mix well and add 33 μl of BCIP stock. Use within 1 hour.

2. Place the washed immunoblot in a suitable container. Add 10 ml of substrate solution per 15 × 15-$cm^2$ membrane.

3. Develop the blot at room temperature with agitation until the bands are suitably dark. A typical incubation with the blot would be approximately 30 minutes.

4. To stop the reaction, rinse the blot with PBS containing 20 mM EDTA, which chelates the $Mg^{++}$ ions.

## Detection method variation 3: Detecting antibodies from multiple species using biotin/streptavidin

An alternative to labeling secondary antibodies with enzymes or iodine is biotinylation. Biotin-labeled antibodies are not detected directly, but need the addition of a third reagent, usually streptavidin coupled with an enzyme or iodinated. A wide range of secondary reagents are available commercially. Although this approach adds a third step to the detection sandwich—antigen/unlabeled primary antibody/biotinylated secondary antibody/enzyme or iodine-labeled streptavidin—the interaction of the biotin/streptavidin is extremely tight ($10^{15}$ liters mol) and adds little time to the procedure. Because the detection is performed using tertiary reagents, multiple batches of streptavidin-conjugated reagents can be used with a variety of secondary antibodies. These then can be detected and compared using a single detection reagent.

Biotinylated antibodies are treated in the same manner as unlabeled antibodies.

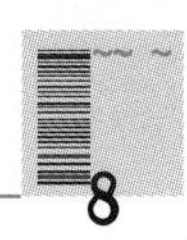


# Variations in the immunoblotting technique

## Determining phosphorylated tyrosine residues using immunoblots

Because specific antibodies to phosphorylated tyrosine residues have been made and are commonly available, they can be used to probe blots for proteins phosphorylated on tyrosine. As this edition was going to press, there were the first reports of antibodies specific for phosphoserine and phosphothreonine (Zymed). If these antibodies prove to be specific and are made available, workers will be able to test proteins for all three phosphorylated residues.

The methods to test for the presence of phosphotyrosines are straightforward. After transfer and blocking of the blot, probe with the anti-phosphotyrosine antibodies and develop by standard methods. This method is particularly powerful when combined with immunoprecipitation to collect the antigen under study before running the blot. This will give excellent specificity to the test and ensure that the band you are examining is the one that is phosphorylated.

## Stripping and reprobing immunoblots

Many researchers have begun the practice of stripping immunoblots and reprobing to detect multiple proteins on the same blot. This is a good method to examine two antigens under identical conditions. However, this approach should not be used for any quantitative comparisons.

If immunoblots do need to be stripped, any method for breaking the antibody/antigen interaction is useful. The recommended treatment for stripping the blot is to treat with 2% SDS, 50 mM DTT in 50 mM Tris-HCl, pH 7.0, for 30 minutes at 70°C, then wash with several changes of a neutral buffer such as PBS. If you know that a blot will be stripped and reprobed, the blot should be blocked in 5% nonfat dry milk prior to developing as long as the blot is not being used with anti-phosphotyrosine antibodies. For reasons that are not entirely clear at present, the use of milk as a blocking solution is the most effective at allowing release of the bound antibodies. After stripping and before reprobing, the blots must be reblocked, so begin again at step 1 (p. 299).

These stripping conditions are relatively harsh, so you should expect that losses of antigens from the filters will occur. We recommend this approach only in certain circumstances. The bonds that hold antigens to nitrocellulose or nylon membranes are noncovalent, and all methods to strip the antibodies from the antigens also remove some of the polypeptides from the filters. Therefore, these methods are never quantitative and should never be used to judge that an antigen is not present. This approach can be used in some cases to confirm that another antigen is present, and stripping and reprobing immunoblots may be effective in these cases. One useful setting would be when archived blots need to be tested for the presence of newly discovered proteins that were unknown when the original samples were run. However, for fresh samples, there are other effective methods to score for the presence of more than one antigen in the same starting preparations. The best method is just to run duplicate blots and probe them individually for the various proteins. When the molecular weights of the

*Blots can be archived by rinsing in water and allowing to dry or by rinsing in PBS and storing in plastic wrap at 4°C.*

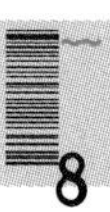



antigens under study are different, the blots can be cut into multiple sections and each probed independently. See p. 285 for advice about how to locate bands and cut the blots after transfer.

## Purifying antibodies from immunoblots

Antibodies that bind to a given polypeptide band can be purified from polyclonal sera by a simple modification of the immunoblotting technique (Olmsted 1981; Smith and Fisher 1984). These band-specific antibodies, although recovered in small amounts, can be useful in studies of complex antigens, often allowing the confirmation of antigen identity. With antigens that are available in larger amounts, such as those isolated from bacterial overexpression systems, this procedure can be scaled up to produce a larger amount of antigen-specific antibodies.

The procedure is to load the antigen into one large preparative well. Run the gel, transfer, and apply the primary antibody as usual. The location of the antigen with the bound antibodies is determined by cutting strips of the blot from the sides. These side strips are processed as normally done for antigen detection. After the localization of the antigen primary antibody complexes on the side strips, align the strips with the untreated portion of the blot. Excise the area of the blot that contains the antigen and primary antibody using a sharp scalpel. Cut this area of the blot into small pieces and transfer the pieces to a test tube. Incubate the blot pieces with 100 mM glycine (pH 2.5) for 10 minutes or with 3 M potassium thiocyanate for 10 minutes. Remove the eluting buffer and neutralize it with one-tenth volume of 1 M Tris (pH 8.0) for the glycine elution or dilute it with 10 volumes of PBS for the potassium thiocyanate elution.

## References

Batteiger B., Newhall W.J., and Jones R.B. 1982. The use of Tween 20 as a blocking agent in the immunological detection of proteins transferred to nitrocellulose membranes. *J. Immunol. Methods* **55:** 297–307.

Beisiegel U. 1986. Protein blotting (review). *Electrophoresis* **7:** 1–18.

Bittner M., Kupferer P., and Morris C.F. 1980. Electrophoretic transfer of proteins and nucleic acids from slab gels to diazobenzyloxymethyl cellulose or nitrocellulose sheets. *Anal. Biochem.* **102:** 459–471.

Bowen B., Steinberg J., Laemmli U.K., and Weintraub H. 1980. The detection of DNA-binding proteins by protein blotting. *Nucleic Acids Res.* **8:** 1–20.

Burnette W.N. 1981. "Western blotting": Electrophoretic transfer of proteins from sodium dodecyl sulfate-polyacrylamide gels to unmodified nitrocellulose and radiographic detection with antibody and radioiodinated protein A. *Anal. Biochem.* **112:** 195–203.

Burridge K. 1976. Changes in cellular glycoproteins after transformations: Identification of specific glycoproteins and antigens in sodium dodecyl sulfate gels. *Proc. Natl. Acad. Sci.* **73:** 4457–4461.

Gershoni J.M. and Palade G.E. 1982. Electrophoretic transfer of sodium dodecyl sulfate-polyacrylamide gels to a positively charged membrane filter. *Anal. Biochem.* **124:** 396–405.

———.1983. Protein blotting: Principles and applications (review). *Anal. Biochem.* **131:** 1–15.

Glenney J. 1986. Antibody probing of western blots which have been stained with india ink. *Anal. Biochem.* **156:** 315–319.

Hancock K. and Tsang V.C.W. 1983. India ink staining of proteins on nitrocellulose paper. *Anal. Biochem.* **133:** 157–162.

Johnson D.A., Gautsch J.W., Sportsman J.R., and Elder J.H. 1984. Improved technique utilizing nonfat dry milk for analysis of proteins and nucleic acids transferred to nitrocellulose. *Gene Anal. Tech.* **1:** 3–8.

Jovin T.M., Dante M.L., and Chrambach A. 1970. Multiphasic buffer systems output, PB 196085–19609, *National Tech. Info. Service.*

Kyhse-Andersen J. 1984. Electroblotting of multiple gels: A simple apparatus without buffer tank for rapid transfer of proteins from polyacrylamide to nitrocellulose. *J. Biochem. Biophys. Methods* **10:** 203–209.

Olmsted J.B. 1981. Affinity purification of antibodies from diazotized paper blots of heterogeneous protein samples. *J. Biol. Chem.* **256:** 11955–11957.

Peferoen M., Huybrechts R., and De Loof A. 1982. Vacuum-blotting: A new simple and efficient transfer of proteins from sodium dodecyl-sulfate-polyacrylamide gels to nitrocellulose. *FEBS Lett.* **145:** 369–372.

Reiser J. and Wardale J. 1981. Immunological detection of specific proteins in total cell extracts by fractionation in gels and transfer to diazophenylthioether paper. *Eur. J. Biochem.* **114:** 569–575.

Renart J., Reiser J., and Stark G.R. 1979. Transfer of proteins from gels to diazobenzyloxymethyl-paper and detection with antisera: A method for studying antibody specificity and antigen structure. *Proc. Natl. Acad. Sci.* **76:** 3116–3120.

Showe M.K., Isobe E., and Onorato L. 1976. Bacteriophage T4 prehead proteinase. II. Its cleavage from the product of gene *21* and regulation in phage-infected cells. *J. Mol. Biol.* **107:** 55–69.

Smith D.E. and Fisher P.A. 1984. Identification, developmental regulation, and response to heat shock of two antigenically related forms of a major nuclear envelope protein in *Drosophila* embryos: Application of an improved method for affinity purification of antibodies using polypeptides immobilized on nitrocellulose blots. *J. Cell Biol.* **99:** 20–28.

Towbin H. and Gordon J. 1984. Immunoblotting and dot immunobinding—Current status and outlook. *J. Immunol. Methods* **72:** 313–340.

Towbin H., Staehelin T., and Gordon J. 1979. Electrophoretic transfer of proteins from polyacrylamide gels to nitrocellulose sheets: Procedure and some applications. *Proc. Natl. Acad. Sci.* **76:** 4350–4354.

# Immunoblotting


## Summary

Detection limit is 2–20 fmoles, or about 0.1–1 ng of a 50-kD protein
Multiple steps over 2 days (or 1 long day)
Detects antigen presence, quantity, size
Semi-quantitative to quantitative
Antigen detection dependent on denaturation-resistant epitope
In general, lower-affinity antibody may work


## Caution

DTT, methanol, SDS, see Appendix IV.

---

1. Solubilize your proteins in Laemmli sample buffer. Final sample buffer conditions should be 2% SDS, 100 mM dithiothreitol (added fresh from a 1 M stock solution, which is kept frozen at –20°C), 60 mM Tris (pH 6.8), 0.01% bromophenol blue, and 10% glycerol. Whole cells can be solubilized directly in sample buffer; purified or partially purified solutions can be diluted 1:1 with 2% sample buffer. Heat to 70°C for 10 minutes. The final protein concentration should not exceed 150 μg/well (15 μg/well for minigels).

2. Run your samples on a SDS polyacrylamide gel, remove the plates, and cut the gel to the desired size for transfer. Mark the gel to establish orientation.

3. Cut one sheet of nitrocellulose paper and four sheets of absorbent filter paper (Whatman 3 MM or equivalent) to the size of the gel.

4. Wet the nitrocellulose membrane in distilled water. Move the membrane to soak in transfer buffer for 5 minutes. Wet the absorbent paper by soaking in transfer buffer. **Transfer buffer 1** (proteins 20,000–400,000 kD): 48 mM Tris, 390 mM glycine, 0.1% (wt/vol) SDS, 20% methanol, and distilled water to 1000 ml. **Transfer buffer 2** (proteins <80,000 kD): 25 mM Tris, 190 mM glycine, 20% methanol, and distilled water to 1000 ml.

5. Immerse gel, membrane, filter papers, and support pads in transfer buffer to ensure that they are thoroughly soaked. Be careful to exclude air bubbles from the support pads.

6. Assemble the transfer sandwich: Support pad | 2 sheets absorbent paper | gel | filter | 2 sheets absorbent paper | support pad. Place the complete sandwich in the transfer tank with the membrane closest to the positive electrode (anode, red electrode).

7. Transfer overnight at 4°C. For proteins over 100,000 kD, transfer at 28 volts for 1 hour, then at 84 volts for 14–16 hours. For proteins under 100,000 MW, transfer at 63 volts for 4–16 hours.

8. After transfer, disconnect the power supply. Disassemble the sandwich and mark the nitrocellulose membrane to retain orientation.

9. Rinse the filter several times with PBS.

10. Incubate the blot in 5% nonfat dry milk/PBS at room temperature with agitation for 2 hours. Then remove the blot from the blocking solution and wash twice for 5 minutes each in PBS.

11. Add the primary antibody solution. Use 10 ml per 15 × 15-cm blot. All dilutions should be done in 3% BSA/PBS.

12. Incubate the blot with antibody for 1 hour at room temperature with agitation. Wash the blot with four changes of PBS for 5 minutes each.

13. Add horseradish peroxidase-labeled secondary reagent. All dilutions should be done in 3% BSA/PBS. Use tissue-culture supernatants either undiluted or diluted up to 1 in 10. This yields an antibody concentration between 1 and 50 μg/ml. For polyclonal sera or ascites fluid, a dilution of 10 μl in 10 ml will normally be sufficient. If the concentration of an antibody solution is unknown, try several dilutions to determine the correct range. If the concentration of an antibody solution is unknown, try several dilutions to determine the correct range.

14. Incubate for 1 hour at room temperature with agitation. Then wash the blot with four changes of PBS for 5 minutes each.

15. Immediately prior to use, prepare fresh chemiluminescence reagent. Prepare only as much reagent as needed, because the reagent has a very short shelf life. Incubate with the blot for 1 minute.

16. Drain the blot and remove excess chemiluminescence reagent by blotting the edge or corner of the filter with a paper towel. Place the blot in plastic wrap to ensure a dry surface for film exposure.

17. Expose the blot to film in the darkroom for 1 minute. Develop the film and determine the correct exposure time for your antigen. Exposure times may range from a few seconds to several hours.

# Immunoaffinity Purification

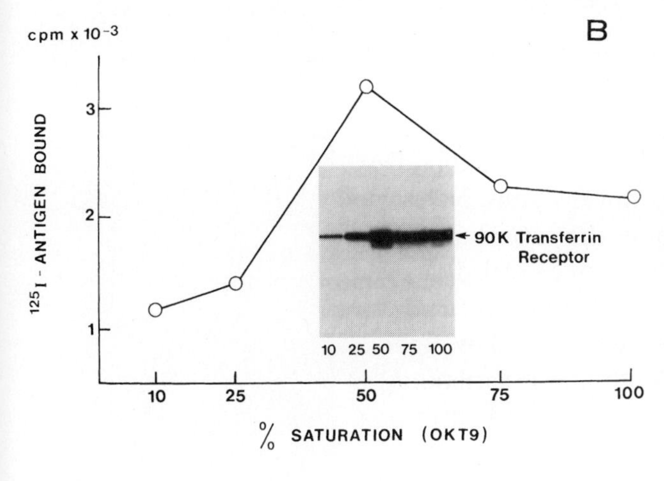


From Schneider C., Newman R.A., Sutherland D.R., Asser U., and Greaves M.F. 1982. A one-step purification of membrane proteins using a high efficiency immunomatrix. *J. Biol. Chem.* **257:** 10766–10769. (Reprinted with permission.)

Fig. 1. Antigen binding as a function of antibody saturation....*B*, Sepharose CL-4B beads were coupled with rabbit anti-mouse Ig at 50% saturation (11 mg/ml beads) and increasing amounts of antibody OKT9 as above. 100% saturation was calculated as a 2:1 ratio (w/w) of monoclonal OKT9 to rabbit anti-mouse Ig respectively; 100% = 22 mg of OKT9, 75% = 16.5 mg of OKT9, 50% = 11 mg of OKT9, 25% = 5.5 mg of OKT9, 10% = 2.2 mg of OKT9/ml of beads. The *inset* shows antigen bound at each concentration point after SDS-polyacrylamide gel electrophoresis. Values are means of three separate experiments.

The time-honored use of affinity chromatography to purify any molecule is one of the most effective methods. The first use of antibodies as a binding agent for immunoaffinity purification relied on the cross-linking of antibodies to themselves to create large multimeric and insoluble matrices for collection of an antigen. This was followed by the covalent coupling of antibodies to inert beads. Although coupling is simple in this approach, much of the antibody reactivity is lost due to the lack of orientation or overcoupling of the antibody. The figure shown here is one of the first to use an orientation method successfully to ensure that the antigen-binding domain of the antibody is available for easy access to the antigen. This same goal is accomplished even more easily by binding and then convalently coupling the antibody to protein A or protein G beads. Finally, widely available monoclonal antibodies that have well-defined binding characteristics for an antigen have made immunoaffinity columns one of the most useful and powerful purification methods.

Immunoaffinity purification takes advantage of the high binding affinity and specificity of an antibody for its antigen to allow large quantities of antigen to be isolated in native or near-native states. Not all antibodies are suitable for immunoaffinity purifications, but when a good antibody is available, the procedure is quick and reliable. The procedure can be scaled to any size, takes no more than a half-day to perform, and can achieve levels of purification unmatched by other methods of chromatography. With simple variations, immunoaffinity methods can also be used to purify antibodies that are antigen-specific.

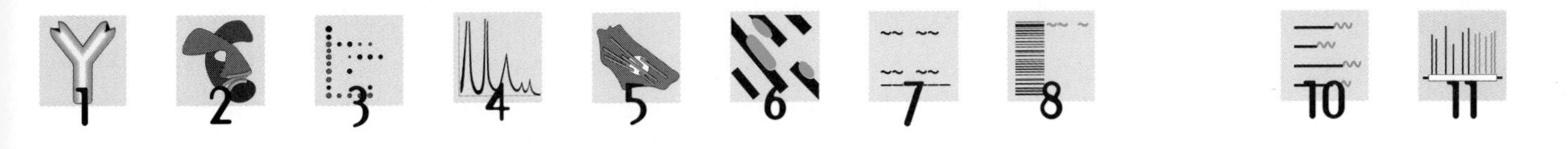


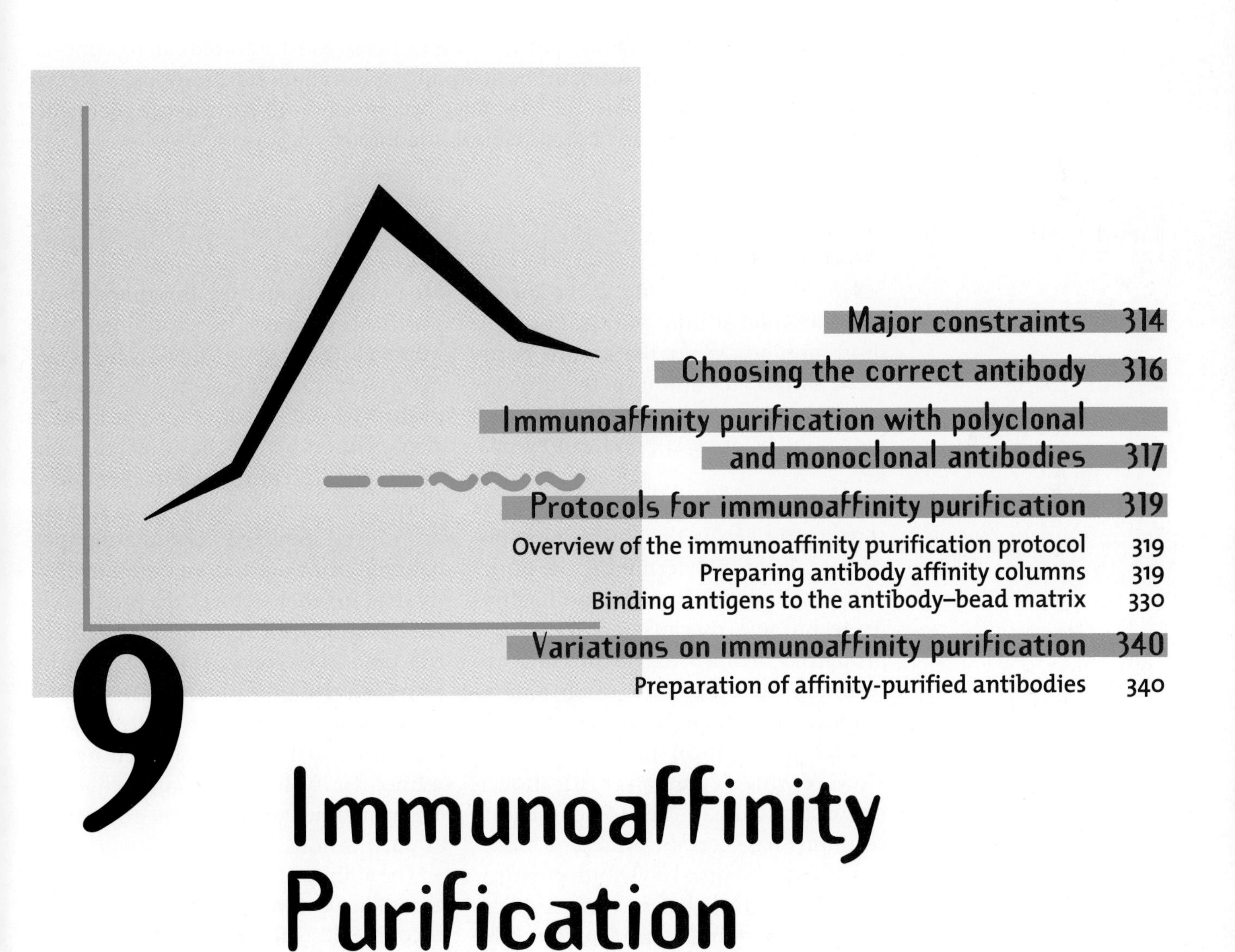



# 9 Immunoaffinity Purification

Immunoaffinity purification is one of the most powerful techniques for the isolation of antigens. In all of the cases discussed below we have used proteins as the example of the antigen under study. However, any molecule that can be bound effectively by an antibody can be purified by these methods. The strategy is simple. Antibodies are covalently bound to an inert bead, and the beads are then mixed with a solution that contains the antigen under study. After the antigen is captured on the antibody–bead matrix, the unwanted antigens are removed by washing. Then the beads are treated with an elution buffer, and the purified antigen is released and available for further study. If elution conditions can be found that are sufficiently mild, the antigen will be released in its native state.

With simple variations in the procedure, immunoaffinity purifications can be used to isolate purified antibodies as well. Here the roles of antibody and antigen are reversed. The antigen is covalently bound to the bead and the antibodies are bound and then released.

Under the proper conditions, purifications of 1,000- to 10,000-fold can be achieved routinely in a single step using immunoaffinity purification. Purifications of greater than 10,000-fold are possible, but this range occurs only with particularly good antibodies or under particularly unique elution conditions.

## Major constraints

Several factors contribute to the success of an immunoaffinity purification. The three most crucial are the starting purity of the antigen, the affinity of the antibody for the antigen, and the ease with which the antibody–antigen bond can be broken.

The relative concentration of the starting antigen is the single most important factor in determining the purity of the final product using immunoaffinity techniques. Because of the unique properties of the antigen–antibody interaction, no other type of chromatographic technique is likely to yield greater purification in a single step. However, the degree of purification is not unlimited, as the use of affinity columns has certain inherent background problems. 1000-fold purifications are routine, and in most applications 10,000-fold purifications are possible. If the protein antigen of interest is rarer than this, immunoaffinity purification must be combined with other methods to achieve a homogeneous product. This may be accomplished by the use of other purification steps either before or after the immunoaffinity column. For example, a common approach would be to run one or more standard chromatography columns prior to using an immunoaffinity step. In other settings, the products of an immunoaffinity column might be run on a SDS-polyacrylamide gel prior to transferring to a membrane for microsequencing. In either of these examples, the purification achieved by immunoaffinity has been augmented by other methods to extend the total range of purification.

The affinity of the antibody for the antigen is the most worrisome of the problems encountered with immunoaffinity purification. The affinity of the antibody will determine the total amount of antigen that can be removed from the antigen-containing solution. For antibodies with high affinities (>$10^8$ liter $mol^{-1}$), quantitative removal can be achieved in less than 1 hour. Even at high antibody concentrations, low-affinity antibodies ($10^6$ liter $mol^{-1}$) will never bind all of the antigen in the solution. Note that all of the times for reaching equilibrium will be considerably longer for immunoaffinity purifications than for techniques such as immunoprecipitation, because the antibodies are bound to a solid support, thus drastically slowing the kinetics of binding. Tricks that can be used to trap antigen more efficiently in other immunochemical techniques, such as using multiple antibodies that recognize multiple epitopes (p. 30) on the same antigen, are not appropriate for most immunoaffinity purifications. As expected, increasing the avidity by these methods will lead to higher antigen binding, but it will also dramatically increase the problems encountered when eluting the antigen. If purification of proteins with native properties is the ultimate goal, antibodies that recognize one epitope or a short peptide sequence are the only useful choice. Only when denatured proteins are the desired end product is the use of antibodies that recognize multiple epitopes suggested.

The third factor that will influence the success of an immunoaffinity purification is the relative ease with which the antigen can be eluted. This is determined solely by the type and number of bonds that form the antibody–antigen interaction, and is, therefore, related to the antibody affinity. However, the affinity does not determine whether the antigen will be easy to elute. The ideal antibody for an immunoaffinity purification is one that has a high affinity for the antigen and whose binding can be reversed by a simple but gentle change in an easily manipulatable variable such as pH. The methods for designing these manipulations are described on p. 335. Often the most important variable to consider when designing an immunoaffinity purification is the choice of antibody and elution conditions. It will be extremely helpful to test several potential antibodies under a number of different elution conditions to find a good combination of high-affinity binding and easy elution conditions.

A common mistake in designing immunoaffinity purification experiments is to equate low affinity with easy elution. Although this may prove to be the case for some low-affinity antibodies, often it is not true. The bonds that hold the antigen to the antibody are of the same basic types for both high-affinity and low-affinity antibodies (see Chapter 2). For example, both high-affinity and low-affinity antibodies may bind an antigen through a salt bridge and a hydrophobic interaction. Eluting the antigen in both cases requires both bonds to be disrupted and, hence, poses similar problems for the choice of elution conditions. In addition, low-affinity antibodies introduce new problems, including low binding capacity, continual leaching from the column during washing, and gradual, rather than sharp, elution profiles.

## Choosing the correct antibody

Finding the best antibody for immunoaffinity purification is an empirical task (Table 9.1). This means that there are no simple shortcuts to enable the worker to choose the best antibody to use in immune purifications. The best approach is to set up several small-scale columns. Use these first to test how well the antibodies perform at collecting the antigen. This could easily be tested by doing immunoprecipitations with the different covalently coupled beads and then testing the amount of antigen bound by immunoblots. Alternatively, the antigen solution could be passed down small columns and the beads collected and eluted with sample buffer for immunoblotting. Once the collection of antibodies that work well at binding the antigen have been determined, the next step will be to test various elution conditions to find an antibody that will give a good elution profile. Various buffers and their use are discussed below on p. 336.

If a useful antibody is not available for immunoaffinity purifications, an excellent alternative is to tag the protein with a well-characterized small epitope that will allow the antigen to be captured with another antibody. The strategy is to prepare an expression vector that will direct the synthesis of a fusion protein between your antigen and a small tag. After the vector is used to produce the newly formed fusion protein, it can be isolated by use of a well-characterized antibody that is specific for the epitope. The use of tags and the available antibodies are discussed in Chapter 10.

Table 9.1 *Antibody choice*

| | **Affinity-purified polyclonal antibodies** | **Monoclonal antibodies** |
|---|---|---|
| **Signal strength (antibody capacity)** | Excellent | Antibody-dependent, but should be excellent |
| **Specificity** | Excellent | Excellent, but some antibodies show cross-reactions |
| **Good features** | Elution profiles known<br>Specificity | Unlimited supply<br>Specificity |
| **Bad features** | Difficult preparation<br>Limited supply | Finding suitable antibody |

We do not recommend the use of unpurified polyclonal antibodies or pooled monoclonal antibodies for immunoaffinity purification.

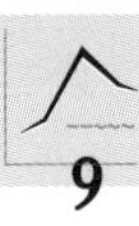



# Immunoaffinity purification with polyclonal and monoclonal antibodies

Most immunoaffinity purifications are done with monoclonal antibodies or affinity-purified polyclonal antibodies. In some cases, total polyclonal antibodies may be appropriate, but almost never will pooled monoclonal antibodies be useful.

## Immunoaffinity purification using polyclonal antibodies

Immunoaffinity purification using polyclonal antibodies has limited applications. Because polyclonal antibodies usually bind to numerous sites on an antigen and therefore bind with high avidity, they are difficult to elute. The harsh conditions needed to elute an antigen when it is bound by several different antibodies usually damages the antibody column and at least partially denatures the antigen. Even when the number of binding sites between the antigen and a polyclonal antibody–matrix is kept low by using saturating amounts of antigen, successful elution is difficult. In this case, the elution conditions for each antibody–antigen interaction are different, so efficient elution cannot be established. Another disadvantage when using polyclonal antibodies is that they contain a number of spurious activities against unrelated antigens. These include all the antibodies in the animal's serum at the time of collection.

Two types of polyclonal antibodies that are useful for immunoaffinity columns are those that have been raised against synthetic peptides or defined regions of an antigen. In both of these cases, because the epitopes for binding the antigen to the column are located in one small region, it may be possible to achieve efficient elution.

One method to make immunoaffinity purifications possible using polyclonal antibodies is to select specific antibodies on an antigen-affinity column (p. 77). This use is limited to cases where sufficient quantities of antigen are available to prepare these columns. However, in some cases, such as purifying a protein from one species with an antibody against an analogous protein from another species, this may be helpful. Affinity-purifying the polyclonal antibodies solves several problems. Only the antibodies that bind to the antigen are collected, and because they have been eluted from the antigen, the exact conditions for releasing the antigen from the immunoaffinity column already have been determined.

## Immunoaffinity purification using monoclonal antibodies

Using monoclonal antibodies for immunoaffinity purifications has a number of advantages compared with other sources of antibodies. Monoclonal antibodies are available in an essentially unlimited supply, and high-affinity monoclonal antibodies can bind to a large proportion of the available antigen. Because all the antibodies are identical and bind to the same epitope, all of the antigen interactions can be broken under similar conditions. Because there are only a limited number of bonds that hold the antigen–antibody complexes together, the conditions to release the antigen are normally gentler than those needed for polyclonal interactions.

The problems that are found when using monoclonal antibodies for immunoaffinity purification normally concern the properties of antigen interaction, commonly low-affinity reactions or cross-reactions. Low-affinity interactions are a problem common to all immunoaffinity purifications and are discussed above. Cross-reactions are particular to monoclonal antibody purifications and are only seen for a subset of antibodies. In these cases, the antibodies bind to other antigens through shared epitopes. These epitopes may be part of a more extensive homology, in which case the monoclonal antibodies may be useful for studying the related proteins but not for purifying the original antigen. On the other hand, the cross-reactions may be limited to the epitope itself. In this case, using other monoclonal antibodies may eliminate the cross-reaction. Another solution would be to purify the antigen away from the spurious protein by some other chromatographic or extraction technique.

## Immunoaffinity purification using pooled monoclonal antibodies

Except in unusual circumstances, there is no reason to pool monoclonal antibodies for preparing immunoaffinity columns. All of the problems of elution discussed in the section on polyclonal antibody columns apply to pooled monoclonal antibodies. The only common use of these reagents is in the purification of antigens that will be denatured before use or in preparing an antigen–antibody–bead complex for immunizations.

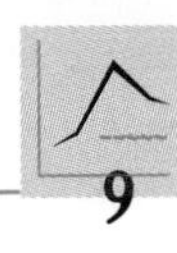


# Protocols for immunoaffinity purification

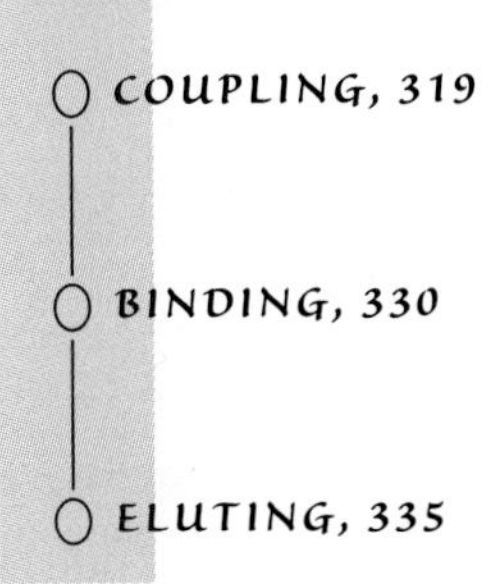


## Overview of the immunoaffinity purification protocol

Immunoaffinity purification can be divided into three steps:

1. Covalent coupling of the antibody to the matrix
2. Binding of the antigen to the antibody–bead matrix
3. Elution of the antigen

In the first step, either monoclonal antibodies or affinity-purified polyclonal antibodies are covalently attached to a solid-phase matrix. Except in unusual settings, we do not recommend using polyclonal antibodies, as the elution of antigen from these columns is very difficult and will normally require conditions that are denaturing to the antigen. There are a large number of different protocols for covalently binding antibodies to a solid phase, but probably the easiest is coupling the antibodies to protein A or protein G beads. Another useful method is to couple the antibody to beads that have been chemically modified to have active groups that will covalently bind the antibody. Techniques for both methods are provided below.

After the preparation of the antibody–bead matrix, the antigen is bound to the antibodies, and contaminating macromolecules are removed by washing. In the third step, the antibody–antigen interaction is broken by treating the immune complexes with strong elution conditions, and the antigen is released into the eluate.

Immunoaffinity purification can be divided conveniently into three steps: (1) the preparation of the antibody column (p. 319), (2) the binding of the antigen to the antibody–bead matrix (p. 330), and (3) the elution of the antigen from the column (p. 335).

Affinity chromatography was first introduced by Cuatrecasas et al. (1968; for general considerations, see Jakoby and Wilchek 1974; Wilchek et al. 1984).

## Preparing antibody affinity columns

A number of methods can be used for covalent attachment of antibodies to solid-phase matrices. Among these, the most convenient rely on two strategies: (1) The most commonly used of these matrices are the protein A and protein G beads. Protein A or protein G binds specifically to the Fc domain of antibodies. After the antibody is bound, the interaction is stabilized by cross-linking the antibody to the protein A or protein G with a bifunctional coupling reagent. (2) The second class of coupling method directly couples the antibody to an activated bead. Beads are activated chemically to contain reactive groups. The beads are mixed with purified antibodies, which interact with the active sites to yield a covalent linkage.

In both cases, the beads for coupling can be purchased from commercial houses. Although activated beads can be prepared in the lab, excellent products can be purchased cheaply and used for these purposes. Hence, we recommend using commercial suppliers for the beads.

The advantages and disadvantages of both methods are summarized in Table 9.2 and are discussed in detail in each section below. If no background information argues against their use, the protein A or protein G columns should be tried first.

Table 9.2 *Methods for coupling antibodies to beads*

| Reagent | Advantages | Disadvantages | Variations | Coupling group on antibody |
|---|---|---|---|---|
| **Protein A** | Antibody oriented correctly; easy | Column retains capacity to bind extraneous antibody; expensive | Direct coupling with dimethyl pimelimidate | $-NH_2$ |
| **Protein G** | Antibody oriented correctly; easy | Column retains capacity to bind extraneous antibody; expensive | Direct coupling with dimethyl pimelimidate | $-NH_2$ |
| **Activated beads** | Cheap; no capacity to bind extraneous antibody | Antibody not oriented; Antibody often damaged by overcoupling | Carbonyldiimidazole | $-NH_2$ |
| | | | Cyanogen bromide | $-NH_2$ |
| | | | Hydroxysuccinimide | $-NH_2$ |
| | | | Iodoacetyl | $-SH_2$ |
| | | | Tresyl chloride | $-NH_2$, $-SH$ |

**Cautions:** Cyanogen bromide, dimethyl pimelimidate, hydroxysuccinimide, tresyl chloride, see Appendix IV.

# Preparing antibody/protein A or/protein G bead columns*



Protein A/protein G bead–antibody columns are one of the most versatile column matrices used for affinity purification of antigens. The columns are easy to prepare, and because the antibody molecules are bound to the matrix via the Fc domain, the antigen-binding site is oriented correctly for maximal interaction with the antigens. The techniques described below are designed for the purification of protein antigens, but analogous strategies could be adapted for any antigen.

Antibodies can be bound directly to protein A or protein G. The choice of either protein A or protein G beads is made based on the affinity of the antibodies for protein A or protein G. In general, we recommend protein A for mouse monoclonal antibodies from the $IgG_{2a}$, $IgG_{2b}$, and $IgG_3$ subclasses and protein G for $IgG_1$. Protein G is recommended for rat monoclonal antibodies. For polyclonal antibodies, protein A should be used for samples from rabbit, human, pig, guinea pig, dog, or cat, whereas protein G is recommended for mouse, rat, sheep, horse, donkey, cow, and goat polyclonal antibodies.

Once the antibodies are bound to the protein A or protein G beads, they are cross-linked to the matrix via a bifunctional coupling reagent. Any bifunctional reagent can be used, but most workers use dimethyl pimelimidate (DMP), which is cheap and easy to handle. Both coupling groups of DMP are identical and bind to free amino groups. Because the carbon backbone has a great deal of flexibility, most antibody/protein A or G pairs have reactive sites within a suitable distance to allow efficient coupling. In the rare cases where coupling is not efficient, other cross-linkers with carbon spacers of different lengths can be used (Table 9.3).

*We do not recommend binding the antibody to the beads by passing the antibody through a column containing the bead, because this will make a gradient of antibody concentrations. The top of the column will have a high concentration, and the bottom of the column will have a low concentration. To avoid this, the antibodies should be bound by mixing in a slurry.*

## Thinking ahead

The major hurdle in using antibody columns for affinity purification of proteins is the ability to elute the antigens from the column under mild enough conditions to retain protein structure and/or function. The ease of elution is determined by the types and number of bonds that hold the antigen to the antibody. Before investing time in building a large-scale column for purification, it is worthwhile to test all available antibody sources to choose the correct antibody to build the column.

## Needed solutions and reagents

Antibody source
Protein A or protein G beads
0.2 M Sodium borate (pH 9.0)
Dimethyl pimelimidate
0.2 M Ethanolamine (pH 8.0)
PBS
Laemmli sample buffer
Coomassie blue (p. 425)

## Special equipment

Rocking platform

*After Gersten and Marchalonis (1978); Schneider et al. (1982); Simanis and Lane (1985).

Table 9.3 *Commonly used cross-linkers*

| Cross-linker | Chemical Name | Homo- or hetero-bifunctional? | Reactive group | Binding group on protein | Photo-activatable | Spacer arm in A |
|---|---|---|---|---|---|---|
| DMA | Dimethyladipimidate | Homo | Imidoester | $-NH_2$ | N | 8.6 |
| DMP | Dimethyl pimelimidate | Homo | Imidoester | $-NH_2$ | N | 9.2 |
| DMS | Dimethylsuberimidate | Homo | Imidoester | $-NH_2$ | N | 11 |
| DSG | Disuccinimidyl glutarate | Homo | *N*-Hydroxysuccinimide | $-NH_2$ | N | 7.7 |
| DSS | Disuccinimidylsuberate | Homo | *N*-Hydroxysuccinimide | $-NH_2$ | N | 11.4 |
| BMH | Bismaleimido-hexane | Homo | maleimide | $-SH_2$ | N | |
| MBS | *m*-Maleimidobenzoyl-*N*-hydroxysuccinimide ester | Hetero | *N*-Hydroxysuccinimide, maleimide | $-NH_2$ $-SH_2$ | N | 9.9 |
| GMBS | *N*[γ-Maleimidobutyryloxy] succinimide ester | Hetero | *N*-Hydroxysuccinimide, maleimide | $-NH_2$ $-SH_2$ | N | 10.2 |
| SMCC | Succinimidyl 4-[*N*-maleimidomethyl]-cyclohexane-1-carboxylate | Hetero | *N*-Hydroxysuccinimide, maleimide | $-NH_2$ $-SH_2$ | N | 11.6 |
| SMPB | Succinimidyl 4-[*p*-maleimidophenyl]-butyrate | Hetero | *N*-Hydroxysuccinimide, maleimide | $-NH_2$ $-SH_2$ | N | 14.5 |
| Sulfo-MBS | *m*-Maleimidobenzoyl-*N*-hydroxysulfosuccinimide ester | Hetero | *N*-Hydroxysuccinimide, maleimide | $-NH_2$ $-SH_2$ | N | 9.9 |
| Sulfo-GMBS | N[γ-Maleimidobutyryloxy] sulfosuccinimide ester | Hetero | *N*-Hydroxysuccinimide, maleimide | $-NH_2$ $-SH_2$ | N | 10.2 |
| Sulfo-SMCC | Sulfosuccinimidyl 4-[*N*-maleimidomethyl]-cyclohexane-1-carboxylate | Hetero | *N*-Hydroxysuccinimide, maleimide | $-NH_2$ $-SH_2$ | N | 11.6 |
| Sulfo-SMPB | Sulfosuccinimidyl 4-[*p*-maleimidophenyl]-butyrate | Hetero | *N*-Hydroxysuccinimide, maleimide | $-NH_2$ $-SH_2$ | N | 14.5 |
| NHS-ASA | *N*-Hydroxysuccinimidyl-4-azidosalicylic acid | Hetero | *N*-Hydroxysuccinimide, photoactivatable hydroxyphenyl azide | $-NH_2$ $-NH_2$ | Y 265–275 nm | 8.0 |
| Sulfo-NHS-LC-ASA | Sulfosuccinimidyl[4-azidosalicylamido]-hexanoate | Hetero | *N*-Hydroxysuccinimide, photoactivatable hydroxyphenyl azide | $-NH_2$ $-NH_2$ | Y 265–275 nm | 18 |
| Sulfo-HSAB | *N*-Hydroxysulfosuccinimidyl-4-azidobenzoate | Hetero | *N*-Hydroxysuccinimide, photoactivatable phenyl azide | $-NH_2$ $-NH_2$ | Y 265–275 nm | 9.0 |
| Sulfo-SAPB | Sulfosuccinimidyl 4-[-*p*-azidophenyl]butyrate | Hetero | *N*-Hydroxysuccinimide, photoactivatable phenyl azide | $-NH_2$ $-NH_2$ | Y 265–275 nm | 12.8 |

**Caution:** Dimethyl pimelimidate, N-hydroxysuccinimide, maleimide, see Appendix IV.
Most of these cross-linkers are also available with cleavable linkages. Data primarily from the Pierce Chemical Catalog.

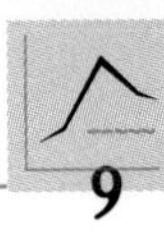


*If it is essential to know the exact concentration of antibodies on the beads. The antibody should be purified prior to binding to the column.*

## Caution

DMP, ethanolamine, SDS, see Appendix IV.

---

1. Bind the antibody to protein A or protein G beads. For general-purpose columns, bind approximately 2 mg of antibody per milliliter of wet beads. Mix the antibodies and protein A/G beads together in a loose slurry, with perhaps 1 ml of bead volume per 10 ml of total solution. Incubate at room temperature for 1 hour with gentle rocking.

   As discussed above, immunoaffinity columns are normally prepared with monoclonal antibodies or affinity-purified polyclonal antibodies. Antibodies can be added from any source including tissue-culture supernatant, ascites, or purified solutions, because the binding to the protein A/G beads will act as a purification step to remove other compounds in the storage buffer or to exchange buffers.

2. Wash the beads twice with 10 volumes of 0.2 M sodium borate (pH 9.0) by centrifugation at 3000*g* for 5 minutes or 10,000*g* for 30 seconds.

*Coupling with DMP must be performed above pH 8.3. If coupling is inefficient, check that the pH is above 8.3 after the addition of the DPM.*

3. Resuspend the beads in 10 volumes of 0.2 M sodium borate (pH 9.0) and remove the equivalent of 10 μl of beads. Add enough dimethyl pimelimidate (solid) to bring the final concentration to 20 mM.

4. Incubate for 30 minutes at room temperature with gentle mixing. Remove the equivalent of 10 μl of the coupled beads.

5. Stop the reaction by washing the beads once in 0.2 M ethanolamine (pH 8.0) and then incubate for 2 hours at room temperature in 0.2 M ethanolamine with gentle mixing.

*The affinity columns are stable for over 1 year when stored at 4°C in buffer containing Merthiolate.*

6. After the final wash, resuspend the beads in PBS with 0.01% Merthiolate.

7. Check the efficiency of coupling by boiling samples of beads taken before and after coupling in Laemmli sample buffer (p. 466). Run the equivalent of 1 μl and 9 μl of both samples on a 10% SDS-polyacrylamide gel (p. 413) and stain with Coomassie blue (p. 425). Good coupling is indicated by heavy-chain bands (55,000 MW) in the "before" but not in the "after" lanes (Fig. 9.1).

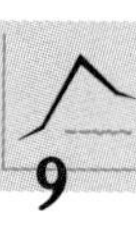

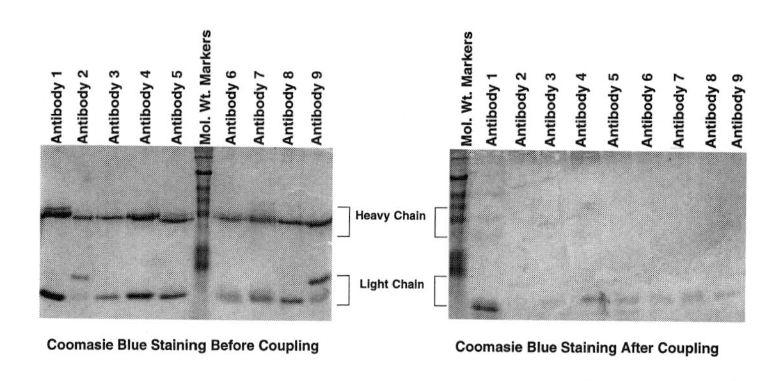


Figure 9.1
Gels for coupling efficiency.

**The beads are now ready for binding of the antigen** (p. 330).

## Common problems

A potential problem with this approach occurs when the antibodies have a free amino group as a key portion of the antigen-binding site. Here the coupling agent will bind to the antigen-binding site and block the interaction with the targeted antigen. This problem can be deduced when coupling is efficient and previous work has shown that the antibody is effective in immunoprecipitations, indicating that the coupling destroys the antibody's ability to bind the antigen. When this occurs, two approaches can be used. Lower amounts of the cross-linking agent can be used to reduce the number of interactions with the antigen recognition site. Alternatively, other bifunctional reagents can be used that do not rely on $-NH_2$ groups. These can be tested easily by coupling antibodies to protein A or G in small-scale procedures that resemble the techniques discussed below.

One experimental caution that should be added when considering the use of these types of affinity columns is that the protein A and protein G molecules remaining on the columns that are not coupled to antibodies will be available for interaction with extraneous antibodies in the antigen preparation. Therefore, when these columns are used with mammalian antigen sources, the columns also purify antibodies that are found in the antigen preparation. These problems will result in contaminating heavy- and light-chain polypeptides in the purified antigen preparations. These can be removed by starting with an antigen source that does not contain the antibodies or removing the contaminating antibodies by passing the preparations through protein A or G columns either before or after the antigen purification steps.

Occasionally the coupling reactions are not complete. This has been reported with older batches of DMP, DMP that has not been carefully stored, or when the antibody preparation contains other compounds that have free amino groups. Incomplete coupling is detected by finding small amounts of heavy chains in the coupling check (step 7). When this occurs, prewash the coupled beads with 100 mM glycine (pH 2.8) to remove any antibodies that are bound only by non-covalent binding to the protein A or G molecules. If the problem is severe, the entire coupling reaction will need to be repeated with controls to find the problem step. It has been our experience that problems normally result from batches of DMP that have been stored improperly or when the pH of the wash and coupling buffers is too low.

## Coupling with activated beads

COUPLING
BINDING, 330
ELUTING, 335

*The antibody preparations must not contain extraneous compounds in the buffer that will combine with reactive groups on the activated beads. Most often, the coupling reactions will target amino groups in the antibody (or thiol groups, if using tosyl chloride). If these compounds have been used during the purification, the antibody preparation should be extensively dialyzed against the binding buffer of 0.5 M sodium phosphate (pH 7.5).*

Another common method of covalently binding antibodies directly to a solid-phase matrix is to activate beads using any of a number of chemical agents and then bind purified antibodies to the beads (for general reviews, see Porath and Axén 1976; Scouten 1987). This approach offers several advantages. The beads normally can be activated in much harsher conditions than proteins can sustain, thus allowing the use of a range of activating protocols. In addition, many of the coupling methods yield a linkage that is stable to a wide range of denaturing conditions. Another advantage is that a number of activated beads are available commercially. Table 9.4 lists five of the commonly used activated beads and recommended commercial products. In general, the commercial beads provide a good source of activated bead for an immunoaffinity purification.

### Thinking ahead

The major hurdle in using antibody columns for affinity purification of proteins is the ability to elute the antigens from the column under mild enough conditions to retain protein structure and/or function. The ease of elution is determined by the types and number of bonds that hold the antigen to the antibody. Before investing the time in building a large-scale column for purification, it will be worthwhile to test all available antibody sources to choose the correct antibody to build the column.

### Needed solutions and reagents

Purified antibodies
0.5 mM Sodium phosphate (pH 7.5)
1 M Sodium chloride, 0.05 M sodium phosphate (pH 7.5)
100 mM Ethanolamine (pH 7.5)
PBS

### Special equipment

Rocking platform

### Caution

Ethanolamine, SDS, see Appendix IV.

1. Prepare a solution of antibody at the desired concentration in 0.5 M sodium phosphate (pH 7.5). Save a small sample to determine the binding efficiency. The amount of antibody to be coupled will vary depending on the individual experiment. For most purposes, 10 mg of antibody per milliliter of beads will yield a high-capacity column.

2. Add the activated beads prepared as described by the manufacturer.

3. Mix gently overnight at room temperature on a rocker.

4. Wash the beads twice with 0.5 M sodium phosphate (pH 7.5). Save the supernatant from the overnight binding. Compare the amount of protein from the "before" and "after" samples of the binding buffers.

5. Wash the beads once with 1 M sodium chloride, 0.05 M sodium phosphate (pH 7.5).

6. Add 10 volumes of 100 mM ethanolamine (pH 7.5). Incubate at room temperature for 4 hours to overnight with gentle mixing.

7. Wash twice with PBS. Add Merthiolate to 0.01%.

   The beads can be stored at 4°C, where they will be stable for several months.

**The beads are now ready for binding of the antigen** (p. 330).

## Common problems

Achieving efficient coupling of antibodies to activated beads is a simple task. However, retaining antibody activity is often difficult. Most of the loss of activity either is due to overcoupling of the antibodies to the beads or results when coupling occurs in the antigen recognition site of the antibody. Either of these outcomes can be seen by a dramatic loss of binding capacity of the antibody–bead matrix compared to the capacity of a similar amount of uncoupled antibody. Retaining 10–50% of the binding activity is common and should be considered a good level of activity. If the activity of the antibodies has been lowered drastically below this during coupling, three approaches can be used to retain antibody activity.

First, an important method to limit inactivation is to stop the reaction before extensive coupling has occurred. The rate of coupling can be determined in an initial experiment. Stop the reaction when no more than 50% of the antibodies are bound. Unbound antibodies are not harmed and can be reused in other experiments. Stopping the reaction early limits the possibilities of each antibody being coupled through many different sites. The correct time to stop the coupling reaction can be determined by a simple time course on small-scale reactions, measuring the amount of unbound antibody by SDS-polyacrylamide gel electrophoresis and Coomassie blue staining of the heavy- and light-chain bands.

A second method to counter overcoupling will be to adjust the pH of the reaction to slow the speed of coupling. Most coupling methods rely on linking through amino groups on the antibody, and the reactivity of amino groups is sensitive to pH. If the antibodies are bound below the pK of the amino groups, most of the amino groups will be protonated and will not be available for coupling at any one time, thus limiting the rate of overcoupling. To help with this problem, the method described below uses a neutral pH. If this still results in overcoupling, a slightly lower pH can be tried. The correct pH to use will have to be determined by empirical tests, as the desired conditions will vary from antibody to antibody. Use decreasing increments of half-pH units to test the new conditions. On the other hand, if the coupling gives too low a yield, raise the pH of the buffer or allow the coupling to proceed longer. For pH values above 8.2, use 0.5 M carbonate buffer in place of the phosphate.

A third method to reduce the problems of overcoupling is to include other amino groups in the coupling reaction with the antibody. In preliminary experiments, test a range of concentrations of small molecules with primary amino groups to block the coupling of the antibody to the beads. The two most commonly used compounds are ethanolamine and glycine. Choose a concentration of the blocking agent that allows only 10% of the antibody to bind during the coupling step. For a reasonable starting point, we would suggest that the final antibody concentration not exceed 10 mg/ml of wet beads.

Finally, it may be that your antibody has an amino group within the antigen-combining site. This site will be particularly sensitive to inactivation following binding to most activated beads. If antigen-binding activity is continually lost in the coupling reaction, an alternative would be to use protein A or protein G beads and linkage with bifunctional cross-linking reagents that do not rely on amino groups.

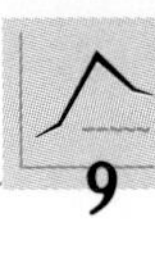


Table 9.4 *Activated beads*

| Coupling mechanism | Binding group on protein | Stability of final linkage | Recommended matrices | Commercial examples |
|---|---|---|---|---|
| **Carbonyldiimidozole** | –$NH_2$ | Avoid pH > 10 | Agarose | CM Bio-Gel A Gel (Bio-Rad)<br>ECH Sepharose 4B (Pharmacia) |
| | | | Cross-linked agarose | Reacti-Gel 6X (Pierce Chemical) |
| | | | Polyacrylic | Reacti-Gel GF-2000 (Pierce Chemical) |
| **Cyanogen bromide** | –$NH_2$ | Good, some leaching | Agarose | CNBr-activated Sepharose (Pharmacia) |
| **Hydroxysuccinimide** | –$NH_2$ | Excellent | Cross-linked agarose | Affigel 10 (Bio-Rad)<br>HiTrap NHS-Activated (Pharmacia) |
| | | | Polyacrylic | AffiPrep 10 (Bio-Rad) |
| **Iodoacetyl** | –$SH_2$ | Excellent | Cross-linked agarose | SulfoLink (Pierce Chemical) |
| | | | Polyacrylic | UltraLink Iodoacetyl (Pierce Chemical |
| **Tresyl chloride** | –$NH_2$<br>–$SH_2$ | Excellent | Cross-linked agarose | Affinica Tresyl (Schleicher & Schuell)<br>Tresyl activated agarose (Pierce Chemical) |

**Caution:** Cyanogen bromide, hydroxysuccinimide, tresyl chloride, see Appendix IV.

## Binding antigens to the antibody-bead matrix

Several different approaches can be taken to allow efficient binding of antigens to immunoaffinity columns. Because the antibody is covalently coupled to the beads and not in solution, the time required for the antibody–bead/antigen interaction to reach completion will be considerably longer than when both the antibody and the antigen are free in solution. Therefore, the binding protocol should maximize the degree of interaction. The two methods we recommend are binding in a constantly mixing slurry of antibody–beads with the antigen solution or by passing the antigen solution down an antibody–bead column, keeping the antigen in contact with the antibody for as long as possible. Unless there are problems, binding in the column should be used as a first choice. If background problems become evident, try the binding in solution protocols. Several small-scale columns can be used to determine the best conditions for binding and collecting the antigen.

### *Affinity*

Although the exact affinity of an antibody for an antigen can be calculated, for most work the crucial criterion is whether the antibodies will remove the antigen from solution quantitatively. The easiest method to test this is to set up small-scale reactions and examine the first wash buffer for the presence of the antigen. If the antibody–bead matrix does not remove most of the antigen within 1–2 hours, several changes in the experimental design may help. The amount of bound antigen may be increased by using higher amounts of antibodies on the beads, by increasing the number of beads, or by increasing the amount of time for binding. Unfortunately, all of these conditions raise the nonspecific background, so a compromise normally results in the highest yields with the lowest acceptable background. On the other hand, using high-affinity antibodies solves the problem of efficiently collecting the antigen. Consequently, they can be used in dilute solutions, at relatively lower concentrations, and for shorter times—all conditions that lead to lower backgrounds.

### *Titrating*

A titration should be performed as a first step in estimating the ratio of column matrix needed to bind a given amount of antigen. This can be handled in a manner similar to immunoprecipitations (see Chapter 7), where an equal volume of the antibody–bead matrix is added to samples containing increasing concentrations of the antigen. The slurry is mixed at 4°C for 1 hour and then processed as for a standard immunoprecipitation. This yields a rough idea of the volume of column matrix needed to collect the desired amount of antigen. If the supernatants from the binding reaction are assayed for the presence of the antigen, the extent of antigen depletion also can be determined.

## Binding in the column

COUPLING, 319

BINDING

ELUTING, 335

The simplest method to bind the antigen to the antibody–bead matrix is to collect the beads in a column and pass the antigen solution down the column. The immobilized antibody captures the antigen as it flows past and holds it until this interaction is broken in the elution step. The efficiency of this method depends on the contact time between the immobilized antibody and the antigen. Therefore, the time of antigen–antibody interaction is extended by using low flow rates.

### Thinking ahead

Before beginning, consider the type and size of the column for collecting the beads. The profile of elution from the column will be sharper if the bed-volume of the beads is wider and shallower than by choosing a narrower and taller size. Also, this arrangement makes it easier to remove the beads if they will be stored in another vessel before their next use. The disadvantage of a too-wide column is the disturbance of the beads while changing buffers for elution.

### Needed solutions

PBS

### Special equipment

Simple chromatography setup

1. Transfer the antibody beads to a suitable column. Wash with 20 bed-volumes of PBS.

2. Apply the antigen solution to the column. Pass the solution through the column with a flow rate of approximately 1 ml/hr per each 1 ml of column volume. This is easiest to control using a pump.

3. Wash the column with 20 bed-volumes of binding buffer.

**The column is now ready for more extensive washing or for elution (p. 335).**

## Common problems

The single biggest problem for this approach is nonspecific binding of proteins to the column. These proteins appear in the eluate and lower the efficiency of the purification. Both the matrix itself and the antibody–matrix complex are surfaces that bind nonspecifically to proteins in your antigen solution. Although these interactions are normally much weaker than the antibody–antigen interaction, the vast excess of the nonspecific proteins in the antigen solution means that there is an inherent background in this procedure. Keeping nonspecific binding to a minimum can be achieved by several approaches.

First, as with all affinity column purifications, the amount of matrix that is used should be adjusted to a level just above saturation. Keeping the volume of the antibody–bead matrix to a minimum keeps the nonspecific background as low as possible. Note, however, that the volume of the antibody–bead matrix needed to capture the bulk of your antigen varies on the flow rate. Slower flow rates use the capacity of the column more effectively, as they allow more time for each antibody-combining site to be filled with an antigen.

A second approach is to lower the amount of nonspecific binding to the column. Many of the proteins that stick to a column matrix are ones that are partially or fully denatured. When preparing the antigen solution, use as little mechanical stress as possible. Avoid excess contact with the air. A good approach to lowering nonspecific binding in the antibody column is to pass the antigen solution through a volume of uncoupled agarose beads equivalent to or larger than the volume of the antibody–bead matrix that will be used. Another source of nonspecific binding comes from small particulate debris that gets caught in the column matrix. Centrifugation of the antigen solution at 100,000*g* for 30 minutes clears most large aggregates from the preparation.

A third approach to lowering the background is to wash the column with buffers that remove nonspecific proteins. Any buffer that does not interfere with the antigen–antibody interaction can be used to remove nonspecific binding. See p. 336 for discussions of appropriate wash buffers.

# Binding in suspension: Antibody-bead slurries

COUPLING, 319
BINDING
ELUTING, 335

A rapid method for capturing an antigen on the antibody–bead matrix is to mix the antigen solution with the beads and rotate or rock the slurry. This method allows the maximum contact between the antigen and the immobilized antibody and so is the quickest method to push the binding reaction to completion. After the binding reaction has been completed, the slurry is passed into a column for collection of the beads and elution of the antigen. This approach gives very good control of the time of interaction and allows the best chance to use the antibody-binding capacity of the matrix to the fullest. It is a little more cumbersome to use than the column capture method described above (p. 331), primarily because of the difficulties of moving the slurry to the column. One other minor disadvantage is that the mixing increases the amount of denaturation of the proteins in the antigen solution and, therefore, the backgrounds may be slightly higher with this approach.

## Thinking ahead

Before beginning, consider the type and size of column for collecting the beads. The profile of elution from the column will be sharper if the bed-volume of the beads is wider and shallower rather than narrower and taller. Also, this arrangement makes it easier to remove the beads if they will be stored in another vessel before their next use. The disadvantage of a too-wide column is the disturbance of the beads while changing buffers for elution.

## Needed solutions

Binding buffer (commonly PBS)

## Special equipment

Rocking platform
Simple chromatography setup

1. Add the antibody–bead matrix to the antigen preparation. The volume of beads to be added should be determined in preliminary test experiments and should be adjusted to a volume that is just sufficient to remove all the antigen in the desired time period of the binding reaction.

   The final bead concentration should be approximately 1 ml of wet bead volume to 10–20 ml of buffer.

2. Incubate the bead–antigen slurry at 4°C with a gentle mixing action. Common methods for mixing include rocking in a closed container or swirling on a platform shaker. The incubation time should be determined in the preliminary bead titration experiments described in step 1. A recommended time to begin these studies would be 2 hours.

3. Transfer the bead slurry into an appropriately sized column. Pour the slurry into the column and use the antigen buffer to rinse the beads from the mixing container. Collect these washes in the column.

4. Wash the beads with 20 bed-volumes of the binding buffer.

**The column is now ready for more extensive washing or for elution** (p. 335).

## Common problems

The single biggest problem for this approach is nonspecific binding of proteins to the beads. These proteins appear in the eluate and lower the efficiency of the purification. Both the matrix itself and the antibody–matrix complex are surfaces that bind nonspecifically to proteins in your antigen solution. Although these interactions are normally much weaker than the antibody–antigen interaction, the vast excess of the nonspecific proteins in the starting antigen preparation means that there is an inherent background in this procedure. Keeping nonspecific binding to a minimum can be helped by several approaches.

First, as with all affinity purifications, the amount of matrix that is used should be adjusted to a level just above saturation. Keeping the volume of the antibody–bead matrix to a minimum keeps the nonspecific background as low as possible. This amount can be determined by doing test titrations of different volumes of antibody–bead matrix and checking for the amount of the antigen captured by the various volumes of beads.

A second approach is to lower the amount of nonspecific binding to the column. Many of the proteins that stick to a column matrix are ones that are partially or fully denatured. When preparing the antigen solution, use as little mechanical stress as possible. The mechanical motion used to keep the beads in suspension during the binding stage should be as gentle as possible. Avoid excess contact with the air. Another source of nonspecific binding comes from small particulate debris that gets caught in the column matrix after the beads are transferred to the column. Before adding the beads to the antigen solution, centrifuge the antigen solution at 100,000*g* for 30 minutes to clear most large aggregates from the preparation.

A third approach to lowering the background is to wash the beads in the column after collection with buffers that remove nonspecific proteins. Any buffer that does not interfere with the antigen–antibody interaction can be used to remove nonspecific binding. See p. 336 for discussions of appropriate wash buffers.

## Eluting antigen from immunoaffinity columns

COUPLING, 319
BINDING, 330
ELUTING

The actual elution of an antigen from an immunoaffinity column is quick and easy. Most of the work is spent in designing and testing the conditions used to achieve an effective elution. Three types of elution are possible. The antigen–antibody interactions can be broken by (1) treating with harsh conditions, (2) adding a saturating amount of a small compound that mimics the binding site, and/or (3) treating with an agent that induces an allosteric change that releases the antigen.

The most commonly used elution procedure relies on breaking the bonds between the antibody and antigen. The elutions may be harsh, denaturing the antibody and the antigen, or mild, leaving both the antigen and antibody in active states.

The relative harshness of the elution conditions depends on the antibody in use. If affinity-purified polyclonal antibodies are being used, the conditions for elution of the antigen will be identical to those used to purify the antibodies. Otherwise, the conditions for elution can be determined only by empirical tests. Developing the elution conditions is done by testing a series of buffers. Commonly used elution conditions are listed in Table 9.5. Strategies for these types of elutions are discussed on p. 336.

When using an antibody raised against a synthetic peptide, the antigen can sometimes be eluted by adding a large molar excess of the synthetic peptide. As the antibody–antigen interaction dissociates, the rebinding of the antigen to the column is inhibited by binding to the excess of the peptide. Although this approach is very attractive for a number of reasons, including the mild elution conditions, getting efficient elution is often difficult. Critical variables include the rate of dissociation of the antigen–antibody binding and the relative affinity of antibody for the peptide compared to the whole antigen. Because the antibodies have been raised against the peptide, they usually bind efficiently to the peptide, so the major problem normally is the off-rate. For elution, the most effective protocols place the peptide in contact with the antigen–antibody column until a new equilibrium is reached. With high-affinity interactions, this takes a significant length of time or an enormous excess of peptide. To test these elution conditions, add increasing amounts of peptide to small columns. Run the elution buffer as slowly as practical to increase the time of peptide contact with the column. If the peptide by itself is not sufficient to give efficient elution, combine a high concentration of the peptide with different elution buffer conditions. These buffers and elution strategies are discussed on p. 336. The conditions from small tests can then be scaled up for elution.

A third method for elution, which can be used only for certain proteins, relies on allosteric changes induced by treating the antigen–antibody column with appropriate ligands. These types of allosteric changes might include treating the antigens with ATP or small cofactors that induce allosteric changes. Antibodies that recognize these allosteric changes or bind to one member of a protein–protein complex that is dissociated by allosteric changes can be used to prepare pure preparations of proteins. Because these types of elution protocols vary from antigen to antigen, they are not discussed in any more detail here, but they can provide an effective and elegant method of elution.

Table 9.5 *Elution reagents*

| Reagent | Suggested buffers | Pre-elution wash | Collection buffer | Column reusable? |
|---|---|---|---|---|
| **High pH** | 100 mM triethylamine, pH 11.5 | 10 mM phosphate, pH 8.0 | 1 M phosphate, pH 6.8 | Often |
| | 100 mM phosphate acid, pH 12.5 | 10 mM phosphate, pH 8.0 | 1 M phosphate, pH 6.8 | Occasionally |
| **Low pH** | 100 mM glycine, pH 2.5 | 10 mM phosphate, pH 6.8 | 1 M phosphate, pH 8.0 | Often |
| | 100 mM glycine, pH 1.8 | 10 mM phosphate, pH 6.8 | 1 M phosphate, pH 8.0 | Occasionally |
| **High salt** | 5 M LiCl, 10 mM phosphate, pH. 7.2 | 10 mM phosphate, pH 7.2 | None required | Often |
| | 3.5 M $MgCl_2$, 10 mM phosphate, pH 7.2 | 10 mM phosphate, pH 7.2 | None required | Often |
| **Ionic detergents** | 1% SDS | Neutral wash buffer | None required | No |
| | 1% DOC | Neutral wash buffer | None required | Seldom |
| **Dissociating agents** | 2 M urea | Neutral wash buffer | None required | Occasionally |
| | 8 M urea | Neutral wash buffer | None required | No |
| | 2 M guanidine HCl | Neutral wash buffer | None required | Seldom |
| **Chaotropic agents** | 3 M thiocyanate | Neutral wash buffer | None required | Seldom |
| **Organic solvents** | 10% dioxane | Neutral wash buffer | None required | Often |
| | 50% ethylene glycol, pH 11.5 | Neutral wash buffer | None required | Often |
| | 50% ethylene glycol pH 8.0 | Neutral wash buffer | None required | Often |
| **Water** | | Neutral wash buffer | None required | Often |

**Caution:** DOC, ethylene glycol, guanidine HCl, lithium chloride, SDS, triethylamine, see Appendix IV.

*If you are experienced with protein chromatography, you may wish to develop the column using a gradient of increasingly harsh elution conditions rather than using the step gradient suggested here.*

## Thinking ahead

The correct conditions for elution are the most difficult point to determine for this procedure. More time spent on testing and adjusting these conditions will pay off in the ability to achieve a sharp elution profile and cleaner antigen preparations.

## Needed solutions

Pre-elution buffer (see Table 9.5)
Elution buffer (see Table 9.5)
Neutralizing buffer (see Table 9.5)

## Special equipment

Simple chromatography setup
Dialysis tubing and setup

## Caution

Deoxycholine, ethylene glycol, triethylamine, see Appendix IV.

1. Change the buffer in the column to the pre-elution buffer by washing with 20 column bed-volumes. See Table 9.5, p. 336, for suggested pre-elution buffer.

2. Using a stepwise elution, sequentially pass 0.5 bed-volumes of the elution buffer (Table 9.5) through the column. Collect each fraction in separate tubes (Fig. 9.2). If either high or low pH is used to elute the column, the collection tubes should contain 0.1 bed-volume of neutralizing buffer (see Table 9.5).

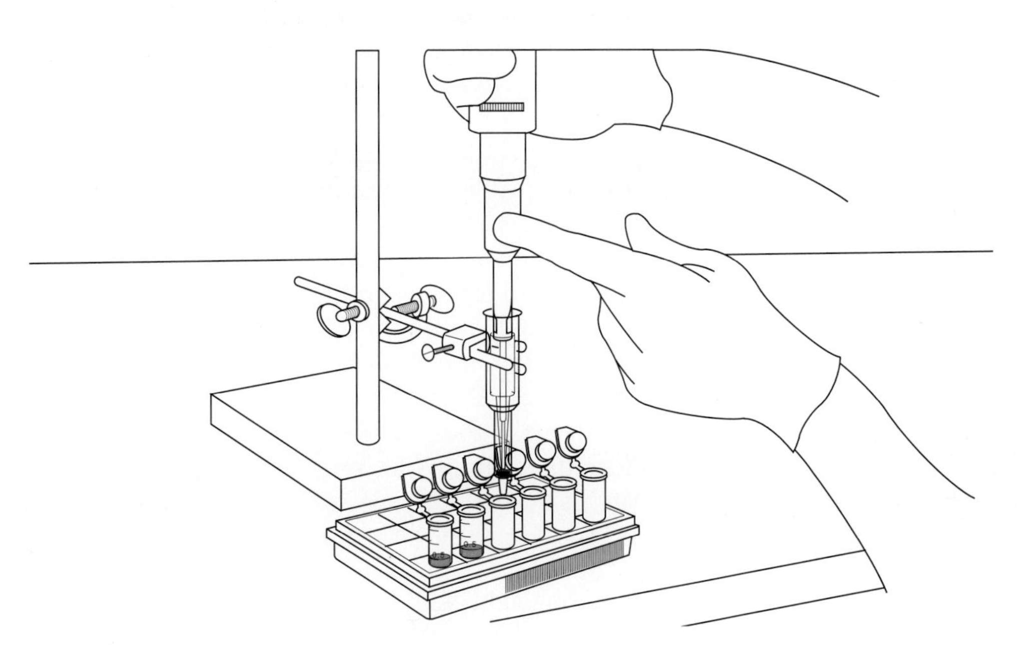

Figure 9.2
Stepwise development of immunoaffinity column.

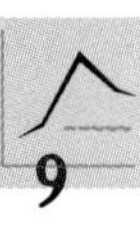


**3** Check each tube for the presence of the antigen. Combine tubes with high concentrations.

Depending on how the antigen will be used, it may be necessary to dialyze the resulting eluted proteins to desalt or change the buffer.

**4** Return the column to the starting buffer by passing 20 column volumes through the matrix. Add 0.01% Merthiolate for long-term storage (4°C).

## Strategies for testing elution conditions

Developing the best elution conditions is an empirical task; potential elution buffers are tested on small-scale columns to determine the proper conditions. There are no good shortcuts nor any guaranteed useful buffers. The best strategy is to test as many antibodies and elution conditions as possible.

An ideal elution profile yields a sharp peak with complete release of the antigen following treatment with a single buffer. Three general points should be considered prior to choosing an appropriate starting point. First, for what techniques will the antigen be used? For many protein chemistry techniques, the antigens will not need to be native, whereas for most enzymatic studies, the elution condition should be as gentle as possible. Second, will the antibody column be reused? If so, mild conditions should be used. Third, make sure the last wash buffer (called the pre-elution buffer in this chapter) is compatible with the elution buffer. For example, the buffering capacity of the pre-elution buffer should be low enough that a sharp change in pH follows the front of the elution buffer.

- If trying for the gentlest elution conditions, start with acid conditions first, then check basic elution buffers. If these conditions do not elute the antigen, try others. A general order to check the various conditions is: acid, pH 3–1.5; base, pH 10–12.5; $MgCl_2$, 3–5 M; LiCl, 5–10 M; water; ethylene glycol, 25–50%; dioxane, 5–20%; thiocyanate, 1–5 M; guanidine, 2–5 M; urea, 2–8 M; SDS, 0.5–2%.
- Use combinations of eluting agents. Antigens that are difficult to elute under the standard elution conditions normally are held by several different types of bonds. Using a combination of several elution conditions can be effective in overcoming these problems.
- If the antigen is difficult to elute under simple conditions, changing antibodies may be easier than testing all conditions.
- Elutions normally are more effective when columns are used rather than batches. As the buffer passes down the column, any antigen–antibody interaction that breathes will be washed away from the remaining antibodies and cannot be rebound. In batch conditions, this is not true. Consequently, batch elutions normally require harsher conditions to elute antigens than column elutions.

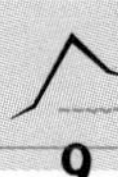


- Try gradient elutions to generate a sharp peak of released antigen.
- Avoid dithiothreitol and other reducing agents, as they will break the disulfide linkages between the heavy and light chains.
- While checking different elution conditions, consider any buffers that fail to elute the antigen as good candidates for wash buffers.
- Some noneluting buffers may, in fact, drive the antibody–antigen equilibrium toward complex formation. For example, high-salt conditions favor hydrophobic interactions. These conditions could be used to make collecting the antigen on the antibody–matrix easier.

# Variations on immunoaffinity purification

## Preparation of affinity-purified antibodies

When purified antigens are covalently bound to beads, immunoaffinity purification techniques can be used to isolate antibodies that are specific for the antigen. This is normally used with polyclonal antibodies that have multiple activities against both your antigen and contaminating antigens. The problems of recognizing multiple antigens can confound many immunochemical techniques. This problem can be solved by purifying the antibodies that are specific for your antigen.

Another application for immunoaffinity purification of antibodies is to concentrate specific antibodies. This is most often used when antipeptide antibodies are prepared. These antibodies are occasionally only usable after affinity purification.

The procedure to purify antibodies is discussed in more detail in Chapter 4, but the methodology and theory are identical to the steps described above, with the antigen being covalently attached to the beads and the antibodies bound and eluted as for antigens.

## References

Cuatrecasas P., Wilchek M., and Anfinsen C.B. 1968. Selective enzyme purification by affinity chromatography. *Proc. Natl. Acad. Sci.* **61:** 636–643.

Gersten D.M. and Marchalonis J.J. 1978. A rapid, novel method for the solid-phase derivatization of IgG antibodies for immune-affinity chromatography. *J. Immunol. Methods* **24:** 305–309.

Jakoby W.B. and Wilchek M., eds. 1974. *Methods in enzymology,* vol. 34: *Affinity techniques* (part B): *Enzyme purification.* Academic Press, San Diego.

Porath J. and Axén R. 1976. Immobilization of enzymes to agar, agarose, and sephadex supports. *Methods Enzymol.* **44:** 19–45.

Schneider C., Newman R.A., Sutherland D.R., Asser U., and Greaves M.F. 1982. A one-step purification of membrane proteins using a high efficiency immunomatrix. *J. Biol. Chem.* **257:** 10766–10769.

Scouten W.H. 1987. A survey of enzyme coupling techniques. *Methods Enzymol.* **135:** 30–65.

Simanis V. and Lane D.P. 1985. An immunoaffinity purification procedure for SV40 large T antigen. *Virology* **144:** 88–100.

Wilchek M., Miron T., and Kohn J. 1984. Affinity chromatography (review). *Methods Enzymol.* **104:** 3–55.

# Immunoaffinity purification

## Summary

Purification factor is 1,000- to 10,000-fold
Rapid antigen purification, columns often reusable
Yields purified antigen
Not useful for quantitation
Efficiency depends on antigen concentration and antibody affinity
Needs moderate affinity antibody

## Caution

DMP, ethanolamine, SDS, see Appendix IV.

1. Bind the antibody to protein A or protein G beads. For general-purpose columns, bind approximately 2 mg of monoclonal antibody or affinity-purified polyclonal antibodies per milliliter of wet beads. Mix the antibodies and protein A or G beads together in a loose slurry, using about 1 ml of bead volume per 10 ml of total solution. Incubate at room temperature for 1 hour with gentle rocking.

2. Wash the beads twice with 10 volumes of 0.2 M sodium borate (pH 9.0) by centrifugation at 3000*g* for 2 minutes or 10,000*g* for 30 seconds.

3. Resuspend the beads in 10 volumes of 0.2 M sodium borate (pH 9.0) and remove and place aside the equivalent of 10 μl of wet bead volume. Add enough dimethyl pimelimidate (solid) to the total bead slurry to bring the final concentration to 20 mM.

4. Incubate for 30 minutes at room temperature with gentle mixing. Remove the equivalent of 10 μl of the coupled beads.

5. Stop the reaction by washing the beads once in 0.2 M ethanolamine (pH 8.0) and then incubate for 2 hours at room temperature in 0.2 M ethanolamine with gentle mixing. The beads can be stored at this stage by washing in PBS and storing in 0.01% Merthiolate in PBS.

6. Check the efficiency of coupling by boiling samples of beads taken before and after coupling in Laemmli sample buffer (p. 465). Run the equivalent of 1 μl and 9 μl of both samples on a 10% SDS-polyacrylamide gel (p. 413) and stain with Coomassie blue (p. 425). Good coupling is indicated by heavy-chain bands (55,000 MW) in the "before" but not in the "after" lanes.

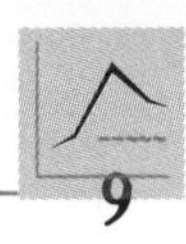

7. Transfer the antibody beads to a suitable column. Rinse the mixing chamber with PBS to collect the remaining beads. If possible, use only as much antibody–bead matrix as needed to bind the total amount of antigen in the preparation.

8. Wash the column with 20 bed-volumes of buffer used to prepare the antigen.

9. Apply the antigen solution to the column. Pass the solution through the column with a flow rate of approximately 1 ml/hour per each 1 ml of column volume. This is easiest to control using a pump.

10. Wash the column with 20 bed-volumes of binding buffer.

11. Change the buffer in the column to the pre-elution buffer by washing with 20 column bed-volumes. See Table 9.5, p. 336, for suggested pre-elution buffer.

12. Using a stepwise elution, sequentially pass 0.5 bed-volume of the elution buffer (Table 9.5) through the column. Collect each fraction in separate tubes. If either high or low pH is used to elute the column, the collection tubes should contain 0.1 bed-volume of neutralizing buffer (see Table 9.5).

13. Check each tube for the presence of the antigen. Combine tubes with high concentrations.

    Depending on how the antigen will be used, it may be necessary to dialyze the resulting eluted proteins to change the buffer.

14. Return the column to the starting buffer by passing 20 column volumes through the matrix. Add 0.01% Merthiolate for long-term storage (4°C).

# Tagging Proteins

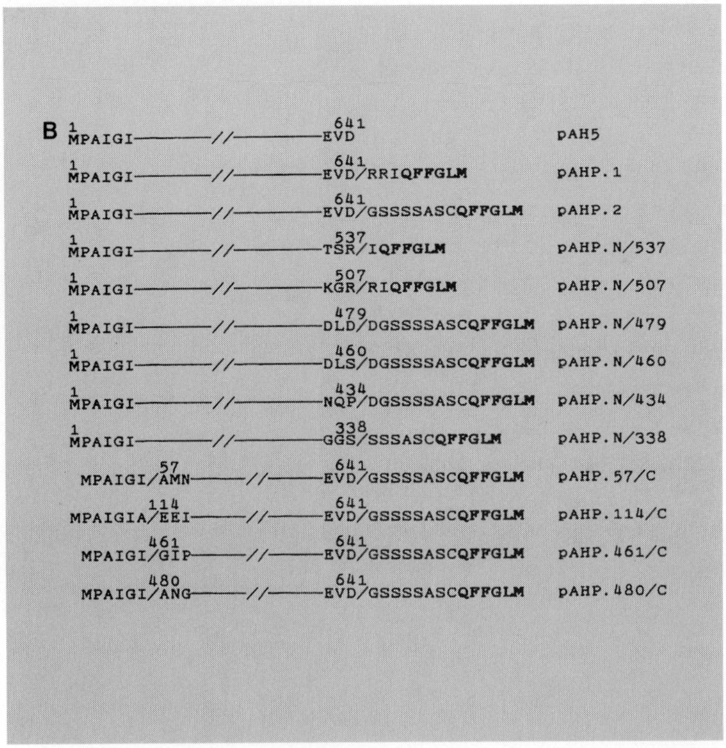

| B | | |
|---|---|---|
| 1 MPAIGI———//——— | 641 EVD | pAH5 |
| 1 MPAIGI———//——— | 641 EVD/RRI**QFFGLM** | pAHP.1 |
| 1 MPAIGI———//——— | 641 EVD/GSSSSASC**QFFGLM** | pAHP.2 |
| 1 MPAIGI———//——— | 537 TSR/I**QFFGLM** | pAHP.N/537 |
| 1 MPAIGI———//——— | 507 KGR/RI**QFFGLM** | pAHP.N/507 |
| 1 MPAIGI———//——— | 479 DLD/DGSSSSASC**QFFGLM** | pAHP.N/479 |
| 1 MPAIGI———//——— | 460 DLS/DGSSSSASC**QFFGLM** | pAHP.N/460 |
| 1 MPAIGI———//——— | 434 NQP/DGSSSSASC**QFFGLM** | pAHP.N/434 |
| 1 MPAIGI———//——— | 338 GGS/SSSASC**QFFGLM** | pAHP.N/338 |
| MPAIGI/AMN (57)——//—— | 641 EVD/GSSSSASC**QFFGLM** | pAHP.57/C |
| MPAIGIA/EEI (114)——//—— | 641 EVD/GSSSSASC**QFFGLM** | pAHP.114/C |
| MPAIGI/GIP (461)——//—— | 641 EVD/GSSSSASC**QFFGLM** | pAHP.461/C |
| MPAIGI/ANG (480)——//—— | 641 EVD/GSSSSASC**QFFGLM** | pAHP.480/C |

From Munro S., and Pelham H.R.B. 1984. Use of peptide tagging to detect proteins expressed from cloned genes: deletion mapping functional domains of *Drosophila* hsp70. *EMBO J.* **3:** 3087–3093. (Reprinted with permission [copyright Oxford University Press].)

Fig. 1. Plasmid structures....(B) Structure of proteins encoded by the various plasmids. Numbers refer to residues of wild-type hsp70; the sequences acound the junctions are shown. A, Ala; C, Cys; D, Asp; E, Glu; F, Phe; G, Gly; I, Ile; K, Lys; L, Leu; M, Met; N, Asn; P, Pro; Q, Gln; R, Arg; S, Ser; T, Thr; V, Val.

The concept of fusing two coding regions together to create a new protein with properties of both starting polypeptides has been a common idea since the beginning of expression cloning. The work in this figure provided a variation on this theme that took advantage of the detailed knowledge of the structure of epitopes from the c-myc protein and created new proteins that could be recognized by already existing antibodies. This approach has now become a staple of molecular cloning. Any newly identified coding region can be recognized by well-characterized antibodies by adding an epitope sequence to the polypeptide. This idea is further enhanced by the possibility of fusing other interesting protein or functional domains to antigens under study. One of the most widely used variations is the fusion to GST, which normally allows the synthesis of a soluble protein in *E. coli* that can be easily purified through binding to glutathione beads. Many other valuable purification tags are in common use today. These approaches have been augmented by the more recent use of GFP fusions, which now allow protein localization to be determined by nonimmunological detection methods. The addition of this approach promises to provide another new avenue to broaden the use of protein tags.

Proteins can be tagged using recombinant DNA techniques to allow their ready purification and their specific detection in different host cell systems. These include tags designed to help specifically with detection (such as green fluorescent protein tags) or with purification (such as the His tags and glutathione-*S*-transferase tags). Epitope tags—short peptide sequences to which strong and specific antibodies have already been produced—can be used for detection and purification using all of the immunological methods described in this book. This chapter describes the different available tag systems, their advantages and disadvantages, and how to choose the right tag for your experiment. The tagging concept is exceptionally versatile and allows many novel approaches for determining protein regulation, structure, and function.

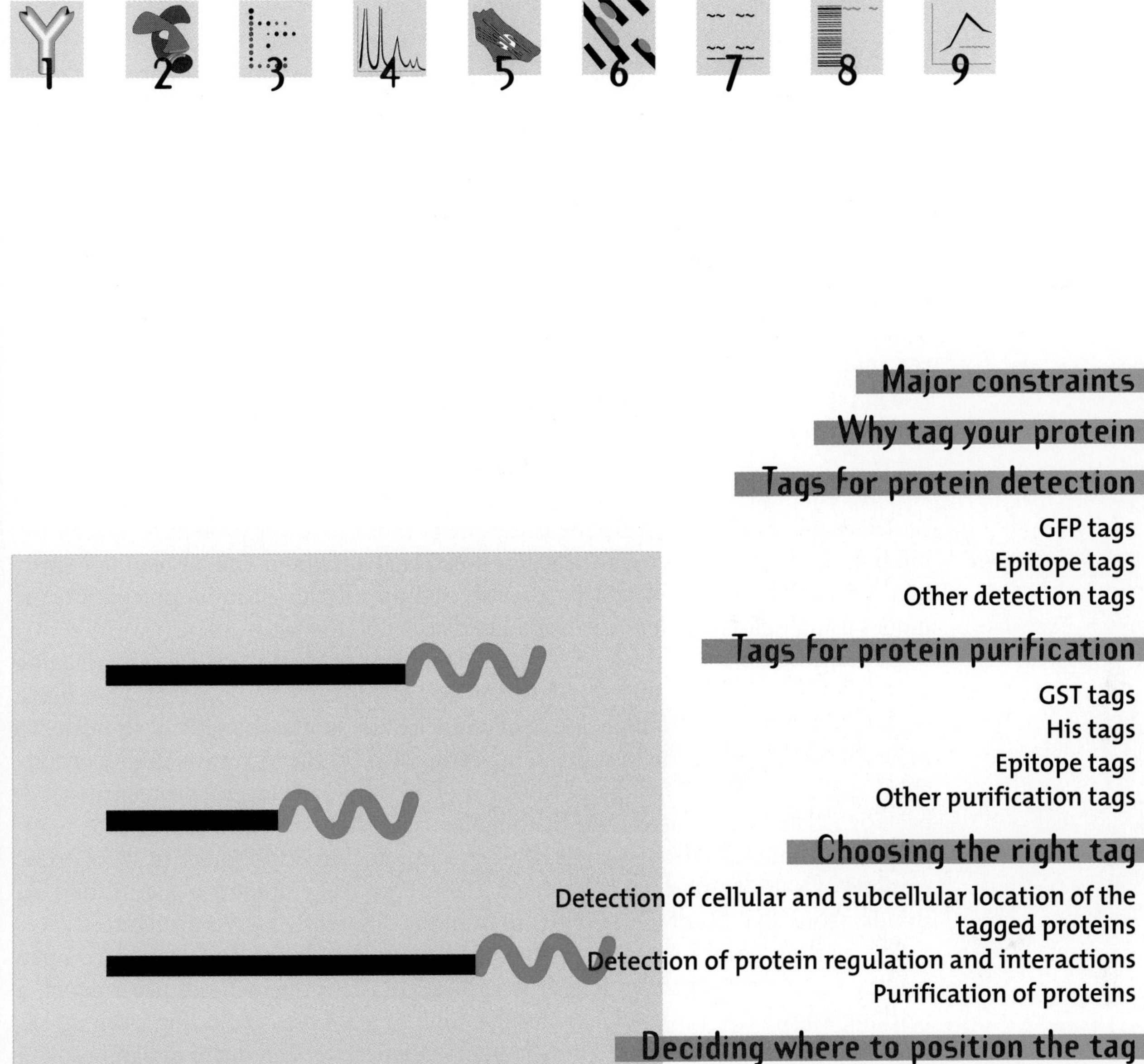




# 10 Tagging Proteins

Historically, proteins have been labeled using radioactive isotopes or fluorescent dyes, procedures that require pure protein. Thus, development of the concept of tagging proteins using recombinant DNA methods has been a major technical advance. In this method, the label, or tag, is attached during synthesis of the protein. The tag itself is a small open reading frame, and fusions of tags with the protein under study are introduced by standard molecular biology methods.

The production of tagged proteins allows them to be produced and detected in a variety of expression systems. The tags permit ready detection and purification of the hybrid protein. Proteins can be tagged by fusion to useful markers, such as green fluorescent protein (GFP) (see Fig. 10.1, below) or the glutathione-*S*-transferase protein (GST) (see Fig. 10.2, below), or they can be tagged by fusion with short peptides that specify interaction with specific ligands, such as the His tag or the streptavidin binding tag.

One variant of this peptide tag approach is epitope tagging, in which a short amino acid sequence is placed within the coding region of the target protein to specify the binding site for a known monoclonal or polyclonal antibody. The tagged target protein can then be readily detected, assayed, and purified in all immunological techniques using well-characterized antibodies directed to the tag.

The tagging concept has been very successful because, despite early doubts, tagging most often does not alter the tagged protein's function. Two developments have made tagging practical: (1) the simple use of oligonucleotide synthesis and PCR strategies to incorporate tags into protein expression vectors and (2) the ready availability of suitable expression vectors for the production of recombinant tagged proteins in viral, bacterial, plant, yeast, insect, and mammalian cell systems. The precise epitope mapping of the binding sites of a large number of monoclonal antibodies to short linear epitopes of 5–15 amino acids has created a large choice of epitope tags, permitting the simultaneous analysis of the activities of multiple differently tagged proteins.

The starting point for tagging is the possession of a cloned and sequenced open reading frame for the protein that is being studied. All of the methods used require a working knowledge of general molecular biology methods, including cloning, sequencing, and PCR reactions. These methods are described in detail in Sambrook et al. (1989).

Tags are used principally for two purposes: (1) protein detection, where the tag is added to allow detection of the tagged protein in cell-based expression systems, thus allowing study of its functions, cellular location, interactions, and biochemical activities and (2) protein purification, where the tag is selected because of its capacity to bind specifically to an immobilized ligand, allowing simple bulk purification of the protein from cell extracts.

Because so many tags are available, strong starting recommendations are made in this chapter for both detection and purification tags, and then alternatives are discussed briefly at the end of each section. Protein tagging is a very effective method and its use will increase dramatically as more novel open reading frames are defined during the course of the various genome projects. For investigators confronted with a protein-encoding gene of unknown function, tagging the protein and then examining its expression in the cell or species of origin is a good approach for making predictions about where the normal untagged protein is located in the cell, what it interacts with, and how it works.

## Major constraints

The major constraint of this system is the possible alteration of the protein's biological activity as a result of adding the tag to the protein, because an essentially new protein is created consisting of the protein of interest fused to the amino acid sequences of the tag. Thus, it is important to realize that the properties of the new protein, rather than the protein of interest, will be evaluated when using this method. Experience suggests that this is often not a problem, however, and information gained by studying the tagged protein can be verified when antibodies to the endogenous untagged protein are eventually produced.

The second constraint, which applies especially to epitope tags, derives from the fact that many of the currently used tags consist of segments of known proteins (for example, the myc gene product). This means that the anti-tag antibody may recognize other cellular proteins besides the tagged protein being analyzed. This problem can be quite serious because antibodies to several of the common tags incorporated into many current expression vectors show considerable cross-reactivity. For this reason, you should perform a quick test of the cross-reactivity of the common anti-tag antibodies in the immunological techniques to be used in studying the tagged protein. These tests are described below (pp. 363–364).

Finally, some of the tag systems are patent protected and only available commercially. This may impose some economic constraints on their use in your lab.

## Why tag your protein

There are many advantages to tagging proteins. Principally, this method provides a powerful way to detect the protein of interest in a range of different cellular contexts.

- Tagging is especially valuable if the open reading frame has been cloned but no antibodies to the protein product exist, either because the protein is novel or because it is a poor immunogen. This is an increasingly common situation as genome projects shift from genomics to proteomics.
- The fact that the tag is not an intrinsic part of the native protein sequence makes it less likely that the tag-binding reagents will affect the protein's function when they are used to isolate it.
- Tagged proteins can be expressed in any cell type given the appropriate expression vector; for example, the same tagged protein can be cloned for high-level expression in bacteria or insect cell systems.
- The tag's localization properties and interactions can be monitored after expression in stably transfected cells, and the tag may be used to detect the protein in cell staining and immunoblotting procedures, where its capacity to distinguish the exogenous product from the endogenous untagged protein is particularly useful.
- Tags can be used in immunoprecipitation experiments where the high specificity of the anti-tag antibody may allow the ready detection of other proteins that bind the tagged protein.

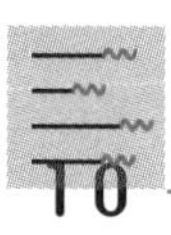


- Tagging may be used to purify the expressed protein where the possibility of very gentle elution methods allowing purification of active protein or protein complexes is a special feature.
- Because each tag is unique, it is possible to use multiple tags simultaneously in the same cell expression system to study protein interactions or colocalization. It is also possible to use multiple tags on the same protein or protein complex, permitting remarkable purifications where both tags are used sequentially in the protocol.

As the widespread utility of these methods has become apparent, an increasing range of commercial products that facilitate this technique have become available. A large number of new tag systems have emerged from the continued success of epitope mapping projects and from studies of novel marker proteins and protein ligand interactions. Even so, it is clear that no universally perfect tag for all purposes has emerged. In many systems, it is often desirable and necessary to be able to use multiple different tags to provide evidence that the tag is not unduly influencing the behavior of the protein.

The two main purposes of the tagging procedure—protein detection and protein purification—place distinct demands on the properties of the tag. Although many tags can be used in both contexts, some are clearly more suitable for only one of the two roles.

## Tags for protein detection

A protein's expression and subcellular location can be detected using tags and cell-staining methods. A wide variety of tags are suitable for protein detection, but two classes are especially important—fluorescent protein tags, which uniquely make it possible to detect the protein in living cells, and epitope tags, which can be used for detection in cell staining, immunoprecipitation, and immunoblotting protocols.

The fluorescent protein tags are unique because they render the fusion protein detectable by immunofluorescence within the living cell in real time; thus, they are especially important in studies of protein and cell location and dynamics. The recent development of more active ones as well as variants that emit light of different colors is greatly extending the range of uses of these protein tags. Antibodies to GFP allow it to be used as a tag for immunostaining, immunoblotting, and immunoprecipitation protocols; however, the large size of this tag makes it more likely to affect the regulation and function of the tagged protein than alternative smaller epitope tags would. The GFP tag presents no serious background problems because most cells used for detection analysis lack fluorescent protein components. But it could present a problem if you work on jellyfish!

Epitope tags can be more difficult to use because here background reactivity of the anti-tag antibody with endogenous components of the host cell needs to be evaluated carefully, and a tag/antibody combination that will minimize these problems must be selected.

## GFP tags

The green fluorescent protein from the jellyfish *Aequorea victoria* is a 238-amino-acid, 27-kD monomeric protein that emits bright green light when exposed to UV radiation, allowing monitoring of its expression and subcellular location in real time in living cells (Prasher et al. 1992). The protein is remarkably stable and retains its fluorescence after exposure to 1.0% SDS, in 8 M urea, and even after heating to 70°C. Important for cellular localization studies, GFP fluorescence persists in formaldehyde-fixed cells. When fused to other proteins, it retains its unique light-emitting properties and does not often interfere with the subcellular localization or biochemical properties of the protein to which it is fused. Therefore, it represents a near-ideal marker for studies of protein expression and localization. In addition, GFP proteins are often expressed at high levels because the GFP segment can protect the complete fusion protein from protein degradation (Fig. 10.1).

The potential of this marker protein has been greatly enhanced by site-directed mutagenesis and structural studies that have allowed the development of a whole series of variants of GFP that are codon-adapted for mammalian cell expression and are both

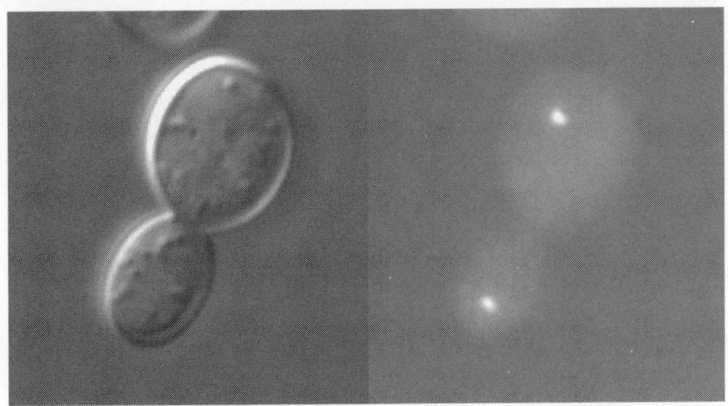


**Figure 10.1**
GFP detection.

*The sequences of variant GFPs at the chromophore site are given below. EGFP is 35 times more active than wild-type GFP, whereas S65T and RSGFP are red-shifted in their emission spectra compared to the wild-type protein.*

| | |
|---|---|
| wtGFP | Phe *Ser Tyr Gly Val Gln* |
| EGFP | *Leu Thr Tyr Gly Val Gln* |
| S65T | *Phe Thr Tyr Gly Val Gln* |
| RSGFP | *Met Gly Tyr Gly Val Leu* |

more intensely fluorescent and red-shifted in their emission spectra. These variants permit double-labeling experiments and fluorescence resonance energy transfer experiments to be devised (Delagrave et al. 1995; Heim et al. 1995; Cormack et al. 1996). An additional variant with an intrinsically shorter half-life in mammalian cells has also been produced. A wide range of vectors allowing fusion of the GFP tag to the open reading frame of interest at either the amino or carboxyl terminus are commercially available, as are polyclonal and monoclonal antibodies to GFP and the pure protein.

## Epitope tags

Epitope tags are useful for labeling proteins for detection using immunostaining, immunoprecipitation, and immunoblotting methods. Because the tags are typically small, they are less likely to affect the protein's biochemical properties than the GFP tag, which is known, for example, to affect protein stability. A wide variety of different epitope tags have been defined and this allows multiple proteins to be labeled and distinguished within the same cellular context, thus allowing the study of protein–protein interactions.

The tags that are most commonly used and are sensible to try first are the myc tag, the HA tag, and the FLAG tag (Table 10.1). These three tags are described below.

Table 10.1 *Most commonly used tags*

| Tag name | Source | Sequence | Antibodies | Reagents available |
|---|---|---|---|---|
| Myc | myc oncogene (Evan et al. 1985) | EQKLISEEDDL | 9E10 | Antibody columns<br>Vectors<br>Peptide |
| HA | Flu hemagglutinin HA-1 protein (Niman et al. 1983; Field et al. 1988) | YPYDVPDYA | 12CA5 | Antibodies<br>Vectors<br>Peptide |
| FLAG | Novel (Hopp et al. 1988) | DYKDDDDK | M1 and M2 | Antibodies<br>Vectors<br>Peptide |

### *Myc tag*

| | |
|---|---|
| **Sequence** | EQKLISEEDL |
| **Antibodies** | 9E10 mouse monoclonal |
| **Supplier** | Sigma |
| **Commercial reagents** | Purified and labeled antibodies<br>Pure peptide |
| **Noncommercial reagents** | Hybridoma cell line. The 9E10 cell line has been deposited by Gerard Evan with the ECACC under ECACC No. 85102202. The fusion partner is SP2/O and the antibody is $IgG_1$ κ (Evan et al. 1985).<br>Multiple vectors for expression in *E. coli*, yeast, insect cells, and mammalian cell systems |

The Myc tag has been perhaps the most widely used epitope tag system. This is due at least in part to its early successful demonstration by Munro and Pelham (1986) and by the generous manner in which the monoclonal antibody cell line 9E10 was distributed (see box above), ensuring wide success to the system. The 9E10 antibody was raised against a synthetic peptide derived from the carboxyl terminus of the human c-myc protein. The immunizing peptide was selected by analysis of the c-myc sequence for regions of hydrophilic character using a Hopp and Woods plot. The peptide was coupled to KLH as a carrier and its sequence AEEQKLISEEDLLRKRREQLKHKLEQL-RNSCA represented residues 408–439 of c-myc. The 9E10 antibody reacted well with the immunizing peptide and detected c-myc particularly well on immunoblotting. However, unlike the other two monoclonal antibodies to this peptide that Evan isolated, it failed to immunoprecipitate the c-myc protein, suggesting that it might show lower backgrounds in detection of the tag (Evan et al. 1985). The myc tag was first demonstrated by Munro and Pelham (1986) who, following their first description of the concept of epitope tagging using the substance P tag (Munro and Pelham 1984), were keen to use a tag that did not require chemical modification for detection and for which an abundant supply of a well-characterized monoclonal antibody was available. Munro and Pelham (1986) used the myc system to tag the p72 (Bip) protein by substituting the carboxy-terminal 60 amino acids with the sequence EQKLISEEDL from myc followed by the sequence D stop. They showed the very clear use of the 9E10 antibody to detect mutant variants of tagged p72 (Bip) that localized to the cell nucleus or the endoplasmic reticulum. Subsequently, the myc tag has been used in almost all vector/expression systems.

## *HA tag*

| | |
|---|---|
| **Sequence** | Tyr Pro Tyr Asp Val Pro Asp Tyr Ala<br>Y P Y D V P D Y A |
| **Antibodies** | 12CA5 monoclonal antibody |
| **Suppliers** | Sigma-Aldrich, Boehringer Mannheim |
| **Commercial reagents** | Purified and labeled (enzyme and fluorescent and biotin) antibodies<br>Pure peptide |
| **Noncommercial reagents** | The hybridoma cell line was widely distributed in the academic community before it was patented. It is not available to the whole academic community in a type culture collection.<br>Multiple vectors for expression in *E. coli*, yeast, insect cells, and mammalian cell systems |

The HA tag is derived from an epitope mapped in the influenza hemagglutinin protein. The production of the antibody is described by Niman et al. (1983), who immunized mice with a large peptide representing amino acids 75–110 of the HA1 protein of the flu virus. The epitope recognized by 12CA5 (then called H26D08) was localized to the smaller peptide YPYDVPDYA by Wilson and colleagues (Wilson et al. 1984), using synthetic peptide analysis. Its use as an epitope tag is described in Field et al. (1988). These investigators used it to tag the amino terminus of the yeast adenyl cyclase gene. Their construction used the sequence GGP as a linker between the amino-terminal tag and the start of the adenyl cyclase gene. This resulted in the following final new amino-terminal sequence leading up to the original initiating methionine of the adenyl cyclase protein.

NH2 M YPYDVPDYASLGGPM

Field et al. (1988) were able to produce the tagged protein in yeast cells and purify the enzyme in active form using peptide elution with the shorter peptide YPYDVPDYA from 12CA5 columns. They achieved a 700-fold purification and a 40% yield but found that they needed to carry out the elution step at 30°C for 15 minutes.

Since then, the HA tag has been successfully used at both amino- and carboxy-terminal sites. Purification using 12CA5 immobilized antibody columns and elution with the epitope peptide has been reported in many cases to result in highly purified active enzymes and DNA-binding proteins and does not always require the 30°C elution condition. The tag has been used effectively to label protein for cell staining, immunoblotting, ELISA, and immunoprecipitation. Its disadvantage is that the anti-HA antibody binds to several cross-reacting cellular proteins in immunoblotting analysis of mammalian cell extracts.

### *FLAG tag*

| | |
|---|---|
| **Sequence** | Asp Tyr Lys Asp Asp Asp Asp Lys<br>D Y K D D D D K |
| **Antibodies** | M1 and M2 mouse monoclonals |
| **Suppliers** | Sigma-Aldrich, and other local distributors |
| **Commercial reagents** | Amino- and carboxy-terminal tagging vectors for *E. coli* and yeast expression systems<br>Purified and labeled antibodies and affinity resins<br>Pure peptide |
| **Noncommercial reagents** | Multiple vectors for expression in *E. coli*, yeast, insect cells, and mammalian cell systems |

The FLAG tag is the only peptide tag that was designed de novo as a tag (Hopp et al. 1988). Thus, it is unique in that the sequence of the tag is not derived from any known protein. This tag is an 8-amino-acid peptide (see box, above) that is hydrophilic and can be placed at both the amino and carboxyl termini of the protein. There are two commerically available antibodies, M1 and M2, that recognize the FLAG tag. The M1 antibody requires the amino terminus of the epitope to be available and is only suitable if the tag is placed at the amino terminus of the protein. Binding of the M1 antibody is promoted by the presence of the divalent cations (preferentially $Ca^{++}$ ions), so that complete or partial disruption of the interaction can be produced by metal-chelating agents like EDTA, allowing very gentle purification.

The power of the system is greatly enhanced by the availability of the M2 antibody, which recognizes the same FLAG epitope when placed internally within a protein or at the carboxyl terminus. M2 recognition of the FLAG epitope does not require divalent cations, but gentle elution of FLAG-tagged protein from M2 antibody has been readily achieved by competitive elution with the free peptide.

A variety of FLAG-tagged proteins have been shown to retain full biochemical activity (for example, transcription factors, growth factors, and enzymes), and this tag has been widely used in cell staining, immunoblotting, and immunoprecipitation protocols. An excellent variety of vectors and detection reagents are available commercially, including antibody affinity resins and directly labeled antibodies, and the widespread success of the system makes a strong case for its use.

Recently, the specificity of the anti-FLAG antibodies has been explored in detail, allowing the use of alternate sequences (Slootstra et al. 1997) and shortened versions of the tag sequence (Knappik and Pluckthun 1994). The anti-FLAG antibodies give generally very low backgrounds, but the M2 antibody has been reported to cross-react with at least one cellular protein (Schäfer and Braun 1995).

## Other detection tags

In addition to the commonly used epitope tags described above, there is a much larger set of alternatives, each of which has potential benefit and may be used by the more experienced investigator. These systems can be adopted if all three of the recommended systems fail, where a particular novel feature is needed, if additional specificities are needed, or where multiple tagged proteins are to be examined in the same expression experiment. These alternatives are listed in Table 10.2.

Table 10.2 *Alternate peptide tags recognized by antibodies*

| Name | Source | Sequence | Antibody | Reference | Comment |
|---|---|---|---|---|---|
| **E tag (glu tag)** | Polyoma middle T | EEEEYMPME | Anti-E tag | Schaffhausen et al. (1982); Grussenmeyer et al. (1985); Schreurs et al. (1995) | |
| **KT3 tag** | Carboxyl terminus of SV 40 large T | TPPPEPET | KT3 | MacArthur and Walter (1984); Kwatra and Walter (1995); Schreurs et al. (1995) | Good peptide elution reported |
| **Tub tag** | Alpha tubulin | EEF | YL1/2 | Skinner et al. (1991); Stammers et al. (1991) | Good peptide elution with EF dipeptide |
| **G tag** | VSV protein | YTDIEMNRLGK | P5D4 | Kries (1986) | Antibody commercially available. Watch out for VSV! |
| **T7 tag** | T7 major capsid protein | MASMTGGQQMG | T7 tag | Novagen | Antibody is only commercial. Tag is incorporated in many T7 vectors |
| **VSV tag** | VSV glycoprotein E | YGDVFKGD | 3B3 | Hatfield et al. (1997) | Watch out for VSV |
| **B tag** | VP7 Bluetongue virus | QYPALT | D11 or F10 | Wang et al. (1996) | Watch out for Bluetongue virus |
| **His tag** | Designed | HHHHHH | 6 HIS Ab | CLONTECH | Cross-reactive? |
| **HSV tag** | HSV glyco-protein D | QPELAPENPEN | | Novagen | |
| **240 tag** | Human p53 protein | RHSVV | PAb240 19.1 | Stephen and Lane (1992) | Cross-reactive on blots. Watch out for p53 |
| **DO1 tag** | Human p53 protein | FSDLWKL | DO-1, DO-7 19.1 | Stephen et al. (1995) | Multiple antibodies commercially available. Very strong. Clean on blots. Watch out for p53 |
| **416 tag** | SV40 T antigen | WEQWW | PAb416 | Harlow et al. (1981); Lindner et al. (1998) | Very strong antibody, commercially available. Few cross-reactions in immunoprecipitation. Watch out for T antigen |

There is a need for further antibody epitope tag systems with the general availability of the Myc system. Because the anti-Myc hybridoma cell line 9E10 has been deposited in a national culture collection, it is available to all investigators who wish to use it for noncommercial purposes. The cost of and limited access to the other antibodies used in tag systems restrict their usefulness to the broad scientific community and consume large amounts of valuable research money. We urge investigators and commercial companies who can to deposit their anti-tag hybridoma cell lines in a national cell culture collection. They will make a lot of friends! Although many labs still prefer to purchase the antibody for the sake of convenience, access to the cell lines allows labs that require large amounts of the antibody to obtain it economically by growing the cell line and preparing the antibody in house. Recently, the first recombinant antibodies to tags were produced in *E. coli* (Lindner et al. 1997). These antibodies may represent an ideal alternate solution to this problem because the clones encoding the recombinant antibody expression constructs can be distributed very economically.

## Tags for protein purification

The use of tags for ready purification of proteins has become an almost universally applied method, and a large number of different tag systems are available. They all depend on a specific interaction between the tag and a solid-phase ligand, allowing the selective binding and elution of the tagged protein from the complex mix of proteins present in the extract. Many of the vectors that incorporate these tags have been designed so that they create a cleavage site for a highly specific protease between the tag segment and the target protein segment of the fusion protein. This permits the separation of the protein from the tag, if needed (Nygren et al. 1994).

Three of the most commonly used tags for purification are GST, His, and epitope tags.

### GST tags

*One of the excellent applications for GST fusions is the production of GST–protein in bacteria, where the GST tag helps to make the protein soluble.*

GST tags (Fig. 10.2) have been one of the most successful tags for purification of proteins from bacterial expression systems. In this system, glutathione-*S*-transferase protein is fused in-frame with the protein to be tagged (Smith and Johnson 1988). The resulting GST fusion proteins can be produced in any expression system. The GST protein binds tightly to the tripeptide glutathione; the protein can be purified on columns of immobilized glutathione and then, after washing away of nonbound proteins, it can be eluted by buffers that contain free glutathione.

This system works exceptionally well, at least in part, because the fusion partner often folds correctly into a functional domain. Rapid and very mild purification of the GST fusion proteins is another key asset of the system, combined with the low cost of the ligand glutathione.

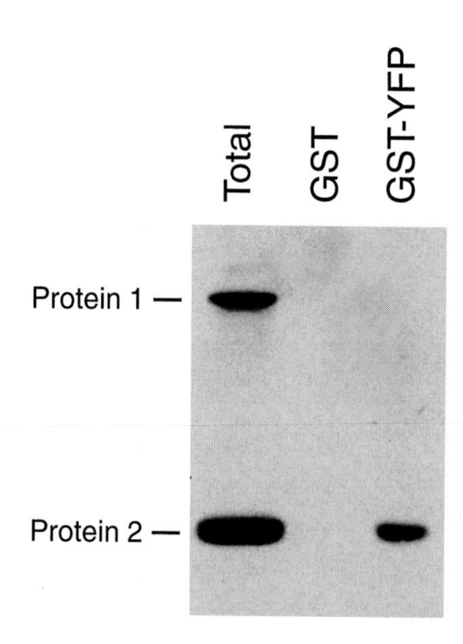


Immunoblot developed with pooled antibodies specific for protein 1 and 2

Figure 10.2
GST pull-down.

## His tags

A second popular and useful tag is polyhistidine, the His tag. This tag consists of a run of 6–10 contiguous histidine residues placed in-frame at the amino or carboxyl terminus of the protein. The His tag has a high specific affinity for metal ions such as nickel. A wide variety of solid-phase columns are available that expose the essential metal coordination sites to which the histidine stretch binds.

A striking feature of the His tag system is that binding of the His-tagged protein to the solid-phase metal is not affected by strong denaturants, allowing the protein to be solubilized and purified in such agents as 8 M urea or 6 M guanidinium. These harsh conditions can, however, result in stripping of the metal from the chelate column. Some of the newer resins that use metals other than nickel offer superior performance because they overcome this problem (Porath 1992). Rapid and very mild elution of the His-tagged proteins is another key asset of the system because the bound protein can be displaced at pH 8.0 in buffers containing 80–100 mM imidazole. Recently, elution with a gradient of L-histidine (0–250 mM in 70 mM Tris HCl, pH 8.2, 100 mM NaCl, 20% vol/vol glycerol) has been shown to be even less harsh, resulting in increased retention of the biological activity of the recovered protein (Gort and Maloy 1998).

## Epitope tags

Epitope tags are widely used in protein purification as well as in protein detection, as discussed above. For a tag to work well in purification, it is important to be able to dissociate the interaction between the antibody and the tag without having to use such severe conditions that the antigen is irreversibly denatured or delivered in poor yield. Release of the tagged protein bound to the solid-phase antibody by competitive elutions with the free peptide is a very attractive option here. Of the epitope tags listed above, the HA tag, the E tag, the tubulin tag (Skinner et al. 1991; Stammers et al. 1991), the KT3 tag (Kwatra et al. 1995), and the FLAG tag have all been used successfully in protein purification using peptide elution.

### Peptide elution from anti-tag antibody columns

One great advantage of immunoaffinity chromatography using anti-tag antibodies is that the bound tagged protein can be eluted by incubating the column in excess amounts of the free epitope peptide. This method is exceptionally gentle because the free peptide can be added in neutral buffers and subsequently separated from the eluted protein by gel filtration. In one variation, the eluting free peptide is synthesized with a biotin group attached so that the free peptide can be removed after elution by using streptavidin-coated beads. To optimize this method of elution, it is important to try to ensure that the initial antibody column is saturated with the tagged antigen so that excess peptide is not needed first to fill unoccupied antibody-binding sites on the column. This can be done by mixing a fixed small amount of the antigen-containing solution with a titration of antibody-coated beads. After 1 hour of incubation, the beads are washed in neutral buffer and the bound and unbound proteins are analyzed by gel electrophoresis and immunoblotting. Use these results to determine the minimum number of antibody beads needed to deplete the antigen completely from the starting extract. The washed antigen-coated beads are then incubated with high concentrations of the free peptide (try 100 μg to 1 mg/ml). The success of the elution depends on the off rate of the bead-bound antigen and the relative avidity of the free peptide and the antigen for the antibody beads. If the antigen is multivalent, elution can be quite inefficient; however, the method works well for monovalent antigens. Attempts are under way to develop variant epitope tags of slightly lower affinity than the original sequence for this specific purpose (Slootstra et al. 1997). The tubulin tag's small size is an advantage here because efficient elution has been achieved with the Asp-Phe dipeptide, which is commercially available at very low cost (Skinner et al. 1991; Stammers et al. 1991).

## Other purification tags

A large number of other purification tags are available as further alternatives to the GST, His, and epitope tags described above. Several of these alternatives having especially attractive features are summarized in Table 10.3.

### *Protein tags for purification*

These alternate protein tags all have distinct advantages for protein purification (Table 10.4). Multiple vectors are available commercially, as are the required solid-phase purification reagents. In all cases, the protein purification tag is quite large, but the vectors incorporate enzyme cleavage sites to allow subsequent removal of the tag. The tag that results in the in vivo labeling of the protein has been used with great success by McMicheal and his colleagues, who mixed the biotin-tagged protein with streptavidin to create a soluble tetravalent form of the T-cell receptor. The streptavidin tag system is very exciting because it is not proprietary, and the short streptavidin tag peptide sequence can be readily fused to the open reading frame of interest using standard methods (see later examples).

Table 10.3 *Alternate peptide tags recognized by other proteins*

| Detection tag | Detection ligand | Tag origin | Sequence | Comments | References |
|---|---|---|---|---|---|
| **S peptide tag** | S protein<br>$K_d = 10^{-9}$M | Pancreatic ribonuclease A | KGTAAAKF ERQHMDS | The 15-amino-acid S peptide when bound by the 104-amino-acid S protein reconstitutes enzymatic activity. S protein is available conjugated to several enzymes and to solid phase. | Richards and Wyckoff et al. (1971); McCormick and Mierendorf (1994) |
| **Strep tag** | Streptavidin $K_d = 2.7 \times 10^{-4}$M | Phage display selection of streptavidin-binding peptide | AWRHPQF GG | Peptide that mimics biotin. Very gentle elution with diaminobiotin is possible. Crystal structure solved. Many forms of solid-phase and labeled streptavidin are available. | Schmidt and Skerra (1993, 1994) |

Table 10.4 *Protein tags for purification*

| Purification tag | Purification ligand | Tag origin | Comments | References |
|---|---|---|---|---|
| **CBD tag** | Crystalline cellulose | Cellulose-binding domain from cellulose-binding protein A (CbpA) of *Clostridium cellulovorans* | Large number of very cheap cellulose matrices available as beads, powders, fibers, and membranes | Goldstein et al. (1993); Tomme et al. (1994) Novagen |
| **Protein A tag** | Immunoglobulin G | Immunoglobulin-binding domain of *Staphylococcus aureus* protein A | Large number of different forms of immobilized IgG available as solid phase, with different levels of affinity for protein A | Pharmacia |
| **Biotin tag** | Avidin/streptavidin | A 386-amino-acid protein domain that is biotinylated in *E. coli* | In vivo addition of biotin only happens in *E. coli*, not insect or mammalian expression systems. Different forms of avidin and streptavidin available to change avidity of binding to solid phase | Promega |

*Innovation*

*It is clear that in modern cell and molecular biology technical innovations, like the development of the GST and GFP systems, have enormous impact. Innovations such as these need to be encouraged, yet it seems that the developers of such systems receive scant academic recognition of their contributions. All of us in the community need to make more effort to support and encourage these academic innovators.*

## Purification of epitope-tagged proteins

Epitope-tagged proteins can be readily purified using the anti-tag antibody column. Such columns are commercially available for the two anti-Flag antibodies M1 and M2. They can be readily produced for the anti-HA and anti-Myc antibodies using the procedures described in Chapter 9. Although one might anticipate being able to develop standard elution conditions for a given anti-tag antibody tag pair, this has not proved to be the case. This is because the exact context of the epitope and the oligomeric state of the tagged protein can profoundly affect the avidity of its interaction with the antibody column. The tag systems do, however, allow very mild elution protocols to be tried using the free peptide tag to displace the bound tagged protein by competition for the solid-phase antibody.

### *Peptide tags for purification*

A recent alternative peptide tag suitable for protein purification has been identified through the use of phage display. A short peptide, AWRHPQFGG, was shown to bind to streptavidin with a moderate affinity. The streptavidin tag system (Schmidt et al. 1996) is not proprietary, and the short streptavidin tag peptide sequence can be fused readily to the open reading frame of interest using standard methods (Table 10.5) (see later examples, p. 371). Streptavidin columns are available commercially. It has been established by X-ray crystallography (Schmidt et al. 1996) that the natural ligand, biotin, and the strep tag peptide bind to the same region of the streptavidin molecule and that streptavidin-tagged proteins can be eluted with free diaminobiotin.

Table 10.5 *Peptide tags for purification*

| Purification tag | Purification ligand | Tag origin | Sequence | Comments | References |
|---|---|---|---|---|---|
| **Strep tag** | Streptavidin<br>$K_d = 2.7$ $10^{-4}$ M | Phage display selection of streptavidin-binding peptide | AWRHPQF GG | Peptide mimics biotin as seen in X-ray structure. Very gentle elution with diaminobiotin is possible. There are many forms of solid-phase streptavidin and avidin commercially available. This is an economic system to use. | Schmidt and Skerra (1993, 1994); Schmidt et al. (1996) |

# Choosing the right tag

A great deal of wasted effort can be avoided by making the correct choice of tag at the start of your study, especially because no tag system is perfect. Thus, the principal goal of the tagging procedure should be considered.

## Detection of cellular and subcellular location of the tagged protein

If the tag is to be used exclusively to monitor protein localization in cells, then the GFP tag has unique advantages, because this system allows direct observation of the location of the protein in living cells in real time. None of the other tags can do this. Thus, if the determination of a protein's cellular "address" is the prime goal of the experiment and you have access to a suitable fluorescence microscope, the GFP system is the tag of choice. If GFP is inappropriate or fails in your tests, the Myc or HA tags should be tried next.

## Detection of protein regulation and interactions

If you want to study the interaction of the protein with components of the host cell using immunoprecipitation and immunoblotting approaches, then the peptide-based tags are the correct choice. Here you need a tag that will not affect the stability or function of the protein and that will be potentially compatible with the use of multiple different tagged proteins in the same cell system.

Most of the problems that arise with these tags are from spurious cross-reactions with host proteins. Thus, a lot of insight can be gained by testing the tag detection system for cross-reactivity with other components of the experimental system you wish to use. We strongly recommend that you carry out control experiments using the anti-tag antibodies or peptide tag-binding proteins in your particular system. The cost of commercial reagents is a consideration, but this has to be balanced against their speed and convenience.

Another important step is to check the anti-tag detection system for background signal in the assay system in which you will be studying the tagged protein. Recently, directly labeled anti-tag antibodies have become available for the FLAG, myc, HA, and VSV-G epitopes. These reagents can help to lower backgrounds, particularly when immunoprecipitations are to be analyzed by immunoblotting. Directly labeled reagents are also available for the detection of S peptide-tagged and streptavidin-tagged proteins.

A sensible starting point is to try out the three most commonly used epitope tags. Test the properties of the commercially available anti-FLAG M1 and M2 antibodies, the anti-HA antibody 12CA5, and the anti-Myc antibody 9E10. Reject the use of those tags where the detecting antibodies show a high background in your system, and select those in which there is a very low or absent background signal. It is important to control for cross-reactions in the detecting reagents as well as in the primary monoclonal antibodies themselves (see Chapter 3). Because all of these antibodies are mouse monoclonal antibodies, they can be compared using the same detection reagents in all of these procedures. An essential step is comparison of the reactions of all four antibodies in your chosen system with a control that is set up with the detecting reagent itself and no primary antibody.

## Testing the anti-tag antibodies for cross-reactions in cell-staining reactions

If the cells in which you wish to express the tagged protein for immunostaining studies grow attached to the tissue-culture dish, a simple staining method can be used.

Fix a 9-cm dish of the cells expressing the epitope-tagged protein using the 50% acetone, 50% methanol method. Draw a grid on the back of the dish using a marker pen. The grid should have seven columns for the seven different antibodies or controls to be titrated and four columns for the different dilutions of each reagent to be examined. Prepare dilutions of the four test antibodies, a positive control antibody (e.g., PC10 anti-nuclear antibody), a negative control antibody (e.g., anti-β-gal antibody BG2), and a no-antibody control solution over the range 10 μg/ml to 0.01 μg/ml with PBS/1%BSA using 10-fold dilutions. Then spot 1-μl drops of each dilution onto the marked grid. Wash and process the plate exactly as described on pp. 115 and 131 using the immunoperoxidase detection method. Compare the staining patterns seen for each antibody using light microscopy. Alternatively, use the immunofluorescence method described on pp. 115 and 136 for higher-resolution studies.

This test is severe for any epitope-tagging system because of the sensitivity of the immunoperoxidase assay. Thus, do not be surprised to see some reactivity with whichever antibody you use. In most cases, the tagged protein will be highly expressed compared to constitutive host components. Nevertheless, this comparative test can provide key guidance in choice of system. Alternative tags should be used if very strong cross-reactions are seen with all four antibodies.

This simple test allows any particular background problem to be defined as being associated with a particular tag system. If all systems give a low background, then the choice can be based entirely on practical factors such as the availability and cost of suitable expression vector systems and their downstream advantages. At the current time, the FLAG system is the most fully developed in terms of sets of protocols, vectors, and detection reagents, but it is not as widely used and is the most expensive. The Myc and the HA systems have the advantage that the hybridoma cells producing the detecting antibodies 9E10 and 12CA5 are available noncommercially.

The value of these initial studies cannot be overemphasized. For example, the E tag, a peptide derived from the polyoma middle-T protein, is widely incorporated into scFv expression vectors. The anti-E tag antibody shows an intense background stain on some mammalian cell lines, perhaps due to reported cross-reactions with microfilaments (Ito et al. 1983), thus precluding its use in the detection of E-tagged proteins in these cells.

## Testing the anti-tag antibodies for cross-reactions in immunoblotting

Prepare a sample extract of the cell system in which you intend to express the tagged protein for SDS gel electrophoresis. Extracts can be soluble protein extracts or total protein extracts of host cell systems. The final extracts should have a protein concentration that does not exceed 10 mg/ml in sample buffer. (Suitable extract preparation methods are described in Chapter 8.) Choose a SDS polyacrylamide gel concentration recipe that will resolve proteins in the predicted molecular-weight range of your tagged protein (see Appendix I). Next, run 5-μl samples of each of three concentrations of the sample (10 mg/ml, 1 mg/ml, 0.1 mg/ml) flanked by molecular-weight marker tracks and adjacent blank tracks loaded with sample buffer alone. You will need six such sets of five gel tracks to test the recommended antibody set.

After gel electrophoresis, transfer the proteins to nitrocellulose using the immunoblotting method described in Chapter 8. After blocking the nitrocellulose, cut the sheet into strips, separating each group of six tracks. Probe each set with one of the four test and two control antibodies at an antibody concentration of 1 μg/ml. Wash and develop the blot using the electrochemiluminescence method. Select an antibody tag system on the basis of the fewest and weakest relative cross-reactive bands seen in the developed blot. Care should be taken to avoid systems that detect cross-reactions with protein components of molecular weights that lie in the range of that expected of the tagged protein.

This test is in many ways the most severe for any epitope-tagging system. Thus, do not be surprised to see some reactivity with whichever antibody you use. Clearly, in most cases, it is expected that the tagged protein will be highly expressed compared to constitutive host components. Nevertheless, this comparative test at a fixed antibody concentration can provide key guidance in choice of system. Only very strong cross-reactions seen with all four antibodies would suggest use of the alternative tags described later.

### *Choosing an alternate peptide tag for detection*

*Should the three common antibody tags prove unsuitable for your system, the alternate peptide tags listed in Table 10.3 can be tried. The VSV-G and 416 tags are good alternatives, whereas if antibody-based detection is the general source of the background problem, the S peptide and streptavidin peptide systems should be evaluated.*

## Testing the anti-tag antibodies for cross-reactions in immunoprecipitation

Use the labeling and extraction method described in Chapter 7 to prepare a labeled extract of the cell system in which you intend to express your tagged protein. Use 1 μg of each of the three tag antibodies in the immunoprecipitation protocol using a preclearance step. Use as controls at least two other monoclonal antibodies and run one immunoprecipitation without adding antibody to establish the background in your cell system. Complete the washing steps and then analyze the composition of the immunoprecipitated proteins by SDS gel electrophoresis and autoradiography. Again, it makes sense to use a gel system that resolves well in the molecular-weight range of your expected tagged protein. The results should be carefully analyzed for background bands immunoprecipitated by the anti-tag antibodies from the cell system you intend to use. Choose the tag whose antibody shows the least background.

## Purification of proteins

Deciding which purification tag to use depends on the use for which the purified protein is required. If the protein is needed in large amounts for immunization or for structural studies, then a small tag or a tag that can be readily removed by enzymatic treatment is desirable. The protein will normally be expressed in *E. coli* for such studies. Because large-scale purification is needed, it is important to choose a tag that binds to a ligand that is economical and readily available. For these reasons, epitope tags are not a good choice here because the antibody columns are expensive and are not readily compatible with large-scale purification from *E. coli.* The best choice is the His tag; the strep tag offers a valuable alternative.

If the protein is needed in smaller amounts for analyzing biochemical activity, examination of protein modification, or analysis of interaction with other cellular proteins, then the tagged protein will be expressed preferentially in the cell system of origin. For many projects, this means expression in mammalian cells or insect cell systems. It may be desirable to express a protein at physiologically more relevant levels, for example, to avoid saturating protein-modifying systems in the host cell. These requirements mean that a high degree of purification is needed and the tags should be small to minimize the chance that they will affect protein function. The His, FLAG, and strep tags are good choices here. They are all small, permit gentle elution from the solid phase, and have all been shown to work in mammalian and insect cell expression systems. Double tagging is a strong recommendation here too because it allows the purification of protein or a protein complex to homogeneity. In choosing the tag, check that the solid phase that will be used in the purification does not bind to any endogenous host cell component.

When the project is focused on protein interactions in vitro, the GST tag is usually the system of choice. GST-tagged proteins are readily produced in good yield in *E. coli*, are soluble, and can be efficiently captured on, and eluted from, glutathione agarose beads. These beads do not show spurious interactions even when incubated with whole-cell extracts of mammalian cells. The GST-tagged proteins often retain their correctly folded structure, and the GST moiety does not interact strongly with other proteins. *E. coli*-produced GST-tagged proteins have found extensive use as reagents to study the interaction of a cloned open reading frame with, for example, labeled mammalian protein extracts in GST-tagged protein precipitation experiments. The availability of good antibodies to GST and the solubility of GST-tagged proteins have allowed the proteins to be used for additional in vitro assay formats. GST-tagged proteins also form excellent substrates for protein kinases and are widely used for this purpose. It is worth remembering that GST is a dimeric protein; therefore, GST fusion proteins are also frequently dimers. Alternative tags that are suitable for this purpose are the cellulose-binding domain tag, the biotin modification tag, and the protein A tag, should any problem be encountered with the GST system.

*Because of the strong immunogenic properties of the GST tag, we do not recommend its use for the purification of proteins for immunization.*

## Testing the anti-tag antibodies for background in immunoaffinity purification

This pretesting of the tags in the system in which you intend to express and analyze your tagged proteins will save enormous amounts of trouble in the long run, and its importance cannot be overemphasized. To test for cross-reactions in immunoaffinity chromatography, prepare small columns of the anti-tag antibodies using protein G beads as described on page 321. Affinity columns of the anti-FLAG antibodies are available commercially. Use the binding in suspension protocol (page 333) to test the antibodies binding to extracts from cells in which you intend to express the tagged protein, for example, *E. coli*, insect cells, and mammalian cells. As a control, use beads to which no antibody has been attached. After thorough washing, collect the beads and analyze the protein eluted by the specific eluting agent (imidazole, glutathione, 2-aminobiotin, or free epitope peptide). By comparison of the level and nature of nonspecific protein binding to the different beads, it is possible to determine if there is a particular contaminating protein present that is specific to one of the anti-antigens. If any substantial amount of protein is eluted by the peptide step alone, then this tag/anti-tag combination cannot be used to purify tagged proteins from this source.

# Deciding where to position the tag

*A very useful method when purifying protein complexes is to tag each protein in the complex with a different peptide tag. In this way, sequential chromatography on the two specific ligand columns will result in the unique recovery of the pure complex because any uncomplexed protein will not be retained by both columns.*

### *Multitags*

*Some groups have found that oligomerizing the tag increases the sensitivity of detection (Nakajima and Yaoita 1997).*

The tag can be placed as an in-frame fusion in any position within the protein (Fig. 10.3). Typically, to minimize the risk that the tag will adversely affect protein function or be buried by the folding of the protein, the tag is placed at the amino or carboxyl terminus of the protein. An additional advantage of placing the tag at the carboxyl terminus of the open reading frame, replacing the endogenous stop codon with a new one, is that only full-length translation products will be detected by the anti-tag reagent. The advantage of placing the tag at the amino terminus is that it can then be incorporated into a standard vector system that has optimized translational initiation signals for successful expression of the tagged fusion protein.

Some workers have placed different tags at each end of the open reading frame to provide a double-tagged protein using, for example, the HA tag at the carboxyl terminus and a His tag at the amino terminus for specific detection and purification. This method combines the advantages of both approaches because only full-length protein will express both tags. However, double tagging does increase the risk that the protein's function may be modified adversely. Several groups have developed combination tags that include, for example, the information of a His purification tag with an epitope tag in a single peptide that can be incorporated at either the amino or carboxyl terminus of the protein to be tagged (Kelman et al. 1995).

Placing the tags elsewhere in the protein is most likely to affect the protein's structure and function. Such internal tags may be useful, for example, in studying protein orientation in the membrane or protein interactions, but these are best undertaken only with some specific predictions of the protein's structure (Canfield et al. 1996).

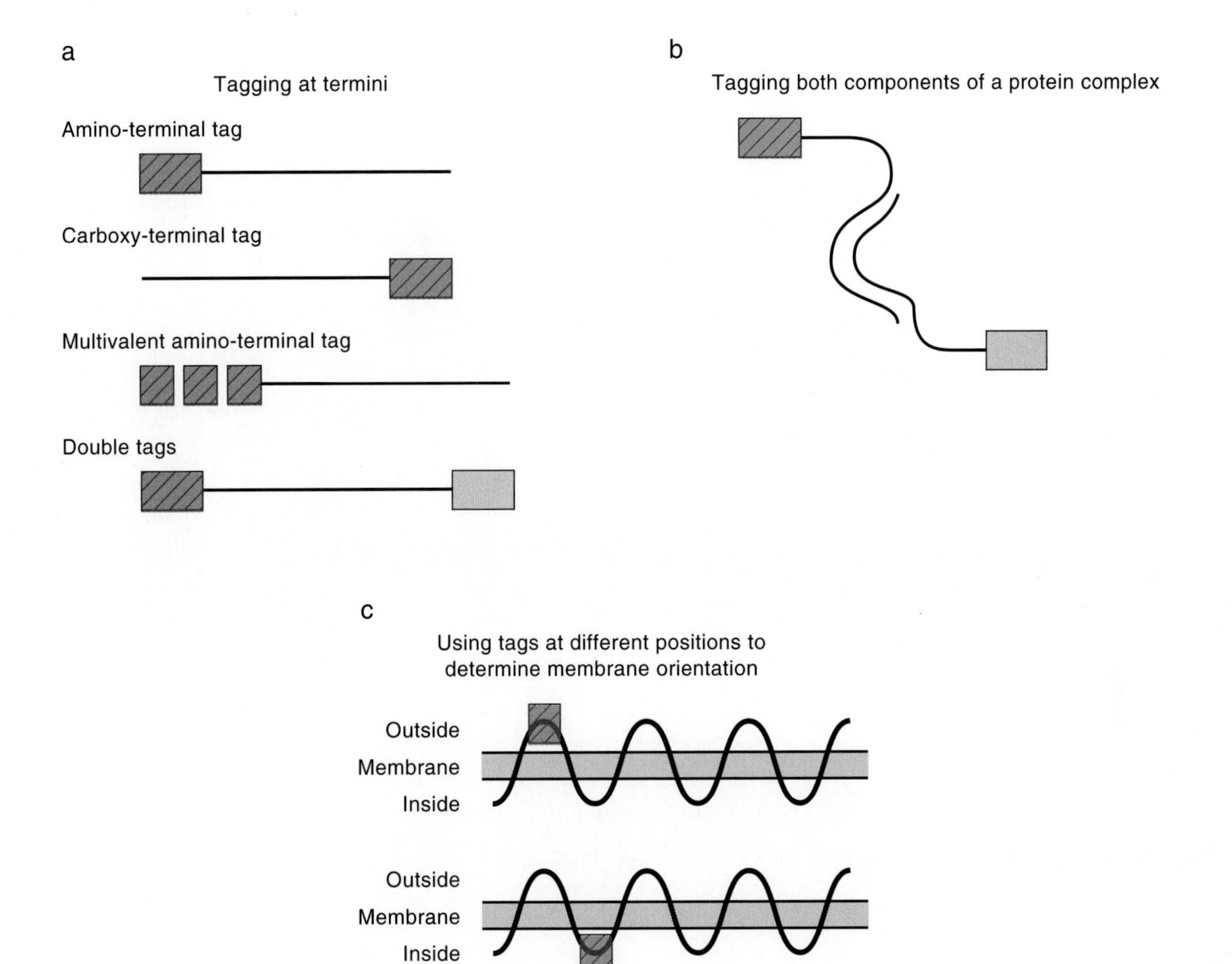


**Figure 10.3**
Different positions to insert tags.

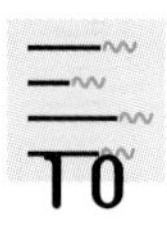



*Removing Gro EL*

*A common contaminant in preparations of affinity-purified GST proteins from* E. coli *is the GroEL protein. This 60,000 MW protein (chaperonin 60, Cpn 60) often binds to abundantly expressed recombinant proteins. However, it can be removed by an additional wash step before specific elution of the affinity column by carrying out a prior additional wash with 20 column volumes of an ATP-containing buffer (add 5 mm ATP to the standard wash buffer). If this is insufficient, then addition of 2.5 mm GroES to the ATP buffer will help to ensure the complete removal of the GroEL protein (Thain et al. 1996).*

### Contamination

When proteins are produced in bacterial expression systems, the full-length protein is often contaminated with amino-terminal and carboxy-terminal truncated fragments. This result arises not only because of proteolysis, but also because of premature termination of translation at the carboxy-terminal end or internal initiation of translation of the highly expressed mRNA at the amino terminus. This problem can be overcome by placing tags for purification at both the amino- and carboxy-terminal ends of the protein. By sequential purification on columns that bind either tag, only full-length protein is isolated. A popular choice is to place the HA tag at the amino terminus and the His tag at the carboxyl terminus. The expressed protein is then purified on a nickel affinity column to purify all His-tagged protein. After washing the column extensively, the His-tagged protein is eluted using imidazole-containing buffers and further purified and concentrated on an anti-HA affinity column using peptide elution to generate the final pure protein.

## How to tag your protein

Tagging of proteins can be performed by recombinant DNA methods. The best method to use depends on the skills of the lab, the exact nature of the construct, and the expression system to be used. In many cases, proprietary vectors are available that allow tagging with proteins or peptides and, in this case, the manufacturer provides detailed protocols. Here we discuss only some theoretical issues to guide vector choice. In other cases, it may be desirable to incorporate a tag into an existing expression system, and we discuss some of the principles involved in making these choices. Two simple example protocols using double-stranded oligonucleotide insertion and PCR-based insertion are also presented.

### Tagging by cloning into a tagging vector

The simplest way to epitope-tag a protein is to clone it into an expression vector that already incorporates the tag as part of the vector and contains a defined multiple

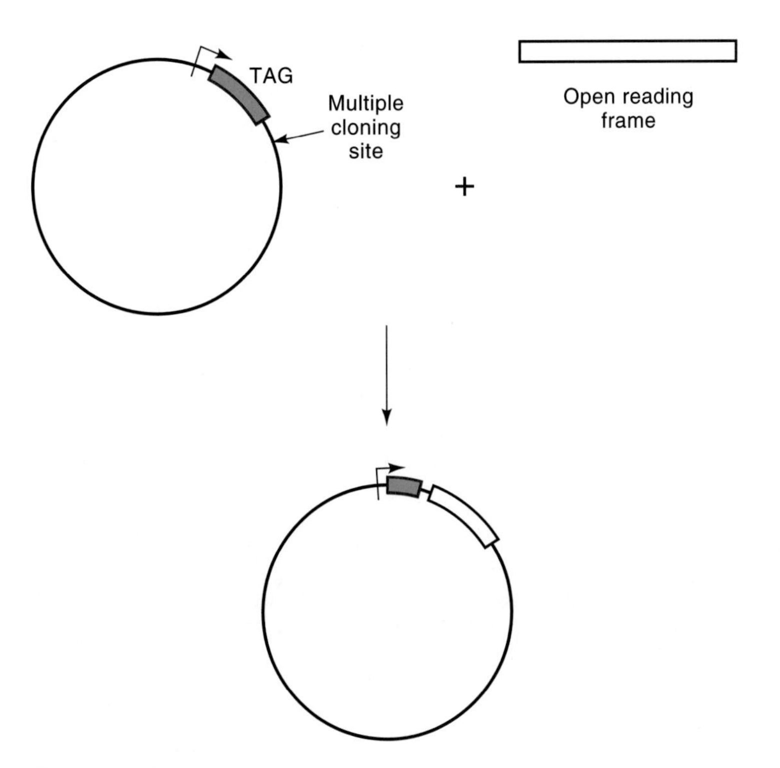


Figure 10.4
Tag by cloning into tagging vector.

cloning site (Fig. 10.4). A large number of commercial and noncommercial vectors of this type are now available.

In designing the cloning strategy, it is important to ensure that the tag is placed in the same reading frame as the protein that is to be tagged. Several of the vectors are available in all three reading frames to aid in this process. Others contain an upstream "shift" sequence that results in frameshifting during protein synthesis so that every potential downstream open reading frame can be translated as an alternate way to overcome this problem. Standard cloning methods can then be used to insert the protein-encoding gene into the expression vector. Many of the best vectors contain unique rare sites flanking the insert and the tag so that the whole tagged protein fragment can be isolated and transferred to other vector systems for expression of the same tagged protein in viral, bacterial, insect, and mammalian cell systems. The fact that the correct protein product is tagged often allows a rapid verification that a protein of the correct size is being produced. When the tagged protein is inserted into a bacterial expression vector, it is often possible to use colony blotting expression protocols to screen the bacterial colonies directly with the tag-binding reagent to identify those that are producing the tag. Cell staining of whole plates of infected insect cells or transfected mammalian cells can also be used as a rapid preliminary screen in these expression systems for expression of the tagged protein.

## Inserting a synthetic tag at a restriction site

In many cases, the open reading frame may have already been inserted into a multiple cloning site of a nontagged expression vector, or you may wish to modify a favorite in-house vector to incorporate an epitope tag. It is straightforward to insert an epitope tag into such a vector by using a suitable pair of oligonucleotides that are designed to encode the epitope in the correct reading frame and insert it at the appropriate unique restriction site (Fig. 10.5). In these cases, consult codon usage tables (see Appendix II) so that the codons selected to encode the particular amino acids of the epitope are commonly used by the organism that will be used to express the tagged protein. Where possible, use two unique sites in the vectors so that the cut vector cannot reanneal to itself. The oligonucleotides that encode the epitope can then be designed to have the appropriate complementary ends. In this case, there is no need to kinase the oligonucleotides, and the vector need not be phosphatased. Because these technologies are described in detail in numerous cloning manuals, only a simple example protocol is given here to illustrate the key considerations.

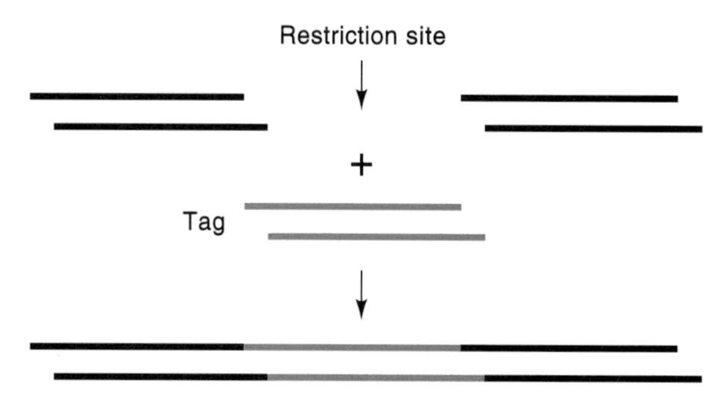


Figure 10.5
Tagging at a restriction site.

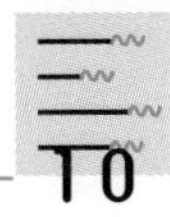

## Example protocol—Inserting a strep tag into an E. coli expression vector for the DNA-binding domain of YFP1

We want to insert a tag at the carboxyl terminus of the DNA-binding domain of protein YFP1. The existing expression vector produces very high levels of the protein fragment in functional form, so we simply want to tag this fragment without changing the vector. Because the system has been optimized for expression, we are anxious not to affect the precise sequence at the promoter at the 5′end (amino terminus) of the construct and so decide to tag the carboxyl terminus. We want to be able to use the tag to purify and immobilize the YFP1 DNA-binding domain, and we expect to analyze the protein fragment for antibody, DNA, and protein-binding properties. We decide that the streptavidin tag is a good choice because it will allow us to purify the protein using monovalent avidin columns, carry out DNA-binding experiments using streptavidin, and immobilize the protein on streptavidin-coated 96-well microtiter plates for protein and antibody interaction analysis. The first step is to examine the vector and determine the site of insertion. In this case, unique sites (*Eco*RI and *Bam*HI) are available within the vector's polylinker at either side of our chosen insertion site. The second step is to design the oligonucleotides to create the appropriate sticky ends for those cloning sites and to encode the strep tag amino acids using appropriate codon choices for the *E. coli* expression system used. Because we are replacing the existing stop codon, we need to incorporate a new stop codon after the carboxyl terminus of the tag. Using these rules, we design the following oligonucleotide pair.

Upper strand

Cloning site 1 A W R H P Q F G G STOP Cloning site 2

*Eco*RI *Bam*HI

5′-AATTC GCA TGG CGT CAT CCG CAG TTC GGC GGC TAG G 3′
3′G CGT ACC GCA GTA GGC GTC AAG CCG CCG ATG CTAG-5′

The two oligonucleotides are annealed and cloned into the appropriately prepared expression vector using standard ligation transformation and screening assays.

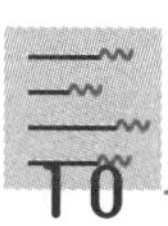



## Inserting an epitope tag by PCR

Often the appropriate restriction sites may not be available in the expression vector to allow the easy cloning of the tag into a restriction site. In these cases, the use of PCR offers an alternate route of the insertion of a peptide tag into a cloned open reading frame. PCR is very flexible, and the forward or reverse primer can be designed with long extensions so that they introduce the peptide tag at the amino terminus or carboxyl terminus of the protein. Codon usage tables (see Appendix II) should be consulted so that the codons selected to encode the particular amino acids of the tag are commonly used by the organism that will be used to express the tagged protein. The primers should be designed to create new restriction sites to facilitate the cloning of the final PCR product. A few extra bases should be added to the primers 5′ to the restriction site. These "add on" bases allow efficient cleavage by the restriction enzymes of the PCR product. Care should also be taken to maintain the correct open reading frame and to create the necessary initiation or stop codons as required. The Kozak consensus translational initiation sequence 5′-CCACCATGG-3′can be used in place of the simple ATG start codon to ensure efficient translation in eukaryotic cells. Slightly more complex PCR protocols permit the insertion of the peptide tag as an in-frame fusion anywhere within the open reading frame. Because these technologies are described in detail in numerous cloning manuals, only a simple example protocol is given here to illustrate the key considerations.

## Example protocol—Using PCR to insert an HA tag at the amino terminus of a cyclin-binding protein for expression in E. coli

The forward PCR primer (for the amino-terminal HA tag) is designed to achieve three objectives.

1. Encode the HA tag
2. Hybridize to the 5′end of the cyclin-binding protein YFP2 open reading frame
3. Create a new restriction site to permit cloning of the new tagged protein encoding PCR product into the preselected expression vector

When we tag the amino terminus, we need to create a new initiating methionine and avoid destroying the correct initiation signals for translation. If we were cloning for expression in a eukaryotic system, we would incorporate the Kozak consensus sequence here, but in this example we will use the existing vector sequences in the expression plasmid that we have selected (pET-5a).

The epitope tag sequence is:

**Tyr Pro Tyr Asp Val Pro Asp Tyr Ala**

**Y P Y D V P D Y A**

We select codon usage that is used frequently by both *E. coli* and humans:

**TAC CCA TAC GAC GTG CCA GAC TAC GCT**

We then select an overlap to place the tag at the amino terminus of YFP2. Usually an 18- to 21-bp overlap is about right. We are aiming for a $T_m$ between 55°C and 80°C. We want to avoid, where possible, runs of three Cs or Gs, and we want to avoid primers that are complementary at their 3′ ends or have significant secondary structure. Correct design of primers can be greatly aided by the use of current software programs, but as a simple rule of thumb, each AT pair contributes 2C, and each GC contributes 4C to the melting temperature.

This is the amino terminus of YFP2:

**ATG GAC CCG GCG GCG GGG AGC**

**M D P A A G S**

We then create the restriction site. In this example, we create a site that is not in the open reading frame: We choose to create an *Nde*I site to encode the initiating methionine and facilitate cloning into the expression vector, and we add a GC extension to help efficient restriction digestion of the PCR product and to prevent fraying of the PCR end.

**GC CATATG**

We create the forward primer by combining these elements and thus order the following oligonucleotide.

**5′-GC CATATGTAC CCA TAC GAC GTG CCA GAC TAC GCT ATG GAC CCG GCG GCG GGG AGC-3′**

A simple reverse primer can be designed to prime the end of the open reading frame and create a suitable restriction site.

The YFP2 sequence at the carboxyl terminus is:

**GGT CCC TCA GAC ATC CCC GAT TGA**
**G P S D I P D ***

So the reverse primer to hybridize to this region of the gene and create an *Eco*RI needed for cloning at the other end of our fragment is:

**GC GAA TTC TCA ATC GGG GAT GTC TGA GGG ACC**

Designing suitable conditions for the PCR using the existing plasmid encoding the YFP2 gene as the template requires careful optimization dependent on the precise apparatus used; such optimization protocols are available in Dieffenbach and Dveksler (1995).

If the correct-sized product is produced, then the PCR product is excised from the gel, purified using a proprietary PCR prep DNA purification system, restriction digested with *Eco*RI and *Nde*I, and ligated into the appropriately prepared vector. In this case, we clone into the pET-5a vector designed for expression in *E. coli* that contains the appropriate sites. The *Nde*I site provides the initiating methionine so that the new amino terminus will be as shown in the diagram.

**MYPYDVPDYAMDPAAGS........**
**!————tag——!——YFP2——-**

*This verification is especially important when the PCR method is used, because it is an error-prone procedure and unexpected mutations may occur.*

## Common problems with peptide tags

Tagging the protein by any of the procedures described is straightforward if your laboratory is experienced in basic molecular biology methods. Problems can arise, of course, and should the tag not be detectable, it is sensible to verify first by sequencing around the site of the tag insertion that the correct construct has been produced.

When using the oligonucleotide insertion method, it is possible, if a single restriction site is used for insertion, to get oligomers of the epitope incorporated, so it is best to use the double-cut strategy detailed in the example.

Sometimes the tag may be successfully incorporated but not recognized by the anti-tag reagent in methods that examine the native protein. This can occur, for example, in immunoprecipitation techniques, immunoaffinity purification, and immunostaining if the folding structure of the protein occludes the tag from the anti-tag reagent used. Because this problem is due to protein folding, it should not affect detection in immunoblotting. Placing the tag elsewhere in the protein, for example at the carboxyl rather than the amino terminus, may overcome this problem.

Finally, the tag may be successfully incorporated but not detected even in the immunoblotting procedure. This can happen if amino acid residues flanking the site of insertion prevent the antibody from binding the epitope. It can be overcome again by placing the tag elsewhere in the protein or by placing spacer residues between the tag sequence and the protein sequence. The sequence SGSG is a suitable spacer.

The final and most difficult problem is the finding that the tag alters the properties of the protein. This is, in many cases, hard to establish unless the untagged protein is already very well characterized. Again, the obvious solutions to reduce this problem are to use different tags and place them in different positions. If all the tagged proteins show the same properties, then it is very unlikely that the tag is responsible for the particular property of the protein, and it is possible to be confident that it is a property of the untagged protein.

## References


Canfield V.A., Norbeck L., and Levenson R. 1996. Localization of cytoplasmic and extracellular domains of Na,K-ATPase by epitope tag insertion. *Biochemistry* **35:** 14165–14172.

Cormack B.P., Valdivia R.H., and Falkow S. 1996. FACS-optimized mutants of the green fluorescent protein (GFP). *Gene* **173:** 33–38.

Delagrave S., Hawtin R.E., Silva C.M., Yang M.M., and Youvan D.C. 1995. Red-shifted excitation mutants of the green fluorescent protein. *Bio/Technology* **13:** 151–154.

Dieffenbach C.W. and Dveksler G.S. 1995. *PCR primer: A laboratory manual.* Cold Spring Harbor Laboratory Press, Cold Spring Harbor, New York.

Evan G.I., Lewis G.K., Ramsay G., and Bishop J.M. 1985. Isolation of monoclonal antibodies specific for human c-*myc* proto-oncogene product. *Mol. Cell. Biol.* **12:** 3610–3616.

Field J., Nikawa J., Broek D., MacDonald B., Rodgers L., Wilson I.A., Lerner R.A., and Wigler M. 1988. Purification of a RAS-responsive adenylyl cyclase complex from *Saccharomyces cerevisiae* by use of an epitope addition method. *Mol. Cell. Biol.* **8:** 2159–2165.

Goldstein M.A., Takagi M., Hashida S., Shoseyov O., Doi R.H., and Segel I.H. 1993. Characterization of the cellulose-binding domain of the *Clostridium cellulovorans* cellulose-binding protein *A. J. Bacteriol.* **175:** 5762–5768.

Gort S. and Maloy S. 1998. Purification of a hexahistidine-tagged protein using L-histidine as the eluent. *Elsevier Trends Journals Technical Tips Online* (http://tto.trends.com/). Document PII: SO168–9525(97) 01389.

Grussenmeyer T., Scheidtmann K.H., Hutchinson M.A., Eckhart W., and Walter G. 1985. Complexes of polyoma virus medium T antigen and cellular proteins. *Proc. Natl. Acad. Sci.* **82:** 7952–7954.

Harlow E., Crawford L.V., Pim D.C., and Williamson N.M. 1981. Monoclonal antibodies specific for simian virus 40 tumor antigens. *J. Virol.* **39:** 861–869.

Hatfield C., Duus K.M., Jones D.H., and Grose C. 1997. Epitope mapping and tagging by recombination PCR mutagenesis. *Bio-Techniques* **22:** 332–337.

Heim R., Cubitt A.B., and Tsien R.Y. 1995. Improved green fluorescence. *Nature* **373:** 663–664.

Hopp T.P., Pricekitt K.S., Price V.L., Libby R.T., March C.J., Ceretti D.P., Urdal D.L., and Conlon P.J. 1988. A short polypeptide marker sequence used for recombinant protein identification and purification. *Bio/Technology* **6:** 1204–1210.

Ito Y., Hamaguchi Y., Segawa K., Dalianis T., Appella E. and Willingham M. 1983. Antibodies against a nonapeptide of polyomavirus middle T antigen: Cross-reaction with a cellular protein(s). *J. Virol.* **48:** 709–720.

Kelman Z., Yao N., and O'Donnell M. 1995. *Escherichia coli* expression vectors containing a protein kinase recognition motif, His6-tag and hemagglutinin epitope. *Gene* **166:** 177–178.

Knappik A. and Pluckthun A. 1994. An improved affinity tag based on the FLAG peptide for the detection and purification of recombinant antibody fragments. *BioTechniques* **17:** 754–761.

Kreis T.E. 1986. Microinjected antibodies against the cytoplasmic domain of vesicular stomatitis virus glycoprotein block its transport to the cell surface. *EMBO J.***5:** 931–941.

Kwatra M.M., Schreurs J., Schwinn D.A., Innis M.A., Caron M.G., and Lefkowitz R.J. 1995. Immunoaffinity purification of epitope-tagged human beta 2-adrenergic receptor to homogeneity. *Protein Expr. Purif.* **6:** 717–721.

Lindner K., Mole S.E., Lane D.P., and Kenny M. 1998. Epitope mapping of antibodies recognising the N terminus of simian virus large tumour antigen. *Intervirology* **41:** 10–16.

Lindner P., Bauer K., Krebber A., Nieba L., Kremmer E., Krebber C., Honegger A., Klinger B., Mocikat R., and Pluckthun A. 1997. Specific detection of his-tagged proteins with recombinant anti-His tag scFv-phosphatase or scFv-phage fusions. *Bio-Techniques* **22:** 140–149.

MacArthur H. and Walter G. 1984. Monoclonal antibodies specific for the carboxy terminus of simian virus 40 large T antigen. J. Virol. 52: 483–491.

McCormick M. and Mierendorf R.1994. S•Tag (TM): A multipurpose fusion peptide for recombinant proteins. In *inNovations* (newsletter), vol. 1, pp. 4–7. Novagen, Inc., Madison, Wisconsin.

Munro S. and Pelham H.R. 1984. Use of peptide tagging to detect proteins expressed from cloned genes: Deletion mapping functional domains of *Drosophila* hsp 70. *EMBO J.* **3:** 3087–3093.

———.1986. An Hsp 70-like protein in the ER: Identity with the 78 kd glucose-regulated protein and immunoglobulin heavy chain binding protein. *Cell* **46:** 291–300.

Nakajima K. and Yaoita Y. 1997. Construction of multiple-epitope tag sequence by PCR for sensitive Western blot analysis. *Nucleic Acids Res.* **25:** 2231–2232.

Niman H.L., Houghten R.A., Walker L.E., Reisfeld R.A., Wilson I.A., Hogle J.M., and Lerner R.A. 1983. Generation of protein-reactive antibodies by short peptides is an event of high frequency: Implications for the structural basis of immune recognition. *Proc. Natl. Acad. Sci.* **80:** 4949–4953.

Nygren P.O., Stahl S., and Uhlen M. 1994. Engineering proteins to facilitate bioprocessing. *Trends Biotechnol.* **12:** 184–188.

Porath J. 1992. Immobilized metal ion affinity chromatography. *Protein Expr. Purif.* **3:** 263–281.

Prasher D.C., Eckenrode V.K., Ward W.W., Prendergast F.G., and Cormier M.J. 1992. Primary structure of the *Aequorea victoria* green-fluorescent protein. *Gene* **111:** 229–233.

Richards F.M. and Wyckoff H.W. 1971. Bovine pancreatic ribonuclease. **4:** 647–806.

Sambrook J., Fritsch E.F., and Maniatis T. 1989. *Molecular cloning: A laboratory manual*, 2nd edition. Cold Spring Harbor Laboratory Press, Cold Spring Harbor, New York.

Schäfer K. and Braun T. 1995. Monoclonal anti-FLAG antibodies react with a new isoform of rat $Mg2^+$ dependent protein phosphatase β. *Biochem. Biophys. Res. Commun.* **207:** 708–714.

Schaffhausen B., Benjamin T.L., Pike L., Casnellie J., and Krebs E. 1982. Antibody to the nonapeptide Glu-Glu-Glu-Glu-Tyr-Met-Pro-Met-Glu is specific for polyoma middle T antigen and inhibits in vitro kinase activity. *J. Biol. Chem.* **257:** 12467–12470.

Schmidt T.G. and Skerra A. 1993. The random peptide library-assisted engineering of a C-terminal affinity peptide, useful for the detection and purification of a functional Ig Fv fragment. *Protein Eng.* **6:** 109–122.

———.1994. One-step affinity purification of bacterially produced proteins by means of the 'Strep tag' and immobilized recombinant core streptavidin. *J. Chromatogr. A* **676:** 337–345.

Schmidt T.G., Koepke J., Frank R., and Skerra A. 1996. Molecular interaction between the Strep-tag affinity peptide and its cognate target, streptavidin. *J. Mol. Biol.* **255:** 753–766.

Schreurs J., Yamamoto R., Lyons J., Munemitsu S., Conroy L., Clark R., Takeda Y., Krause J.E., and Innis M. 1997. Functional wild-type and carboxyl-terminal-tagged rat substance P receptors expressed in baculovirus-infected insect Sf9 cells. *J. Neurochem.* **64:** 1622–1631.

Skinner R.H., Bradley S., Brown A.L., Johnson N.J., Rhodes S., Stammers D.K., and Lowe P.N. 1991. Use of the Glu-Glu-Phe C-terminal epitope for rapid purification of the catalytic domain of normal and mutant *ras* GTPase-activating proteins. *J. Biol. Chem.* **266:** 14163–14166.

Slootstra J.W., Kuperus D., Pluckthun A., and Meloen R.H. 1997. Identification of new tag sequences with differential and selective recognition properties for the anti-FLAG monoclonal antibodies M1, M2 and M5. *Mol. Divers.* **2:** 156–164.

Smith D.B. and Johnson K.S. 1988. Single-step purification of polypeptides expressed in *Escherichia coli* as fusions with glutathione S-transferase. *Gene* **67:** 31–40.

Stammers D.K., Tisdale M., Court S., Parmar V., Bradley C., and Ross C.K. 1991. Rapid purification and characterisation of HIV-1 reverse transcriptase and RnaseH engineered to incorporate a C-terminal tripeptide α-tubulin epitope. *FEBS Lett.* **283:** 298–302.

Stephen C.W. and Lane D.P. 1992. Mutant conformation of p53. Precise epitope mapping using a filamentous phage epitope library. *J. Mol. Biol.* **225:** 577–583.

Stephen C.W., Helminen P., and Lane D.P. 1995. Characterisation of epitopes on human p53 using phage-displayed peptide libraries: Insights into antibody-peptide interactions. *J. Mol. Biol.* **248:** 58–78.

Thain A., Gaston K., Jenkins O. and Clarke A.R. 1996. A method for the separation of GST fusion proteins from co-purifying GroEL, *Elsevier Trends Journals Technical Tips Online* (http://tto.trends.com/). Document PII: S0168–9525(96)40018X.

Tomme P., Gilkes N.R., Miller Jr., R.C., Warren A.J., and Kilburn D.G. 1994. An internal cellulose-binding domain mediates adsorption of an engineered bifunctional xylanase/cellulase. *Protein Eng.* **7:** 117–123.

Wang L.F., Yu M., White J.R., and Eaton B.T. 1996. BTag: A novel 6 residue epitope tag for surveillance and purification of recombinant proteins. *Gene* **169:** 53–58.

Wilson I.A., Niman H.L., Houghten R.A., Cherenson A.R., Connolly M.L., and Lerner R.A. 1984. The structure of an antigenic determinant in a protein. *Cell* **37:** 767–778.

# Epitope Mapping

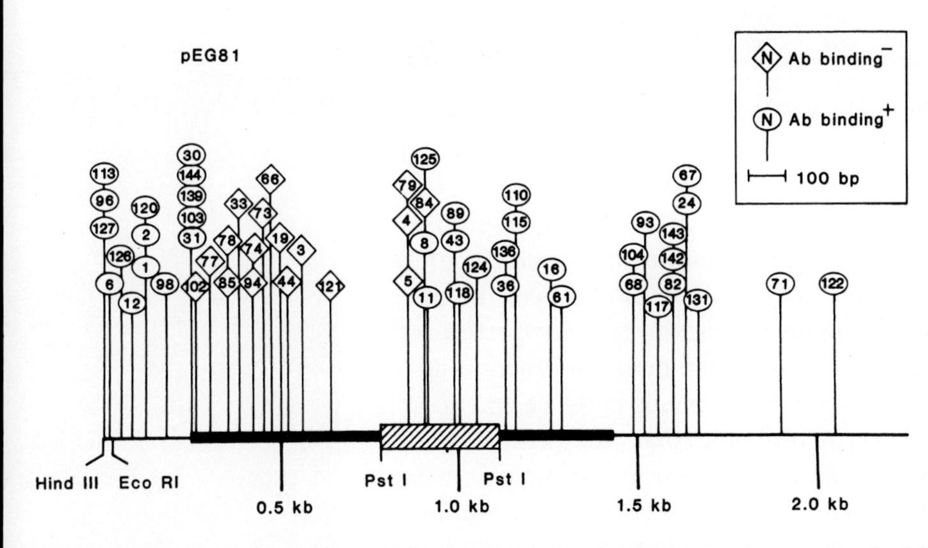


Lupski J.R., Ozaki L.S., Ellis J., and Godson G.N. 1983. Localization of a *Plasmodium* surface antigen epitope by Tn5 mutagenesis mapping of a recombinant cDNA clone. *Science* **220:** 1285–1288. (Reprinted with permission [copyright American Association for the Advancement of Science].)

Fig. 1. A transposon Tn5 map of plasmid pEG81. The map shows the physical location of 57 independent Tn5 inserts (*13*). The insertion mutations were mapped with respect to the unique HindIII site of pEG81 by HindIII digest of purified plasmid DNA. Inserts on the right side of pEG81::Tn5-121 were digested with PvuII plus BamHI to demonstrate they were in the proper ($Ap^r$ gene) side of pEG81. The Tn5 hops into the cDNA inserts were confirmed by PstI digestion; the disappearance of the 340-bp restriction fragment generated from PstI digestion of pEG81 was judged as being due to Tn5 insertion into this fragment. The circled numbers indicate inserts that had no effect on the ability of lysate from cells bearing this plasmid to bind 2G3; lysates from cells containing plasmid with inserts indicated by numbers enclosed in diamond shape no longer bound antibody (also see Table 1).

Early epitope mapping experiments relied on elegant, but painstaking, protein chemistry approaches. These methods relied primarily on protein modification and proteolysis. Amino acids were selectively marked by chemical modification of the side chains, and binding loss was measured. Protein antigens were also cleaved and then sequenced to identify small antibody binding domains. The results were beautiful examples of the best in protein chemistry, but the determination of the full set of epitopes for an antigen was a full life's work. Molecular cloning and advances in peptide synthesis have dramatically changed epitope mapping. Epitopes can now be identified by mutagenesis, by protein synthesis, or by protein competition. And with the identification of epitope sequences come all of the advantages of knowing the site of antibody binding. Epitope mapping can be used for such disparate needs as to localize protein functional activities or to have binding domains that can be used for specific tags.

Determining the binding sites (epitopes) for monoclonal and polyclonal antigens on protein antigens often provides extremely useful information that greatly extends the power of immunochemical analysis. Epitope mapping is used to examine the specificity of the immune response or to distinguish between different antibodies. It can also determine such properties as the sites of protein modification, origin of protein fragments, or orientation of proteins in the cell membrane. The use of antibodies that bind defined epitopes can enhance understanding of protein domain structure, protein function, and protein interactions. Panels of mapped antibodies have proved to be a key resource in many fields, allowing unequivocal identification of the protein in different cellular contexts and, in some cases, allowing specific determination and modification of their function.

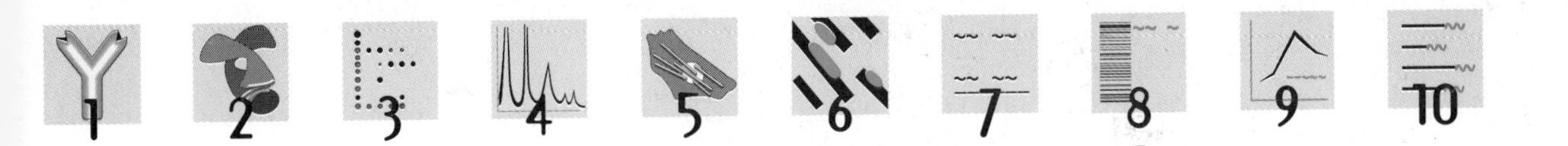


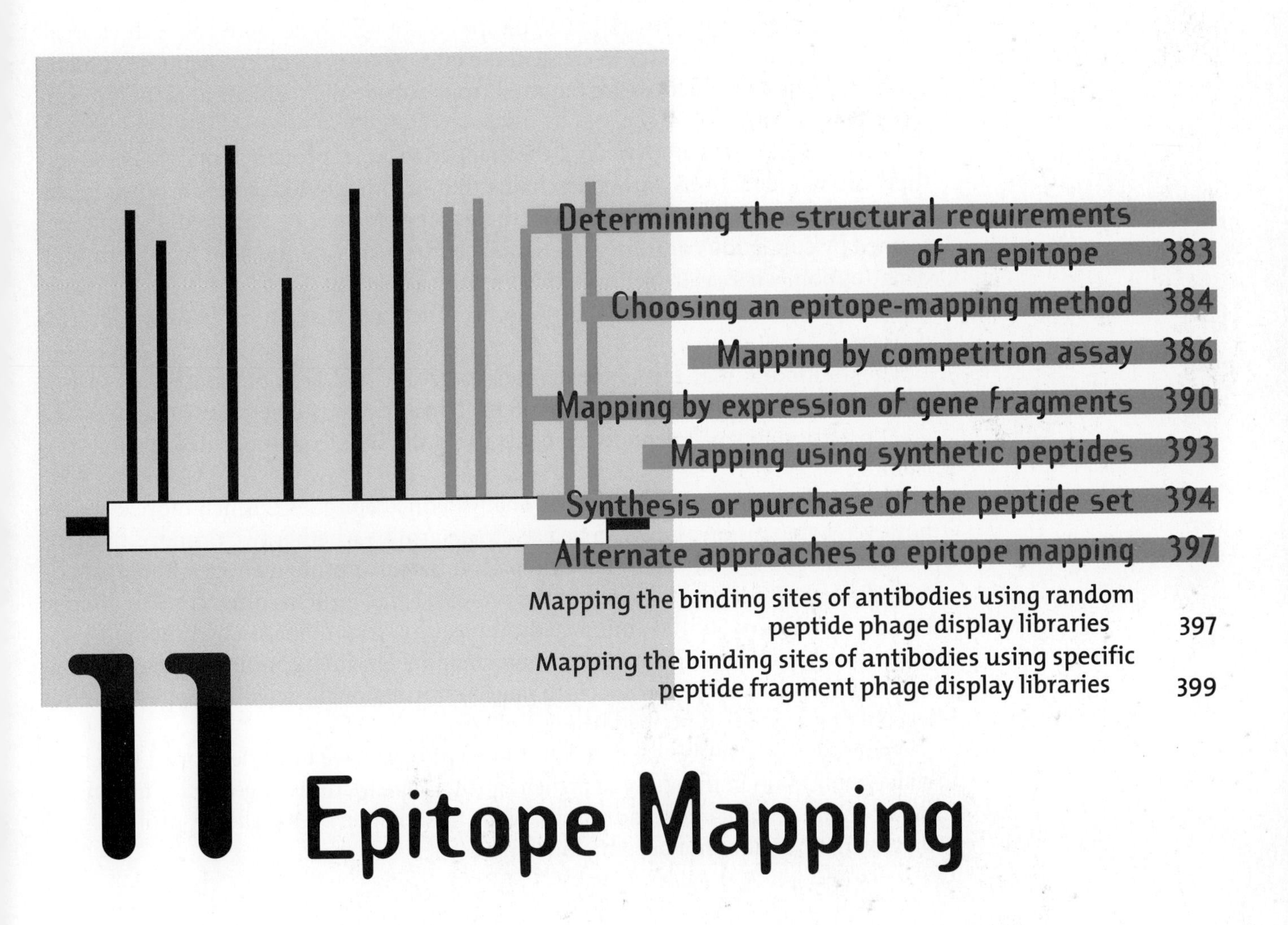



# 11 Epitope Mapping

Epitope mapping is used to examine the specificity of the immune response or to distinguish between different antibodies. It can also determine such properties as the sites of protein modification, origin of protein fragments, or orientation of proteins in the cell membrane.

Two classes of epitopes can be distinguished functionally: linear epitopes, which can be mapped to small linear peptide sequences of 5–20 amino acids, and conformational epitopes, which are formed by the folding of proteins in larger domains. Structural studies of antibody–antigen cocrystals explain these two types of epitopes (see Chapter 2).

Linear epitopes form highly structured multiple interactions between the antibody combining site and multiple amino acid side chains and backbone contacts within a contiguous peptide sequence. These epitopes are also called continuous epitopes. They may, in fact, require some local structural distortion or involve closely spaced but noncontiguous amino acids such as those found on one face of an amphipathic $\alpha$ helix so that the description as linear epitopes is not wholly accurate. Nevertheless, all of the information necessary to create these epitopes is present in a peptide segment, and no additional sequences are required from outside the segment to form the antibody-binding site.

Conformational epitopes can only be mapped to larger protein domains. These epitopes show interactions with side chains that, although close to each other in the folded protein, are widely separated in the linear sequence. As expected, the epitopes formed by contiguous or nearly contiguous amino acids are resistant to loss through denaturation, whereas those formed from noncontiguous amino acids are lost when the protein unfolds. This provides a useful functional distinction between the two classes.

The antibodies that recognize denaturation-resistant epitopes work well in immunoblotting, and their binding sites on protein antigens can be readily mapped with great precision to small peptide segments using the simple methods described in this chapter.

The precise mapping of conformationally defined epitopes is much more difficult; however, competition assays can be used to determine whether two or more antibodies that recognize conformational epitopes on the same protein antigen bind to sterically discrete or overlapping sites on the protein. Large proteins often contain discrete folding domains of 50–100 amino acids; thus, using recombinant DNA methods, it is now often possible to localize such conformation-sensitive epitopes at least to fragments of this size. Simple protocols to map conformationally sensitive epitopes to this level of precision are described below.

Many very innovative ways to determine epitopes have been developed that have wider application in the study of protein–protein interactions in general. These novel methods are summarized and discussed in this chapter, but detailed protocols for these variations have not been included here.

## Determining the structural requirements of an epitope

When choosing an epitope-mapping method, it is first important to determine what the goals of the study are. If the goal of the study is simply to determine whether two different antibodies recognize sterically discrete epitopes, all that is needed is to compare the binding of the antibodies in a competition binding assay. This method will determine if the antibodies are able to block each other's binding to the antigen. If, however, the goal of the study is to map the binding site of the antibody on the protein, then determining the antibody's ability to react with defined large fragments of the antigen is the next step. These procedures work with antibodies that recognize either conformational or linear epitopes. If the antibody recognizes the antigen in immunoblotting protocols, the precise mapping of the epitope can be established by the use of synthetic peptides corresponding to small linear segments of the protein antigen.

In designing an epitope-mapping project, it is very helpful to determine the structural class of epitope with which your antibody reacts. This can be done by carrying out the immunoblotting procedure described in Chapter 8 using an extract that contains the protein to be studied. If your antibody gives a positive reaction in this method, then you have a linear epitope capable of closer mapping. If it does not react with the antigen in the immunoblotting method, then its epitope is lost on denaturation, is conformational, and can only be mapped to a larger domain. In either case, you will be able to determine whether different antibodies bind to the same site on the protein using the competition assay. Table 11.1 summarizes the properties of linear and conformational epitopes and how they behave in immunoblotting, immunoprecipitation, and immunostaining procedures.

Table 11.1 *Properties of linear and conformational epitopes*

| Epitope class | Immunoblotting | Cell staining | Immunoprecipitation | Epitope size | Structural requirements |
|---|---|---|---|---|---|
| **Linear** | Antibody always binds | Antibody usually binds | Antibody may not bind | 5–20 amino acids | Short linear amino acid sequence |
| **Conformational** | Antibody never binds | Antibody usually binds | Antibody usually binds | | Folded protein domain |

# Choosing an epitope-mapping method

There are many potential methods for mapping and characterizing the location of epitopes on proteins, ranging from solving the crystal structure of the antibody–antigen complex to analysis of vast libraries of random peptide sequences. These variants are discussed below. Three of the simplest, most widely applicable, and most robust assays are competition assays, gene expression assays, and synthetic peptide-based assays (Table 11.2).

Mapping by competition assay is a very widely used method that can rapidly determine whether two different monoclonal antibodies are able to bind independently to the same protein antigen or whether their binding sites on the protein overlap in such a way that both are not able to bind to the antigen at the same time. The assay can be configured in a large number of different formats using either labeled antigen or labeled antibody. Commonly, the antigen is immobilized on a 96-well plate. The ability of unlabeled antibodies to block the binding of labeled antibodies is measured using radioactive or enzyme labels.

Using this kind of assay with a panel of monoclonal antibodies allows the number of sterically discrete epitopes on the protein antigen to be determined. The method is very versatile and remarkably accurate. For example, we used this kind of assay to map 10 or more independent epitopes on SV40 large T antigen (Gannon and Lane 1990). It is particularly useful in determining if a new monoclonal antibody to a particular protein is distinct from other antibodies to the same protein (Wagener et al. 1983,

**Table 11.2** *Application and requirements of recommended epitope-mapping methods*

| Method | Conformational epitope | Linear epitope | Requirements | Precision |
|---|---|---|---|---|
| **Competition assay** | Yes | Yes | Labeled antibody; antigen | Determines steric competition only |
| **Gene fragment expression** | Often but not always | Yes | cDNA must be cloned (gene sequence known) | Conformational 50–200 amino acid domains. Linear 10–20 amino acids |
| **Synthetic peptide library** | Never | Yes | Peptide library must be made but cDNA clone not required | Complete description of epitope 3–15 amino acids |

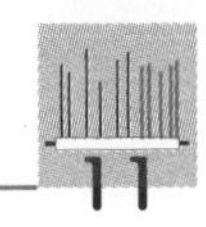


1984; Kuroki et al. 1990, 1992a,b). The assay can be used with antibodies that bind both conformational and linear epitopes.

The second approach to mapping an epitope is based on the concept of cutting the protein into smaller fragments and then examining whether the antibody will react with any of these pieces. Historically, these fragments were produced by chemical or proteolytic cleavage of the protein antigen. These remain powerful methods, but the advent of systems for the expression of recombinant proteins has allowed an alternative genetic approach to protein fragmentation. In these procedures, the open reading frame encoding the protein is fragmented either randomly or by specific genetic construction, and the reactivity of the expressed fragments of the protein with the test antibody is determined.

The versatility of DNA fragmentation protocols combined with the vast range of available systems for the expression of recombinant protein has created an almost infinite number of variants on this theme. These range from the entire synthesis of gene segments (Alexander et al. 1992) to the cloning of random fragments of the open reading frame generated by digestion with DNase for expression on the surface of bacteriophage particles (Petersen et al. 1995; Fack et al. 1997).

All of these variants are effective, because only small amounts of protein need to be expressed to determine whether an antibody can bind to it. Thus, even if only a small fraction of the expressed protein fragment folds correctly, it may still be sufficient to give a strong antibody-binding signal, making this method useful for mapping the binding sites of antibodies to both conformation-sensitive and linear epitopes.

A useful example protocol where defined gene fragments are produced by PCR and then transcribed and translated into protein in vitro in the presence of radioactive amino acids is outlined below (p. 391). Binding of the antibody to the labeled protein fragments is then determined by immunoprecipitation and gel electrophoresis.

The third approach to epitope mapping is only applicable to antibodies that work in immunoblotting and react with short linear peptide epitopes. The identification of the epitopes with which these antibodies react has been done using large libraries of random peptide sequence displayed on the surface of phage particles. Alternatively, vast libraries of random synthetic peptides have been analyzed. A much simpler approach in cases where the amino acid sequence of the protein or gene fragment contains the epitope is to synthesize (or order) a defined library of overlapping peptide segments of the protein. These peptide set libraries can then be easily tested for binding to the test antibody in simple binding assays and will define the linear epitope to a stretch of 5–15 amino acids.

## Mapping by competition assay

The simplest way to determine whether two monoclonal antibodies bind to distinct sites on a protein antigen is to carry out a competition assay, which will determine the capacity of one antibody to inhibit the binding of another antibody. If there is competition, then the two antibodies recognize identical or sterically overlapping epitopes. In contrast, if the two antibodies do not interfere with each other's binding and can both bind simultaneously to the antigen, then the antibodies must be different from each other and recognize discrete epitopes (Fig. 11.1).

This test is most useful in the analysis of monoclonal antibody specificity because polyclonal sera typically recognize multiple different epitopes. There are many assay designs that measure the competition of antibodies for binding to protein antigen. Most of these techniques require at least one of the antibodies to be directly labeled. The method also requires a source of reasonably pure antigen. In this simple protocol, an ELISA protocol is used, and the antibodies to be tested are labeled by biotinylation (Wagener et al. 1984). This example protocol examines the ability of two newly derived monoclonal antibodies, XH1 and XH2, to compete for binding to the target anti-

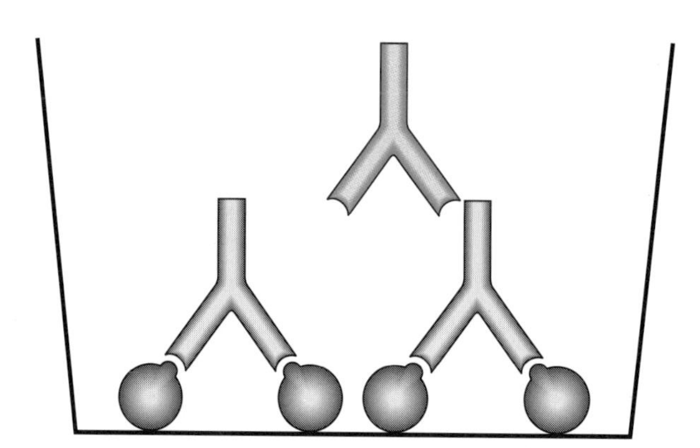


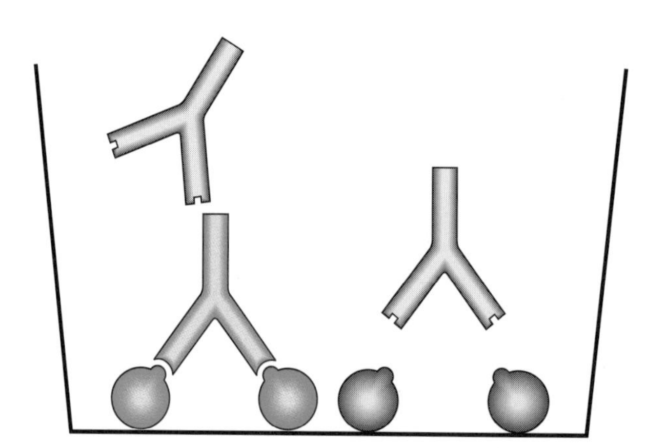


Figure 11.1
Competition assay.

gen YFP1 with the well-characterized ZO-1 anti-YFP1 antibody. In the first step, 96-well plates are coated with the YFP1 antigen and direct binding assays are run to determine that all of the antibody preparations are active and able to react with the immobilized antigen. These antibody preparations are also titrated so that sensitive conditions can be established for the competition assay. In the second step, the competition analysis itself is carried out to compare the ability of unlabeled XH2, XH1, and ZO-1 to block the binding of the biotin-labeled ZO-1 antibody to YFP1.

### Needed reagents and solutions

PBS
PBS Tween (0.05%)
PBS BSA (PBS with 1% BSA), no azide
0.1 M Sodium bicarbonate buffer, pH 9.6
Streptavidin peroxidase conjugate
Rabbit anti-mouse IgG peroxidase conjugate
YFP1
Biotin-labeled ZO-1 antibody
Unlabeled ZO-1 antibody
Unlabeled XH1 and XH2 antibodies
Unlabeled control monoclonal antibody PC10
TMB substrate (50 ml of 50 g/l stock in 5 ml of 0.1 M sodium acetate, pH 6.6, with 1 ml of $H_2O_2$)

### Cautions

Biotin, hydrogen peroxide, sulfuric acid, see Appendix IV.

## Determination of the activity and titer of the test and control antibodies

1. Prepare a stock solution of YFP1 at 20 µg/ml in 0.1 M sodium bicarbonate buffer, pH 9.6 (or PBS). Add 50 ml to the wells of a 96-well microplate and incubate for 2 hours at room temperature or overnight at 4°C.

2. Wash the wells three times in PBS Tween.

3. Fill the wells (200 µl) with PBS BSA and incubate at room temperature for 1 hour.

4. Wash twice in PBS Tween.

5. In a separate 96-well plate, prepare a titration series of the biotin-labeled ZO-1 and the unlabeled ZO-1, XH1, XH2, and control PC10 antibodies over five 10-fold dilutions using PBS BSA as a diluent. The starting concentration of the antibody solutions should be about 10 µg/ml. Hybridoma supernatants can be used neat.

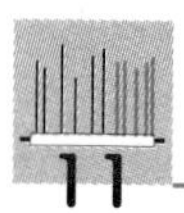



6. Transfer 50 µl of each dilution onto the antigen-coated plate and incubate for 2 hours at room temperature.

7. Wash the plate four times in PBS Tween.

8. Add 50 µl of rabbit anti-mouse peroxidase conjugate (diluted 1 in 5000 in PBS BSA) to all the wells containing unlabeled antibody. Add the streptavidin-peroxidase conjugate (diluted 1 in 5000 in PBS BSA) to the wells that contain the biotinylated ZO-1 antibody.

9. Incubate for 2 hours at room temperature or overnight at 4°C; then wash the plate four times in PBS Tween.

10. Add 50 µl of freshly prepared TMB substrate to each test well and incubate at room temperature for 5–15 minutes as the blue color develops in the wells containing the highest concentration of specific antibody.

11. After development of the blue color, stop the reaction by adding 50 µl of 100 mM sulfuric acid. Determine the absorbance of the now-yellow product read at 450-nm wavelength in a microplate reader.

    The positive antibodies should give a clear strong signal, which diminishes through the latter part of the dilution series. This establishes that the specific unlabeled antibodies are able to bind to the target antigen and identifies any of those having very weak activity. This dilution series also establishes a suitable concentration to use of the labeled antibody in the competition assay.

**This assay determines that the ELISA protocol is suitable for running the competition assay.**

## The competition assay

1. Prepare antigen-coated plates as in steps 1–4 above.

2. Incubate the wells with the dilution series of unlabeled antibodies as above for 2 hours at room temperature.

3. Without washing the wells, add 50 µl of the dilution of the biotin-labeled ZO-1 antibody that gave the strongest signal before the next point in the

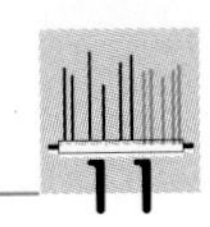


*Competition assays can be established in many different formats. For example, they can be used where the antigen is a fixed monolayer culture of cells that express the protein. The key requirements remain the same, however: a demonstration that all of the antibodies are able to bind the test antigen in the assay and the labeling of one of the antibodies that allows it to be distinguished from the competitor antibody. Some antigens are partially denatured on absorption to plastic, and in these cases, alternate means of immobilizing the antigen may be explored.*

titration curve showing a strongly reduced signal, as determined in the previous procedure.

4. Wash the plate four times in PBS Tween.

5. Add streptavidin-peroxidase conjugate (diluted 1 in 5000 in PBS BSA) to all of the wells.

6. Incubate for 2 hours at room temperature or overnight at 4°C and then wash the plate four times in PBS Tween.

7. Add 50 μl of freshly prepared TMB substrate to each test well and incubate at room temperature for 5–15 minutes. The blue color develops in the wells containing the highest concentration of specific antibody.

8. After development of the blue color, stop the reaction by adding 50 μl of 100 mM sulfuric acid. Determine the absorbance of the now-yellow product read at 450-nm wavelength in a microplate reader.

   A strong reduction in the signal of the binding of the labeled ZO-1 should be seen by the highest concentrations of the unlabeled ZO-1 (homotypic competition). The PC10 antibody should not inhibit the signal at any concentration. The novel competing antibody XH2 reduces the signal, whereas the other new antibody XH1 does not. Therefore, XH2 and ZO-1 recognize sterically competitive epitopes, whereas the XH1 epitope is clearly unique.

The use of surface plasmon resonance for competition mapping is very effective (Johne et al. 1993). Here total mass bound to the antigen-coated chip is determined optically as antibody solution is pumped past it. There is no need to label or even purify the antibodies to be tested in this method. The equipment required and the need to use specially coated chips do mean that this technique can be expensive.

## Mapping by expression of gene fragments

Many protocols, as well as one commercial kit (Novatope), have been devised to express random or defined segments of an open reading frame in an expression vector system. The library of gene fragments is then tested for reaction with the antibody to be mapped, and the nature of the gene fragment(s) that reacts with the antibody is determined either by sequence analysis or by virtue of the previously defined nature of the fragment of the gene present in the vector. In many cases, investigators may already have libraries of gene fragments cloned into expression vectors by virtue of previous studies. These may represent incomplete cDNA constructs or fragments derived from expression libraries. All of these libraries can be used in simple immunochemical tests to determine whether they contain the relevant epitope. If the antibody reacts well with the target antigen in immunoblotting methods, it makes sense to use this same procedure to analyze any expressed gene fragments.

If the antibody does not work on immunoblots of expressed protein fragments, it is still worthwhile attempting to probe these gene fragments in direct blotting analysis of the bacterial colonies. In this direct blotting assay, for example, all of the monoclonal antibodies to SV40 large-T antigen that did not work in immunoblotting could still be epitope-mapped by examining their reactivity with fragments of SV40 expressed as fusion proteins to β-galactosidase. Thus, many denaturation-sensitive epitopes can be mapped using these kinds of expression constructs.

If no previous library of gene fragments has been prepared in an expression vector, and epitope mapping is the primary goal of preparing the library, we recommend selecting a method that is fast, simple, and adaptable; does not require extensive cloning and sequencing; and has a good chance to map, at least partially, denaturation-sensitive epitopes.

A good choice is a method that is based on the principle of expression PCR in which a PCR product is designed to incorporate the key DNA control elements necessary for efficient in vitro transcription and translation. It has been widely used and refined for the detection of truncation mutations that affect the production of proteins involved in human genetic diseases such as APC and BRCA2. There is wide technical support and ready availability of the key component kits.

Using the expression PCR procedure, it is possible to produce a series of defined gene fragments, which can then be expressed using in vitro transcription and in vitro translation kits. No cloning step is required beyond the initial cloning of the open reading frame into the transcription translation vector, because the PCR product itself acts as the template for the transcription translation reaction. Translation of the PCR-encoded transcription product also means that any errors due to the inaccuracy of the PCR are not isolated by cloning. Sufficient labeled in vitro translation product is produced to permit analysis of the fragments for antibody reactivity by direct immunoprecipitation.

The aim of the procedure is to use the PCR to produce a series of linear DNA fragments that include the promoter fragment for in vitro transcription and the appropriate signals for the efficient initiation of translation. The series is designed to produce a set of overlapping truncations from both the carboxyl terminus and the amino terminus of the cloned open reading frame. These linear PCR fragments can then be

*When analyzing the results of any epitope-mapping project, it is essential that only positive reactions with protein fragments are used in the assignment. Absence of reactivity with a particular fragment should not be interpreted to mean that the epitope is not contained within it because local folding changes could have disguised the epitope. Although this is an especially prevalent problem with the mapping of conformation-dependent epitopes, it is still logical to abide by this rule in all cases.*

used directly as templates for the in vitro transcription and translation reactions. Radioactive amino acids are included in the translation reaction so that the protein products can be identified and analyzed by immunoprecipitation. This method has many advantages over alternative expression strategies in which each product must be cloned before analysis is possible. Protein fragments produced by in vitro translation are soluble and often fold into their correct native conformation.

The production of the carboxy-terminal truncation set is straightforward, because here no alteration is required to the amino terminus of the protein or to the promoter element. The 5′ PCR primer is designed to ensure that the PCR product contains the complete promoter element, whereas the series of 3′ antisense primers defines the new ends of the protein truncation fragments.

Producing the set of truncations from the amino terminus is more difficult because of the need to preserve the transcription and translation initiation signals at the 5′ end of the PCR product. This can be achieved by the use of a universal promoter element cassette that contains the necessary signals for successful in vitro transcription and translation, that is, an RNA polymerase-binding region, an untranslated leader sequence, a Kozak sequence, and a translation initiation codon. This universal promoter element can be joined to any open reading frame containing the PCR product by a technique known as splicing by overlap extension (SOE), essentially a PCR without added primers. The splicing reaction creates a fused product that brings together all of the elements necessary for transcription and translation starting at any selected point within the open reading frame (Kain et al. 1991; Burch et al. 1993; Tropak and Roder 1994; Farley and Long 1995)

**The [$^{35}$S]methionine-labeled products of translation can now be analyzed by immunoprecipitation and gel electrophoresis.**

If the expression PCR approach is not appropriate because of the cost of the in vitro transcription/translation kits or because of restrictions on the use of radioisotopes, a valuable alternative is to use PCR to clone defined fragments of the open reading frame into the multicloning site of a simple and powerful bacterial expression vector. It is best to use a vector where the fragments will be produced as gene fusions; suitable vectors are the GST fusion vectors and the β-galactosidase expression vectors. Both of these systems produce large amounts of the fusion protein and contain suitable restriction sites. These sites can be created in the correct reading frame by incorporating them into the PCR primer sequences (see Chapter 10). The fusion proteins can be examined for antibody reactivity by direct blotting of bacterial colonies or by immunoblotting of extracts derived from bacterial cells expressing the fusion protein.

## Mapping using synthetic peptides

In this method, a set of overlapping synthetic peptides is synthesized, each corresponding to a small segment of the linear sequence of the protein antigen and arrayed on a solid phase. The panel of solid-phase peptides is then probed with the test antibody, and bound antibody is detected using an enzyme-labeled secondary antibody. This method is very rapid and can be extraordinarily successful, usually yielding unequivocal results with antibodies that work well in immunoblotting and that recognize denaturation-resistant epitopes. In our experience, it does not work at all with antibodies that only react with nondenatured native protein.

### Design of the peptide set

***What to do at the carboyxl terminus***

*If you are designing a pepscan set that includes the extreme carboxyl terminus of a protein antigen, it is best to complete the series with two shorter peptides, because some antibodies may recognize the free COOH at the terminus.*

If time and money were not constraints, the optimal peptide set would consist of peptides long enough to encompass the biggest possible contiguous epitope (probably 15–20 amino acids) and staggered by a single amino acid. Such a set would map precisely the largest possible number of antibodies; however, it requires 500 peptides to cover a 500-amino-acid protein. A practical compromise is to design sets in the range of 15-amino-acid-long peptides with 5-amino-acid overlaps or 20-amino-acid-long peptides with 10-amino-acid overlaps. This requires 100 peptides for the 15-amino-acid series and 50 for the 20-amino-acid series. If the gene fragment analysis has successfully localized the epitope to a region of 100 amino acids or less, a library of only 10–15 amino acid peptides would be needed (Fig. 11.2).

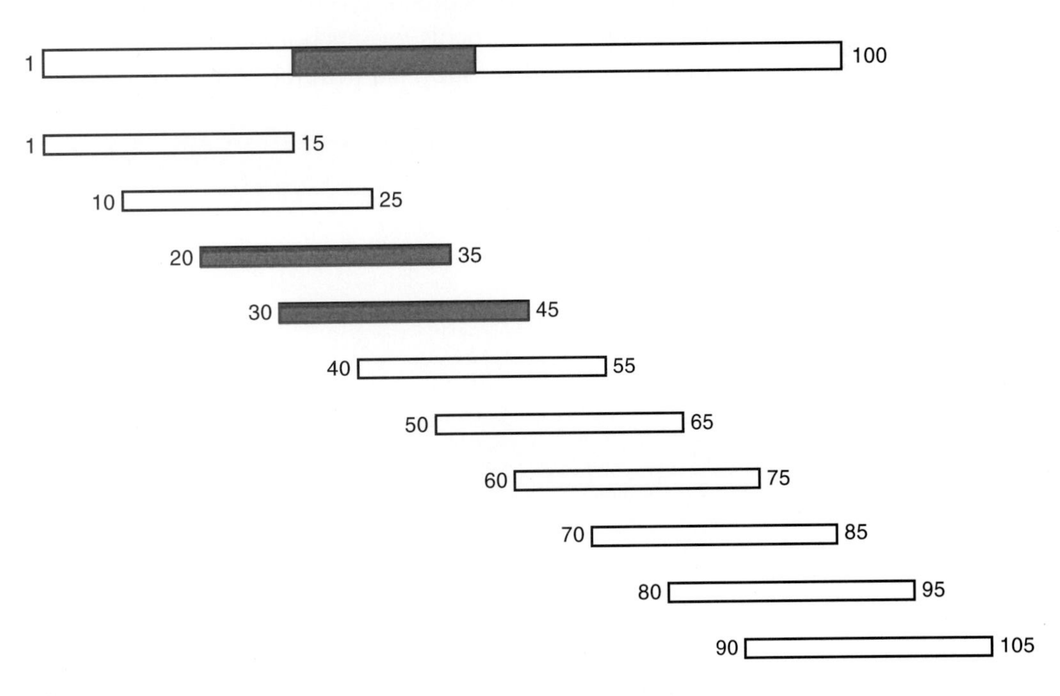


**Figure 11.2**
Design of peptide set.

## Synthesis or purchase of the peptide set

A large number of companies now perform custom synthesis or market kits or machines for synthesis in the lab. However, these options are expensive.

Peptides can also be synthesized on pins in plastic microtiter trays or on paper supports. The peptide arrays can be probed directly with antibody on the solid support, or the peptides can be cleaved from the solid support and prepared for assay. If a simple yes/no mapping answer is required for only one or two antibodies, then the paper system is adequate and the most economical. If the antigen is a major topic of research in the lab, we recommend purchasing the peptides as free biotin-conjugated peptides with a 4-amino-acid spacer group between the biotin and the cognate peptide sequence. In this approach, the master stock of peptide, typically 1 mg, allows 4000 or more assays of the peptide set. The peptide concentration can be controlled for affinity measurements; its purity can be analyzed, and sufficient peptide is available if needed to prepare solid phases for surface plasmon resonance analysis, for affinity columns, or for immunogens.

*The process of peptide synthesis is very suitable for complete automation, and small chip-based arrays of peptides are being produced in the private sector. These arrays could dramatically increase the speed and reduce the cost of pepscan analysis. It would be worthwhile for one of the synthesis firms to make pepscan sets available at low cost for some of the key protein antigens.*

Nominally cheaper methods in which the peptide is synthesized on the solid phase and then analyzed directly lack this degree of flexibility. The synthesis cannot be readily analyzed and the plates must be stripped of antibody and detection reagent for reuse. Although this will work a few times, it is not practical for more than a few assays.

In addition, the cost of a peptide set needs to be placed in context. Although it may cost $6,000 to cover a 400-amino-acid domain, this option does not have any labor cost and provides key information for many experiments. Sharing of the use and cost of peptide sets among a few labs quickly brings the cost within the normal range of lab expenditures. The protocol used for analysis of such biotin-labeled peptides is described below. Protocols for sets bound to the paper or to the solid phase are similar in principle and are supplied with the commercial products.

## Running the assay using biotin-tagged peptides

### Thinking ahead

The assay is run in plastic 96-well microtiter plates. These are precoated with streptavidin, and the peptide array is then gridded out and probed with the antibody to be mapped.

### Needed reagents and solutions

Tween 0.1%/PBS
2% BSA/PBS
0.1% (wt/vol) BSA/PBS
Peptide
Peroxidase-conjugated second antibody
TMB substrate (50 μl of 50 g/l stock in 5 ml of 0.1 M sodium acetate, pH 6.6, with 1 μl of hydrogen peroxide)
100 μM sulfuric acid

### Cautions

DMSO, hydrogen peroxide, sulfuric acid. see Appendix IV.

1. Dissolve each dry peptide in 100% DMSO at 10 mg/ml to prepare master stock. Prepare a working stock by diluting each master stock 1/10, and store both stocks at –70°C.

2. Coat sufficient 96-well plates for a duplicate determination with 50 μl/well of streptavidin (5 μg/ml in deionized water). Incubate overnight at 37°C.

3. Wash the plates four times with Tween 0.1%/PBS and then block nonspecific protein-binding sites by incubating the plates for 2 hours at room temperature with 2% BSA/PBS. Wash with Tween 0.1%/PBS.

4. Dilute each peptide into 0.1% (wt/vol) BSA/PBS to a concentration of 5 μg/ml (a 1/200 dilution from the working stock), and add 50 μl of peptide per well. Incubate for 2 hours or overnight in a humid chamber.

5. Aspirate the peptides from the wells, then wash the plate four times with Tween 0.1%/PBS.

6. Add the test antibody to the plate. Hybridoma supernatants should be tested neat and at 1/10 dilution in Tween 0.1%/PBS. Polyclonal sera should be tested at 1/200 and 1/2000 dilution in Tween 0.1%/PBS. Purified antibodies should be tested at 1 and 10 μg/ml.

7. After 2 hours or overnight incubation, aspirate the antibody-containing wells and wash four times with Tween 0.1%/PBS. Then add peroxidase-conjugated second antibody (rabbit anti-mouse IgG 1/1000 in 5% FCS/PBS for monoclonal primary antibodies). Incubate for 2 hours at room temperature.

8. Wash the plate four times, and then detect the bound antibody using the TMB substrate (50 ml of 50 g/l stock in 5 ml of 0.1 M sodium acetate, pH 6.6, with 1 ml of hydrogen peroxide) at 50 ml/well.

9. After development of the blue color, stop the reaction by adding 50 μl of 100 mM sulfuric acid. Determine the absorbance of the yellow product read at 450-nm wavelength in a microplate reader, or determine by eye.

In a successful experiment, very strong signals will be obtained for one, two, or three peptides in the series according to the selected degree of overlap and the size of the epitope. For example, with a 15-amino-acid-long peptide having a 5-amino-acid stagger, some antibodies will give strong signals with three peptides localizing their binding site to 5 amino acids, whereas others will signal on two peptides localizing the epitope to 10 amino acids. Some (more rarely) will only show a signal with a single peptide, meaning that amino acids crucial for the epitope are scattered through the 15-amino-acid region of the antigen.

The background for all of the other peptides should be very low, which provides an excellent internal control. It should be confirmed from the control plate that the positive peptides do not give any specific signal with the detection reagents alone in the absence of the primary test antibody. The epitope can be further defined, if needed, by analysis of new sets of peptides containing amino acid substitutions (typically alanine substitutions of each residue, but in some cases analysis of all 19 other possible amino acids), truncated peptides, or closer overlaps.

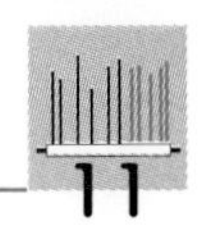

# Alternate approaches to epitope mapping

There are many alternate procedures by which epitopes can be mapped, ranging from cocrystallization of the antibody and the antigen to analysis of random peptide libraries by phage display procedures. These are shown in Table 11.3.

One of the most powerful of these commonly used procedures is random peptide libraries, which often work well with antibodies that recognize short linear epitopes. The rationale of this method differs from the others described because it defines the specificity of the antibody independently of knowledge of its target antigen. The reagents for this kind of epitope mapping are now more widely available, as are specialist manuals describing the method. Its basis is described below.

## Mapping the binding sites of antibodies using random peptide phage display libraries

An attractive novel route to determining the epitope specificity of antibodies is the use of phage display libraries. These libraries are constructed by cloning complex mixtures of peptide-encoding oligonucleotides into the amino terminus of the minor coat protein gene (gene 111) of f1-type ssDNA phage.

A vast library of recombinant phage is created, each one of which expresses at its surface a peptide sequence fused to the gene 111 coat protein. Libraries with inserts

Table 11.3 *Alternate approaches to epitope mapping*

| Mapping method | Conformational epitope | Linear epitope | Requirements | Advantages | Disadvantages |
|---|---|---|---|---|---|
| Antibody selection from random synthetic peptide library | No | Yes | Purchase of library; need mass spectrometer or sequencer to deconvolute | Universal library for all antibodies<br>No knowledge of antigen required | Small amounts of bound peptide must be sequenced |
| Antibody selection from random phage display peptide library | No (one published exception) | Yes | Purchase of library<br>Slow | Universal library for all antibodies<br>No knowledge of antigen required | Bound phage must be purified and sequenced |
| Protein fragmentation by proteolysis or chemical cleavage | Possible | Yes | Requires reasonable amounts of antigen | Do not need cloned gene encoding antigen | Protein fragments must be sequenced to determine precise origin |

encoding 6, 12, 15, and 20 amino acids are available from the developers of the libraries in return for shipping costs. Recently 8- and 12-amino-acid libraries have also become available commercially (New England Biolabs).

The libraries are amplified as stocks, and then an aliquot sufficient to represent multiple copies of each independent clone is mixed with the specific antibody. Antibody-bound phage are collected by an immunoaffinity selection procedure known as biopanning, and unbound phage are removed. The bound phage are then eluted and used to infect bacteria; the selected stock is amplified. The selection procedure is repeated, usually for two more rounds.

Individual plaques of the final selected stock are grown and checked for specific antibody reactivity by ELISA, and the DNA around the insert site is sequenced. Analysis of the sequence encoding the peptide defines the specificity of the antibody.

The method is very powerful, because no prior knowledge of the specificity of the antibody is needed, and comparison of the sequence of individual isolated phage can give a very detailed definition of the critical residues defining the antibodies' specificity. Commonly, if the antigen is known, this consensus sequence can be located within its primary sequence defining the location of the epitope.

For this method to be successful, a number of conditions must be met. First, the library must be of sufficient size and diversity to contain a specific reactive phage. Practical constraints mean that libraries containing about $10^8$ independent clones are the maximum that can be achieved. Thus, although the hexapeptide library could in theory be complete ($6.4 \times 10^7$), those containing larger inserts cannot be. However, the nature of antibody interactions with peptides permits considerable degeneracy, and so the incomplete libraries can still be very powerful.

Analysis of positive clones shows that only two or three residues within the epitope are absolutely specified, in that no substitution is tolerated and that at other positions a variably constrained range of substitutions is permitted. In some cases, absolutely specified residues are spaced by several less tightly constrained positions. This means that some antibodies will fail to select clones from the 6-mer libraries, but will do so from libraries with larger inserts. Libraries with inserts that are between 10 and 15 amino acids provide the best compromise. The techniques required for manipulation of the libraries are described below and are familiar to those who use the M13 phage for sequencing purposes. Because useful libraries are readily available, the preparation of the libraries is not described here. A full account is given in Smith and Scott (1993).

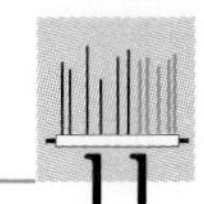


## Mapping the binding sites of antibodies using specific peptide fragment phage display libraries

In this powerful variation of the use of phage display libraries, a specific library of peptide fragments of the target antigen is created using partial DNase digestion of a DNA molecule encoding the target gene to create random fragments of the open reading frame. These fragments are then cloned as gene fusions to the gene 111 protein and used to create a phage display library or small peptide fragments of the open reading frame. Because these libraries are very highly enriched for reactive peptides, only one round of selection is needed to isolate reactive phage (Petersen et al. 1995; Fack et al. 1997). Because of the random nature of the insert fragments, sequencing the reactive phage defines a set of overlapping reactive segments and the minimum overlap can then be used to determine the minimum epitope length. Although the method has the disadvantage that a new library must be made for each protein antigen to be evaluated, the variable length of the insert and the fact that the sequences are derived from the target open reading frame suggest that this method will be successful in a wider variety of cases than the random libraries. It will also not detect mimotope sequences that are sometimes discovered using the random peptide libraries.

Table 11.4 *Comparison of epitope mapping strategies*

| Mapping method | Conformation epitopes | Linear epitopes | Requires antigen? | Accuracy | Requires labeled antibody | Requires cloned antigen ORF |
|---|---|---|---|---|---|---|
| Competition assay | Yes | Yes | Yes | Very accurate; but assay only distinguishes that epitopes are different | Yes, unless Biacore | No |
| X ray | Yes | Yes | Yes | Complete | No | Usually, as a lot of pure antigen needed |
| Gene fragment | Yes, if protein contains multiple folding domains | Yes | Yes | 10 amino acids for linear epitopes; folding domain for conformational epitopes | | |
| Synthetic peptide fragment | No | Yes | No | 5–15 amino acids | No | No, but must know sequence |

## References


Alexander H., Alexander S., Getzoff E.D., Tainer J.A., Geysen H.M., and Lerner R.A. 1992. Altering the antigenicity of proteins. *Proc. Natl. Acad. Sci.* **89:** 3352–3356.

Burch H.B., Nagy E.V., Kain K.C., Lanar D.E., Carr F.E., Wartofsky L., and Burman K.D. 1993. Expression polymerase chain reaction for the in vitro synthesis and epitope mapping of autoantigen. Application to the human thyrotropin receptor. *J. Immunol. Methods* **158:** 123–130.

Fack F., Hugle-Dorr B., Song D., Queitsch I., Petersen G., and Bautz E.K. 1997. Epitope mapping by phage display: Random versus gene-fragment libraries. *J. Immunol. Methods* **206:** 43–52.

Farley P.J. and Long C.A. 1995. Plasmodium yoelii yoelii 17XL MSP-1: Fine-specificity mapping of a discontinuous, disulfide-dependent epitope recognized by a protective monoclonal antibody using expression PCR (E-PCR). *Exp. Parisitol.* **80:** 328–332.

Gannon J.V. and Lane D.P. 1990. Interactions between SV40 T antigen and DNA polymerase α. *New Biol.* **2:** 84–92.

Johne B., Gadnell M., and Hansen K. 1993. Epitope mapping and binding kinetics of monoclonal antibodies studied by real time biospecific interaction analysis using surface plasmon resonance. *J. Immunol. Methods* **160:** 191–198.

Kain K.C., Orlandi P.A., and Lanar D.E. 1991. Universal promoter for gene expression without cloning: expression-PCR. *BioTechniques* **10:** 366–374.

Kuroki M., Fernsten P.D., Wunderlich D., Colcher D., Simpson J.F., Poole D.J., and Schlom J. 1990. Serological mapping of the TAG-72 tumor-associated antigen using 19 distinct monoclonal antibodies. *Cancer Res.* **50:** 4872–4879.

Kuroki M., Wakisaka M., Murakami M., Haruno M., Arakawa F., Higuchi H., and Matsuoka Y. 1992a. Determination of epitope specificities of a large number of monoclonal antibodies by solid-phase mutual inhibition assays using biotinylated antigen. *Immunol Invest.* **21:** 523–538.

Kuroki M., Arakawa F., Haruno M., Murakami M., Wakisaka M., Higuchi H., Oikawa S., Nakazato H., and Matsuoka Y. 1992b. Biochemical characterization of 25 distinct carcinoembryonic antigen (CEA) epitopes recognized by 57 monoclonal antibodies and categorized into seven groups in terms of domain structure of the CEA molecule. *Hybridoma* **11:** 391–407.

Petersen G., Song D., Hugle-Dorr B., Oldenburg I., and Bautz E.K. 1995. Mapping of linear epitopes recognized by monoclonal antibodies with gene-fragment phage display libraries. *Mol. Gen. Genet.* **249:** 425–431.

Smith G.P. and Scott J.K. 1993. Libraries of peptides and proteins displayed on filamentous phage. *Methods Enzymol.* **217:** 228–257.

Tropak M.B. and Roder J.C. 1994. High-resolution mapping of GenS3 and B11F7 epitopes on myelin-associated glycoprotein by expression PCR. *J. Neurochem.* **62:** 854–862.

Wagener C., Fenger U., Clark B.R., and Shively J.E. 1984. Use of biotin-labeled monoclonal antibodies and avidin-peroxidase conjugates for the determination of epitope specificities in a solid-phase competitive enzyme immunoassay. *J. Immunol. Methods* **68:** 269–274.

Wagener C., Yang Y.H., Crawford F.G., and Shively J.E. 1983. Monoclonal antibodies for carcinoembryonic antigen and related antigens as a model system: A systematic approach for the determination of epitope specificities of monoclonal antibodies. *J. Immunol* **130:** 2308–2315.

## Further readings


### NMR and crystallographic studies

Bizebard T., Gigant B., Rigolet P., Rasmussen B., Diat O., Bosecke P., Wharton S.A., Skehel J.J., and Knossow M. 1995. Structure of influenza virus haemagglutinin complexed with a neutralizing antibody. *Nature* **376:** 92–94.

Lawrence M.C. and Colman P.M. 1993. Shape complementarity at protein/protein interfaces *J. Mol. Biol.* **234:** 946–950.

Zvi A., Kustanovich I., Hayek Y., Matsushita S., and Anglister J. 1995. The principal neutralizing determinant of HIV-1 located in V3 of gp120 forms a 12-residue loop by internal hydrophobic interactions. *FEBS Lett.* **368:** 267–270.

### Peptide approaches

Geysen H.M., Barteling S.J., and Meloen R.H. 1985. Small peptides induce antibodies with a sequence and structural requirement for binding antigen comparable to antibodies raised against the native protein. *Proc. Natl. Acad. Sci.* **82:** 178–182.

Geysen H.M., Meloen R.H., and Barteling S.J. 1984. Use of peptide synthesis to probe viral antigens for epitopes to a resolution of a single amino acid. *Proc. Natl. Acad. Sci.* **81:** 3998–4002.

Geysen H.M., Rodda S.J., Mason T.J., Tribbick G., and Schoofs P.G. 1987. Strategies for epitope analysis using peptide synthesis. *J. Immunol. Methods* **102:** 259–274.

Geysen H.M., Tainer J.A., Rodda S.J., Mason T.J., Alexander H., Getzoff E.D., and Lerner R.A. 1987. Chemistry of antibody binding to a protein. *Science* **235:** 1184–1190.

Kordossi A.A. and Tzartos S.J. 1987. Conformation of cytoplasmic segments of acetylcholine receptor alpha- and beta-subunits probed by monoclonal antibodies: Sensitivity of the antibody competition approach. *EMBO J.* **6:** 1605–1610.

### Chemical modification of side chains

Atassi M.Z. 1975. Antigenic structure of myoglobin: The complete immunochemical anatomy of a protein and conclusions relating to antigenic structures of proteins. *Immunochemistry* **12:** 423–438.

Burnens A., Demotz S., Corradin G., Binz H., and Bosshard H.R. 1987. Epitope mapping by chemical modification of free and antibody-bound protein antigen. *Science* **235:** 780–783.

Gudmundsson E.M., Young N.M., and Oomen R.P. 1993. Characterisation of residues in antibody binding sites by chemical modification of surface-adsorbed protein combined with enzyme immunoassay. *J. Immunol. Methods* **158:** 215–227.

Imoto T. and Yamada H. 1989. Chemical modification. In *Protein function: A practical approach* (ed. T.E. Creighton), pp. 247–277, IRL press, Oxford, United Kingdom.

### Protein footprinting

Morris G.E., Frost L.C., Newport P.A., and Hudson N. 1987. Monoclonal antibody studies of creatine kinase. Antibody-binding sites in the N-terminal region of creatine kinase and effects of antibody on enzyme refolding. *Biochem J.* **48:** 53–59.

Nguyen thi Man, Cartwright A.J., Morris G.E., Love D.R., Bloomfield J.F., and Davies K.E. 1990. Monoclonal antibodies against defined regions of the muscular dystrophy protein, dystrophin. *FEBS Lett.* **262:** 237–240.

Sheshberadaran H. and Payne L.G. 1988. Protein antigen-monoclonal antibody contact sites investigated by limited proteolysis of monoclonal antibody-bound antigen: Protein “footprinting”. *Proc. Natl. Acad. Sci.* **85:** 1–5.

Suckau D., Kohl J., Karwath G., Schneider K., Casaretto M., Bitter-Suermann D., and Przybylski M. 1990. Molecular epitope identification by limited proteolysis of an immobi-

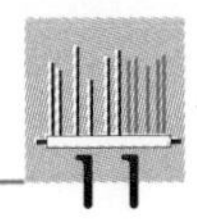


lized antigen-antibody complex and mass spectrometric peptide mapping. *Proc. Natl. Acad. Sci.* **87:** 9848–9852.

Zhao Y., Muir T.W., Kent S.B., Tischer E., Scardina J.M., and Chait B.T. 1996. Mapping protein-protein interactions by affinity-directed mass spectrometry *Proc. Natl. Acad. Sci.* **93:** 4020–4024.

## Positional scanning of synthetic combinatorial libraries

Appel J.R., Buencamino J., Houghten R.A., and Pinilla C. 1996. Exploring antibody polyspecificity using synthetic combinatorial libraries. *Mol. Divers.* **2:** 29–34.

Houghten R.A. 1985. General method for the rapid solid-phase synthesis of large numbers of peptides: Specificity of antigen-antibody interaction at the level of individual amino acids. *Proc. Natl. Acad. Sci.* **82:** 5131–5135.

Houghten R.A., Pinilla C., Blondelle S.E., Appel J.R., Dooley C.T., and Cuervo J.H. 1991. Generation and use of synthetic peptide combinatorial libraries for basic research and drug discovery. *Nature* **354:** 84–86.

Picksley S.M., Vojtesek B., Sparks A., and Lane D.P. 1994. Immunochemical analysis of the interaction of YFP1 with MDM2: Fine mapping of the MDM2 binding site on YFP1 using synthetic peptides. *Oncogene* **9:** 2523–2529.

Pinilla C., Appel J.R., and Houghten R.A. 1993. Functional importance of amino acid residues making up peptide antigenic determinants. *Mol. Immunol.* **30:** 577–585.

Pinilla C., Appel J.R., Blanc P., and Houghten R.A. 1992. Rapid identification of high affinity peptide ligands using positional scanning synthetic peptide combinatorial libraries. *BioTechniques* **13:** 901–905.

## Phage display libraries

Bottger V., Bottger A., Howard S.F., Picksley S.M., Chene P., Garcia-Echeverria C., Hochkeppel H.K., and Lane D.P. 1996. Identification of novel mdm2 binding peptides by phage display. *Oncogene* **13:** 2141–2147.

Bottger A., Bottger V., Garcia-Echeverria C., Chene P., Hochkeppel H.K., Sampson W., Ang K., Howard S.F., Picksley S.M., and Lane D.P. 1997. Molecular characterization of the hdm2-YFP1 interaction. *J. Mol. Biol.* **269:** 744–756.

Daniels D.A. and Lane D.P. 1994. The characterisation of YFP1 binding phage isolated from phage peptide display libraries. *J. Mol. Biol.* **243:** 639–652.

McConnell S.J., Kendall M.L., Reilly T.M., and Hoess R.H. 1994. Constrained peptide libraries as a tool for finding mimotopes. *Gene* **151:** 115–118.

Stephen C.W. and Lane D.P. 1994. Mutant conformation of YFP1. Precise epitope mapping using a filamentous phage epitope library. *J. Mol. Biol.* **225:** 577–583.

Stephen C.W., Helminen P., and Lane D.P. 1995. Characterisation of epitopes on human YFP1 using phage-displayed peptide libraries: Insights into antibody-peptide interactions. *J. Mol. Biol.* **248:** 58–78.

## Homolog scanning

Cunningham B.C., Jhurani P., Ng P., and Wells J.A. 1989. Receptor and antibody epitopes in human growth hormone identified by homolog-scanning mutagenesis. *Science* **243:** 1330–1336.

Horton R.M., Hunt H.D., Ho S.N., Pullen J.K., and Pease L.R. 1989. Engineering hybrid genes without the use of restriction enzymes: Gene splicing by overlap extension. *Gene* **77:** 61–68.

Lee C., Luck M.D., Juppner H., Potts Jr., J.T., Kronenberg H.M., and Gardella T.J. 1995. Homolog-scanning mutagenesis of the parathyroid hormone (PTH) receptor reveals PTH-(1–34) binding determinants in the third extracellular loop. *Mol. Endocrinol.* **9:** 1269–1278.

Wang L., Hertzog P.J., Galanis M., Overall M.L., Waine G.J., and Linnane A.W. 1994. Structure-function analysis of human IFN-α. Mapping of a conformational epitope by homologue scanning. *J. Immunol.* **152:** 705–715.

### *Construct a synthetic gene and manipulate the fragments*

Alexander H., Alexander S., Getzoff E.D., Tainer J.A., Geysen H.M., and Lerner R.A. 1992. Altering the antigenicity of proteins. *Proc. Natl. Acad. Sci.* **89:** 3352–3356.

Alexander H., Alexander S., Heffron P., Fieser T.M., Hay B.N., Getzoff E.D., Tainer J.A., and Lerner R.A. 1991. Synthesis and characterization of a recombinant myohemerythrin protein encoded by a synthetic gene. *Gene* **99:** 151–156.

Ikeda M., Hamano K., and Shibata T. 1992. Epitope mapping of anti-recA protein IgGs by region specified polymerase chain reaction mutagenesis. *J. Biol. Chem.* **267:** 6291–6296.

### *Random fragment library in yeast*

Madaule P., Gairin J.E., Benichou S., and Rossier J. 1991. A peptide library expressed in yeast reveals new major epitopes from human immunodeficiency virus type 1. *FEMS Microbiol. Immunol.* **3:** 99–107.

### *Random fragment libraries in lambda phage*

Mehra V., Sweetser D., and Young R.A. 1986. Efficient mapping of protein antigenic determinants. *Proc. Natl. Acad. Sci.* **83:** 7013–7017.

Porzig H., Li Z., Nicoll D.A., and Philipson K.D. 1993. Mapping of the cardiac sodium-calcium exchanger with monoclonal antibodies. *Am. J. Physiol.* **265:** C748–C756.

### *Random libraries in filamentous phage*

Cwirla S.E., Peters E.A., Barrett R.W., and Dower W.J. 1990. Peptides on phage: A vast library of peptides for identifying ligands. *Proc. Natl. Acad. Sci.* **87:** 6378–6382.

Devlin J.J., Panganiban L.C., and Devlin P.E. 1990. Random peptide libraries: A source of specific protein binding molecules. *Science* **249:** 404–406.

Scott J.K. and Smith G.P. 1990. Searching for peptide ligands with an epitope library. *Science* **249:** 386–390.

### *Expression of PCR fragments or restriction enzyme fragments in plasmids*

Lenstra J.A., Kusters J.G., and van der Zeijst B.A. 1990. Mapping of viral epitopes with prokaryotic expression products. *Arch. Virol.* **110:** 1–24.

### *Expression PCR*

Burch H.B., Nagy E.V., Kain K.C., Lanar D.E., Carr F.E., Wartofsky L., and Burman K.D. 1993. Expression polymerase chain reaction for the in vitro synthesis and epitope mapping of autoantigen. Application to the human thyrotropin receptor. *J. Immunol. Methods* **158:** 123–130.

Kain K.C., Orlandi P.A., and Lanar D.E. 1991. Universal promoter for gene expression without cloning: Expression-PCR. *BioTechniques* **10:** 366–374.

### *Transposon mutagenesis*

Sedgwick S.G., Nguyen T.M., Ellis J.M., Crowne H., and Morris G.E. 1991. Rapid mapping by transposon mutagenesis of epitopes on the muscular dystrophy protein, dystrophin. *Nucleic Acids Res.* **19:** 5889–5894.

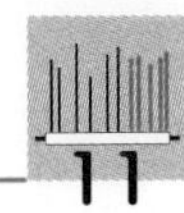


### *Inference of epitopes by evolutionary conservation*

Nguyen thi Man, Cartwright A.J., Osborne M., and Morris G.E. 1991. Structural changes in the C-terminal region of human brain creatine kinase studied with monoclonal antibodies. *Biochim. Biophys. Acta* **1076:** 245–251.

Ping L.H. and Lemon S.M. 1992. Antigenic structure of human hepatitis A virus defined by analysis of escape mutants selected against murine monoclonal antibodies. *J. Virol.* **66:** 2208–2216.

# Appendixes

# Appendix I
# Electrophoresis

## SDS-polyacrylamide gel electrophoresis[*]

### Caution

Acrylamide, SDS, bisacrylamide, TEMED, ammonium persulfate, β-mercaptoethanol, DTT, see Appendix IV.

---

If using a commercial apparatus, assemble the gel plates following the manufacturer's instructions. If not, arrange gel plates as below. The plates should be clean and free of detergents. Silicon rubber tubing can be placed between the glass plates to make a good, watertight seal.

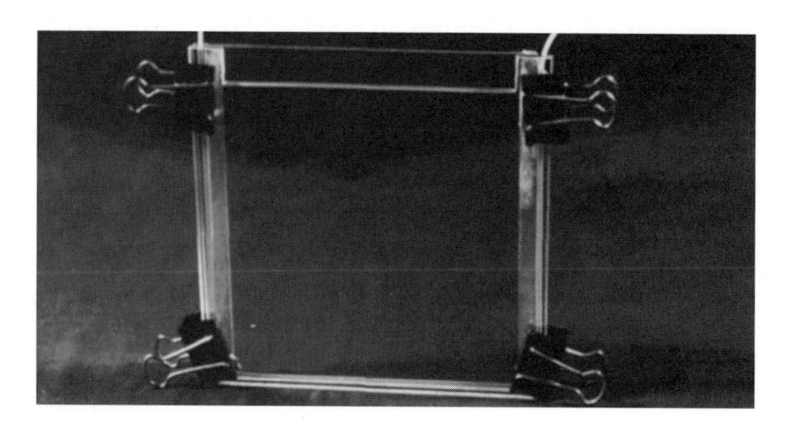

2. Prepare the acrylamide solution for the separating gel using the values given on p. 413.

---

3. Pour the acrylamide solution between the plates. The meniscus of the acrylamide solution should be far enough below the top of the notched plate to allow for the length of the teeth on the comb plus 1 cm. Carefully overlay the acrylamide solution with isobutanol or water. For gels made with acrylamide concentrations lower than 8% use water; for gels of 10% or greater use isobutanol (or water-saturated isobutanol). The overlaying solution creates a barrier to oxygen, which inhibits the polymerization of the acrylamide. Place the gel in a vertical position at room temperature.

---

4. After the gel has set (about 20–30 minutes), pour off the overlay and wash the top of the separating gel several times with distilled water. Drain well or dry with the edge of a paper towel.

*Laemmli (1970), based on Smithies (1955), Raymond and Weintraub (1959), Davis (1964), Ornstein (1964), Summers et al. (1965).

5. Prepare the acrylamide solution for the stacking gel from the values on p. 413. Pour the solution for the stack directly onto the polymerized separating gel. Place the appropriate comb into the gel solution, being careful not to trap any bubbles. To clean the comb, wash with water and ethanol. Place the gel in a vertical position at room temperature. The stacking gel will set in approximately 10 minutes.

6. Heat samples in sample buffer at 85°C for 10 minutes.

7. After the stacking gel has set, carefully remove the comb. Wash the wells immediately with distilled water to remove unpolymerized acrylamide. Straighten the teeth of the stacking gel, if necessary, and place in an appropriate gel box with running buffer in the bottom reservoir. Add running buffer to top reservoir. Any bubbles caught between the plates at the bottom of the gel can be removed by squirting running buffer through a syringe fitted with a bent needle.

8. Load samples into the bottom of the wells. The samples can be conveniently loaded using either (1) a microliter syringe (washed by pipetting in the bottom reservoir buffer between each sample), (2) a micropipettor fitted with a long narrow tip, or (3) Teflon tubing fixed to the end of a microliter syringe (24-gauge, thin-walled spaghetti tubing fits snugly on 22-gauge needles; discard each piece after a single use).

9. Start electrophoresis at 100–125 V. After the dye front has moved into the separating gel, increase to 200 V. The plates will become warm to the touch, but should not be hot. If the plates are too warm to touch easily, lower the voltage.

10. When the dye front reaches the bottom of the gel, turn off the power pack. Remove the gel plates and gently pry the plates apart. Use a spatula or similar tool to separate the plates (not at an ear). Cut a corner from the bottom of the gel that is closest to the number 1 well.

    **The gels are now ready for fixing (p. 430), staining (p. 424), transfer (p. 284), fluorography (p. 422), or autoradiography (p. 432).**

## Notes

i. Spacers can be glued directly onto the glass plates. Two good choices of glues are 3M Scotch epoxy 2216 B/A and quick-drying CA9. Be sure both the gel plates and the spacers are clean before gluing. Clamp the spacers tightly to the plates before the glue hardens. This will prevent the hardened glue from increasing the thickness of the gel.

ii. If protein samples are resuspended in sample buffer lacking any reducing agents and the gels are run as normal, proteins that are linked by disulfides will run as discrete multimers. Comparing samples, plus and minus reduction, can then be used to study protein complexes held by disulfide bridges. **Note:** β-Mercaptoethanol or dithiothreitol (DTT) will diffuse between lanes, and if samples with and without reducing agents are to be compared, they should be separated by several lanes or run on different gels.

iii. Effective separation of some proteins can be enhanced by varying the ratio of the bisacrylamide cross-linker (*N,N'*-methylene-bisacrylamide) to the acrylamide monomer. The gel formulations described on p. 413 yield 30% total acrylamide composed of 29.2% monomer and 0.8% cross-linker, or a ratio of 36.5:1. Higher ratios allow most proteins to migrate faster and also promote easier transfer for immunoblots. Lower ratios yield firmer gels and slower rates of migration. Not all proteins are affected equally, and changing the ratio of monomer to cross-linker can be used to gain better separation between some proteins.

iv. When proteins are difficult to elute from gels, the cross-linker can be changed to one that can be cleaved by simple chemical modifications. Common cleavable cross-linkers are BAC (*N,N'*-bisacrylylcystamine) and DATD (*N,N'*-diallyltartardiamide). For additional information on BAC, see Hansen (1976) and Hansen et al. (1980); for additional information on DATD, see Anker (1970).

v. When studying two or more proteins with widely differing molecular weights, gels can be prepared with higher acrylamide concentrations at the bottom of the gel compared with the top. These gradient gels can be prepared from any combination of acrylamide concentrations and are poured by using a gradient maker using standard recipes. Be certain to clean the gradient maker before using and to wash the gradient maker before the remaining acrylamide polymerizes in the apparatus.

vi. In addition to the Tris/glycine buffers suggested here, many different combinations of buffers can be used. For a partial list, see p. 414; for a more detailed list, see Jovin et al. (1970).

vii. For greater reproducibility from day to day, the acrylamide and bisacrylamide can be prepared in large batches and either stored at 4°C for 1 month or frozen in aliquots and used indefinitely. Remove the required amount, warm to room temperature, and add ammonium persulfate and TEMED immediately before use.

*Solutions for Tris/glycine SDS-polyacrylamide gel electrophoresis*

| 6% | 5 ml | 10 ml | 15 ml | 20 ml | 25 ml | 30 ml | 40 ml | 50 ml |
|---|---|---|---|---|---|---|---|---|
| $H_2O$ | 2.6 | 5.3 | 7.9 | 10.6 | 13.2 | 15.9 | 21.2 | 26.5 |
| 30% Acrylamide mix[a,e] | 1.0 | 2.0 | 3.0 | 4.0 | 5.0 | 6.0 | 8.0 | 10.0 |
| 1.5 M Tris (pH 8.8) | 1.3 | 2.5 | 3.8 | 5.0 | 6.3 | 7.5 | 10.0 | 12.5 |
| 10% SDS[b,e] | 0.05 | 0.1 | 0.15 | 0.2 | 0.25 | 0.3 | 0.4 | 0.5 |
| 10% APS[c,e] | 0.05 | 0.1 | 0.15 | 0.2 | 0.25 | 0.3 | 0.4 | 0.5 |
| TEMED[d,e] | 0.004 | 0.008 | 0.012 | 0.016 | 0.02 | 0.024 | 0.032 | 0.04 |
| **8%** | **5 ml** | **10 ml** | **15 ml** | **20 ml** | **25 ml** | **30 ml** | **40 ml** | **50 ml** |
| $H_2O$ | 2.3 | 4.6 | 6.9 | 9.3 | 11.6 | 13.9 | 18.5 | 23.2 |
| 30% Acrylamide mix | 1.3 | 2.7 | 4.0 | 5.3 | 6.7 | 8.0 | 10.7 | 13.3 |
| 1.5 M Tris (pH 8.8) | 1.3 | 2.5 | 3.8 | 5.0 | 6.3 | 7.5 | 10.0 | 12.5 |
| 10% SDS | 0.05 | 0.1 | 0.15 | 0.2 | 0.25 | 0.3 | 0.4 | 0.5 |
| 10% APS | 0.05 | 0.1 | 0.15 | 0.2 | 0.25 | 0.3 | 0.4 | 0.5 |
| TEMED | 0.003 | 0.006 | 0.009 | 0.012 | 0.015 | 0.018 | 0.024 | 0.03 |
| **10%** | **5 ml** | **10 ml** | **15 ml** | **20 ml** | **25 ml** | **30 ml** | **40 ml** | **50 ml** |
| $H_2O$ | 2.0 | 4.0 | 5.9 | 7.9 | 9.9 | 11.9 | 15.8 | 19.8 |
| 30% Acrylamide mix | 1.7 | 3.3 | 5 | 6.7 | 8.3 | 10.0 | 13.3 | 16.7 |
| 1.5 M Tris (pH 8.8) | 1.3 | 2.5 | 3.8 | 5.0 | 6.3 | 7.5 | 10.0 | 12.5 |
| 10% SDS | 0.05 | 0.1 | 0.15 | 0.2 | 0.25 | 0.3 | 0.4 | 0.5 |
| 10% APS | 0.05 | 0.1 | 0.15 | 0.2 | 0.25 | 0.3 | 0.4 | 0.5 |
| TEMED | 0.002 | 0.004 | 0.006 | 0.008 | 0.01 | 0.012 | 0.016 | 0.02 |
| **12%** | **5 ml** | **10 ml** | **15 ml** | **20 ml** | **25 ml** | **30 ml** | **40 ml** | **50 ml** |
| $H_2O$ | 1.6 | 3.3 | 4.9 | 6.6 | 8.2 | 9.9 | 13.2 | 16.5 |
| 30% Acrylamide mix | 2.0 | 4.0 | 6.0 | 8.0 | 10.0 | 12.0 | 16.0 | 20.0 |
| 1.5 M Tris (pH 8.8) | 1.3 | 2.5 | 3.8 | 5.0 | 6.3 | 7.5 | 10.0 | 12.5 |
| 10% SDS | 0.05 | 0.1 | 0.15 | 0.2 | 0.25 | 0.3 | 0.4 | 0.5 |
| 10% APS | 0.05 | 0.1 | 0.15 | 0.2 | 0.25 | 0.3 | 0.4 | 0.5 |
| TEMED | 0.002 | 0.004 | 0.006 | 0.008 | 0.01 | 0.012 | 0.016 | 0.02 |
| **15%** | **5 ml** | **10 ml** | **15 ml** | **20 ml** | **25 ml** | **30 ml** | **40 ml** | **50 ml** |
| $H_2O$ | 1.1 | 2.3 | 3.4 | 4.6 | 5.7 | 6.9 | 9.2 | 11.4 |
| 30% Acrylamide mix | 2.5 | 5.0 | 7.5 | 10.0 | 12.5 | 15.0 | 20.0 | 25.0 |
| 1.5 M Tris (pH 8.8) | 1.3 | 2.5 | 3.8 | 5.0 | 6.3 | 7.5 | 10.0 | 12.5 |
| 10% SDS | 0.05 | 0.1 | 0.15 | 0.2 | 0.25 | 0.3 | 0.4 | 0.5 |
| 10% APS | 0.05 | 0.1 | 0.15 | 0.2 | 0.25 | 0.3 | 0.4 | 0.5 |
| TEMED | 0.002 | 0.004 | 0.006 | 0.008 | 0.01 | 0.012 | 0.016 | 0.02 |
| **STACK** | **1 ml** | **2 ml** | **3 ml** | **4 ml** | **5 ml** | **6 ml** | **8 ml** | **10 ml** |
| $H_2O$ | 0.68 | 1.4 | 2.1 | 2.7 | 3.4 | 4.1 | 5.5 | 6.8 |
| 30% Acrylamide mix | 0.17 | 0.33 | 0.5 | 0.67 | 0.83 | 1.0 | 1.3 | 1.7 |
| 1.0 M Tris (pH 6.8) | 0.13 | 0.25 | 0.38 | 0.5 | 0.63 | 0.75 | 1.0 | 1.25 |
| 10% SDS | 0.01 | 0.02 | 0.03 | 0.04 | 0.05 | 0.06 | 0.08 | 0.1 |
| 10% APS | 0.01 | 0.02 | 0.03 | 0.04 | 0.05 | 0.06 | 0.08 | 0.1 |
| TEMED | 0.001 | 0.002 | 0.003 | 0.004 | 0.005 | 0.006 | 0.008 | 0.01 |

[a]Commonly 29.2% acrylamide and 0.8% *N,N′*-methylene-bisacrylamide; [b]sodium dodecyl sulfate; [c]ammonium persulfate; [d]*N,N,N′,N′*-tetramethylethylenediamine; [e] see Appendix IV for caution.

*Alternative buffer systems for discontinuous polyacrylamide gel electrophoresis*

| System | Running buffer | Separating gel buffer | Stacking gel buffer | Sample buffer[a] |
|---|---|---|---|---|
| SDS[b]/phosphate[c] | 100 mM sodium phosphate (pH 7.2) 0.2% SDS | 100 mM sodium phosphate (pH 7.2) 0.2% SDS | No stack | 100 mM sodium phosphate (pH 7.2) 1% SDS 10% glycerol 0.001% bromophenol blue[b] |
| Urea/glycerol[b,d] | 50 mM Tris, 100 mM glycine[b] (pH 8.7) | 0.375 M Tris, 40% glycerol (pH 9.1) | 0.12 M Tris, 8.5 M urea (pH 6.8) | 0.12 M Tris (pH 6.8) 8.5 M urea 0.001% bromophenol blue |
| Tris/borate[e] | 65 mM Tris, 0.1% SDS, (pH to 8.3 with boric acid) | 0.375 M Tris, (pH to 8.3 with sulfuric acid)[b] | 75 mM Tris, (pH to 8.3 with sulfuric acid) | 75 mM Tris, 2% SDS 10% glycerol 0.001% bromophenol blue (pH to 8.3 with sulfuric acid) |
| Tris/tricine[f] | **Cathode buffer:** 0.1 M Tris, 0.1 M tricine, 0.1% SDS (pH about 8.5; do not adjust) **Anode buffer:** 0.2 M Tris (pH to 8.9 with HCl) | 10 ml of acrylamide solution: 48% (wt/vol) acrylamide, 1.5% bis-acrylamide; makes 16.5% T (monomer and cross-linker), 6% C (cross-linker) acrylamide mix Add to 10 ml of gel buffer; 3.0 M Tris-HCl (pH 8.45), 0.3% SDS. Add 4 g of glycerol and bring to 30 ml with $H_2O$ For optional spacer gel: 6.1 ml of acrylamide solution plus 3.1 ml of gel buffer; bring to 12.5 ml with $H_2O$ | 1 ml of acrylamide solution plus 3.1 ml of gel buffer, bring to 12.5 ml with $H_2O$ | 50 mM Tris, 2% β-mercaptoethanol, 0.1% bromophenol blue (pH to 6.8 with HCl) |

[a] All samples buffers can be supplemented with 100 mM dithiothreitol, if desired.
[b] See Appendix IV for caution.
[c] Weber and Osborn (1969).
[d] Sobieszek and Jertschin (1986).
[e] J. Brugge (pers. comm.).
[f] Schagger and von Jagow (1987).

## Partial proteolytic peptide maps—V8 protease*

Treating identical samples of a protein with the same protease, but at different concentrations, generates a series of products ranging in size from fully digested to undigested. When the products of these individual reactions are run side by side on lanes of a one-dimensional SDS-polyacrylamide gel, a ladder of digestion products is displayed that gives a diagnostic fingerprint of the polypeptide backbone. When two proteins are identical or closely related, these partial proteolytic maps can be used to confirm their relationship. Although partial proteolytic maps can confirm that two proteins are related, only minor changes in the polypeptide sequence are needed to produce a vastly different pattern. Therefore, partial maps should only be used to test for identity or close relationships.

To prepare samples for enzyme treatment, run multiple lanes of the antigen on a preliminary gel. Each band will then become the substrate for a different digest, normally being exposed to one of a range of enzyme concentrations.

### Caution

DTT, polyacrylamide, radioactive substances, SDS, see Appendix IV.

---

1. Run the preliminary SDS-polyacrylamide gel as normal. **If the protein bands of interest are radiolabeled:** Rinse the gel in water and dry without fixing. Place labels near three corners of the dry gel. Mark the labels with radioactive ink to serve as guides when aligning the film after developing. Expose the gel to X-ray film as normal. Develop the film and use the film as a template to locate and excise the bands of interest. **If the proteins of interest are not labeled:** Locate the bands by staining the gel with one of the Coomassie or silver staining methods on pp. 424–428. Dry as normal, and excise the bands of interest.

2. Remove the backing paper from each slice with a scalpel.

3. Prepare a polyacrylamide gel as described on p. 410 but with these changes: (1) Include 1 mM EDTA in all the gel mixes, and (2) make the stacking gel about twice the normal depth (about 3 cm from the bottom of the well to the top of the separating gel). Usually a 12–15% separating gel is appropriate. After the stacking gel has polymerized, transfer to the gel tank. Add running buffer to the bottom chamber and remove any bubbles between the plates at the bottom of the gel.

4. Fill the wells of the stacking gel with 0.1% SDS, 1 mM EDTA, 2.5 mM DTT, and 0.125 M Tris (pH 6.8).

*Cleveland et al. (1977); Fischer (1983).

5. Push the dried gel slices into the appropriate wells. Align the gel slice along the bottom of the well. Incubate for 10 minutes.

6. Add running buffer to the top chamber.

7. Overlay the slice with 20 μl of 20% glycerol, 0.1% SDS, 1 mM EDTA, 2.5 mM DTT, and 0.125 M Tris (pH 6.8).

8. Overlay the 20% glycerol mix with 10 μl of 10% glycerol, 0.1% SDS, 1 mM EDTA, 2.5 mM DTT, 0.001% bromophenol blue, and 0.125 M Tris (pH 6.8) containing a dilution of V8 protease. In preliminary tests, 10-fold dilutions between 50 ng and 5 μg of protease per lane are used to establish the range of protease concentrations that will be used in the final experiment.

9. Run the gel at 125 V until the bromophenol blue forms a sharp line and has migrated about two-thirds of the distance into the stacking gel.

10. Turn off the power pack and allow the proteins to digest for 30 minutes.

11. Turn on the power pack and run the gel until the bromophenol blue reaches the bottom of the separating gel.

12. Turn off the power pack. Disassemble the gel plates and process as needed for the various samples (radioactive samples for autoradiography or fluorography and nonradioactive samples for staining).

## Note

Depending on the protein, V8 protease can be substituted with other proteases or chemical cleavage agents using a similar technique.

## Two-dimensional isoelectric focusing/SDS-polyacrylamide gel electrophoresis*

 **Caution**

Acrylamide, ammonium persulfate, bisacrylamide, β-mercaptoethanol, sodium hydroxide, TEMED, see Appendix IV.

Prior to electrophoresis, prepare the following solutions:

### Urea/NP-40 solution

| | |
|---|---|
| Urea | 120 g |
| NP-40 | 4.2 ml |
| Distilled $H_2O$ | 90 ml |

### Acrylamide

| | |
|---|---|
| Acrylamide | 9.0 g |
| Bisacrylamide | 0.54 g |
| Distilled $H_2O$ | 30 ml |

### Ampholyte mixture

| | |
|---|---|
| Ampholyte, pH 6.0–8.0 (or other narrow range) | 80% |
| Ampholyte, pH 3.5–10.0 (or other wide range) | 20% |

### Ammonium persulfate 10%

### Phosphoric acid 34%

### Sodium hydroxide 2.4%

### Sample buffer

| | |
|---|---|
| Urea | 9 M |
| NP-40 | 4% |
| β-Mercaptoethanol | 2% |

For high reproducibility between different gels, all these solutions should be dispensed in appropriate volumes, sealed, and frozen at –20°C.

### *Sample preparation*

1. For sample preparation, immune complexes collected on SAC or protein A beads (p. 244) can be resuspended in 25 μl of sample buffer. Samples of other proteins can be diluted into sample buffer. Dried proteins can be resuspended in sample buffer.

*Knowles (1987).

2. Heat at 50°C for 30 minutes. Spin to remove the solid-phase matrix or any debris. Carefully transfer to clean tubes. Ready for loading. Samples may be stored at –20°C prior to electrophoresis.

### *First dimension*

1. To prepare the first dimension (isoelectric focusing gel), add 3.0 ml of the acrylamide solution (at room temperature) to 18.8 ml of the urea/NP-40 solution (the urea/NP-40 solution can be heated to 37°C to increase the solubility of the urea). Mix gently. Add 1.25 ml of the Ampholyte solution (room temperature), and mix gently. Add 75 µl of 10% ammonium persulfate and 20 µl of TEMED. This yields a final volume of 23.15 ml.

2. Pour the first-dimension tube gels. There are many different two-dimensional gel apparatuses. Follow the manufacturer's instructions for pouring the first dimension.

3. After the first dimension has polymerized (about 15 minutes for the initial stages), allow the gel to sit at room temperature for a further 30 minutes.

4. Remove the tube gels from the casting apparatus. Wash the bottom ends of the tube gels with distilled water. Insert the tube gels into the electrophoresis apparatus. The bottom running buffer is prepared by diluting 1 volume of 34% phosphoric acid to 400 volumes of distilled water. Check to ensure that no bubbles are found at the interface of the bottom of the tube gel and the running buffer. Completely assemble the apparatus and add the top running buffer. Top running buffer can be prepared by adding 1 volume of 2.4% sodium hydroxide to 30 volumes of distilled water. Using a syringe fitted with a 1.5-in. needle, wash the top of each tube gel with top running buffer. This will remove any unpolymerized acrylamide and any air bubbles.

5. Carefully layer the samples onto the top surface of the isoelectric focusing gel. Approximately 20 µl/gel is appropriate. Samples can be applied using either (1) a microliter syringe (washed by pipetting in distilled water between each sample), (2) a micropipettor fitted with a long narrow tip, or (3) Teflon tubing fixed to the end of a microliter syringe (24-gauge, thin-walled spaghetti tubing fits snugly on 22-gauge needles; discard each piece after a single use).

6. Attach the electrodes to the isoelectric focusing apparatus: the positive (red) electrode to the bottom and the negative (black) electrode to the top. Consult the manufacturer's instruction for the appropriate running conditions.

7. After the run is complete, turn off the power pack and disassemble the apparatus. Remove the tube gel.

8. Remove the gels from the glass tubes by applying even gentle pressure from the 1-ml syringe filled with distilled water applied to one end of the tube. As the gel emerges, be careful to align it in such a way that the positive and negative ends are known.

   The isoelectric focusing gel can be immediately loaded on the second dimension or stored at –70°C.

### *Second dimension*

1. Cast an SDS-polyacrylamide slab gel using the protocol described on p. 413. The choice of acrylamide percentage depends on the protein under study. The separating gel is poured and allowed to polymerize as usual. **For isoelectric focusing gels of 1 to 2 mm in diameter**: The separating gel should be poured to within approximately 1 mm of the top. Overlay with isobutanol. After polymerization, go directly to step 3. The tube gel will be placed directly onto the separating gel, with no stacking gel. **For thicker isoelectric focusing gels:** A stacking gel is needed. The meniscus of the separating gel should be approximately 1 cm below the top. For these gels, go on to step 2.

2. Wash the top of the separating gel with water. Drain well or dry with the edge of a paper towel. Prepare the stacking gel solution as described on p. 413. Pour on top of the separating gel. The stacking gel solution should come to approximately 1 mm below the top of the glass plates. Overlay with isobutanol-saturated water. Allow the gel to polymerize (approximately 15–30 minutes).

3. Wash the top of the gel with water. Drain well or dry with the edge of a paper towel. Prepare a 0.5% agarose solution in 1× Laemmli gel running buffer (p. 465). Add bromophenol blue to 0.001%. Melt in a boiling water bath or in a microwave oven. Cool to 50°C. Layer over the separating gel, completely filling the remaining space. Carefully lay the isoelectric focusing gel into the agarose, being careful to avoid any bubbles. Mark the positive end. Allow the agarose to harden at room temperature (~10 minutes).

Place the gel plates in an electrophoresis tank and run as usual.

The gels can be processed for staining, autoradiography, fluorography, or blotting as usual.

## Note

i. Many protocols need good internal markers for both molecular weights and pI. Commercially produced prestained markers are the best that are available at present.

## Alkylation of proteins prior to running on a gel*

### Caution

DTT, β-mercaptoethanol, NEM, SDS, see Appendix IV.

1. If using proteins from immunoprecipitations, wash immune complexes as usual. Remove the final wash as completely as possible. If using other sources of proteins, transfer them to 20 mM phosphate (pH 7.0), or resuspend the proteins directly in 20 μl of water. Protein concentrations should be under 1 mg/ml.

2. Add 20 μl of 1.5% SDS with 20 mM DTT.

3. Heat to 85°C for 10 minutes. Carefully transfer the supernatant to a fresh tube.

4. Add 10 μl of freshly prepared 0.2 M *N*-ethylmaleimide (NEM) (12.5 mg/ml of water; this should be a saturated solution). Make up the solution just prior to using. The 10-minute, 85°C incubation is a good time to try to get the NEM into solution. An ultrasonic water bath helps, but repeated pipetting is sufficient. Because the solution is saturated, complete dissolution is impossible. Alternatively, dissolve the NEM in 20 mM sodium acetate (pH 6.0).

5. Incubate for 60 minutes on ice.

6. Add 10 μl of 50% glycerol, 0.5 M β-mercaptoethanol with 0.001% bromophenol blue.

   **The sample is now ready for electrophoresis.**

*L. Crawford (pers. comm.); Riordan and Vallee (1972).

## PPO fluorography*

### Caution

Diphenyloxazole (PPO), DMSO, glacial acetic acid, methanol, radioactive substances, see Appendix IV.

1. After electrophoresis or staining, place the gel in destain (7% glacial acetic acid, 25% methanol) for 30 minutes with shaking. Carefully pour off the destain, rinse in dimethylsulfoxide (DMSO) waste solution (see step 3 for the origin of DMSO waste), and drain. Add 5 gel volumes of DMSO waste solution.

2. Incubate for 45 minutes with shaking at room temperature. Discard the DMSO waste and add 5 gel volumes of fresh DMSO.

3. Incubate for 45 minutes with shaking at room temperature. Decant the DMSO into the DMSO waste solution container. Add 5 gel volumes of 22% (wt/vol) diphenyloxazole (PPO) in DMSO.

4. Incubate for 45 minutes with shaking at room temperature. Decant the PPO/DMSO back into its container. For routine work this solution can be used again. (A 500-ml stock can be used for 10–15 gels when [$^{35}$S]methionine is the radioisotope).

5. Place the PPO-impregnated gel in a gentle flow of water. It should immediately turn white as the PPO begins to come out of solution.

6. Wash under a gentle stream of fresh water for 30 minutes to 1 hour. Remove the gel and dry as normal.

   Fluorographed gels should be exposed at –70°C (p. 432).

## Notes

i. For gels using $^{3}$H radioisotopes, film should be preflashed to maintain a linear relationship between amount of radioactive decay and film darkening. For details, see Laskey and Mills (1975). An excellent description of fluorography can be found in a pamphlet available from Amersham plc written by Ron Laskey (Radioisotope detection by fluorography and intensifying screens; Review 23).
ii. Several companies supply commercial alternatives to PPO. They are simpler to use, but are considerably more costly than PPO.

*Bonner and Laskey (1974).

## Phosphor imaging

### Caution

Radioactive substances, see Appendix IV.

The analysis of the distribution of radioactively labeled molecules by phosphor imaging offers advantages over the use of X-ray film. Phosphor imaging for $^{32}P$ is up to 250× more sensitive than straight autoradiography and up to 15× more sensitive for X-ray film exposures at –70°C with intensifying screens. Another major advantage is that the dynamic range of the phosphor imaging plate is considerably wider than X-ray film darkening, and so the method is especially suited for quantitation. Finally, because the results are fed directly to a computer, the quantitative analysis of the results is much faster and easier.

The imaging plate must be handled with care because it consists of fine crystals of a phosphor. When exposed to high-energy radiation, the energy in the radiation is trapped in an excited form in the phosphor. It is this energy that is released as luminescence when the plate is subsequently scanned with the imaging laser. The released luminescence is then detected by a photomultiplier tube, and the resulting electrical signal is used to construct the final image of the distribution of the original radiation source.

To use this method, the gel or blot should be completely dried down onto 3MM filter paper. It is then placed in contact with the imaging plate, and exposure is carried out at room temperature. It is very important to achieve close and even contact between the dried gel and the screen. Once sufficient time has elapsed, the plate can be quickly transferred to the imaging machine. If a dilution series of small spots of isotope dried onto paper are used to create a control image on the same plate, then absolute calculations of the amount of isotope in a given band or spot on the test gel or blot can be calculated from a standard curve.

Workers should consult the instructions for their phosphor imager for suggested operating methods.

## Counting $^{35}S$, $^{14}C$, or $^{3}H$ from polyacrylamide gel slices

### Caution

Ammonium hydroxide, hydrogen peroxide, radioactive substances, toluene, see Appendix IV.

1. Using an autoradiogram as a template, excise the region of the gel that contains the radioactive protein of interest. This can be most easily done from a dried, but unfixed, gel.

2. Place the gel slice in a counting vial.

3. Swell the gel slice in a minimal amount of water (20 µl per 1 × 5-mm slice) for 30 minutes at room temperature.

**Either:** Dissolve the gel slice in 1.0 ml of 19 parts 30% hydrogen peroxide, 1 part 14.8 M ammonium hydroxide by incubation at 37°C overnight.* Add aqueous-based scintillant.

**Or:** Add 10 ml of freshly prepared ammonia/solubilizer/scintillant (prepared by adding 0.5 ml of 14.8 M ammonium hydroxide to 10 ml of NCS solubilizer [Amersham] or Solusol [National Diagnostics], mix, and add to 100 ml of toluene-based scintillant). Incubate overnight at room temperature with shaking.**

Count.

## Counting $^{32}P$ or $^{125}I$ from polyacrylamide gel slices

### Caution

Radioactive substances, see Appendix IV.

1. Using an autoradiogram as a template, excise the region of the gel that contains the radioactive protein of interest.

2. Place the gel slice in a counting vial. $^{32}P$ samples can be counted using Cerenkov counting, and $^{125}I$ samples in a gamma-counter.

### Note

i. The efficiency of Cerenkov counting will depend on the volume of the sample, and comparisons should be made from similar-sized gel slices.

## Coomassie Blue staining—Standard method

### Caution

Acetic acid, methanol, see Appendix IV.

After electrophoresis, transfer the gel to a clean glass or plastic container. Add 5 gel volumes of 0.25% Coomassie Brilliant Blue R-250, 50% methanol, and 10% acetic acid.

*Bonner and Laskey (1974).
**Ward et al. (1970).

2. Incubate 4 hours to overnight at room temperature with shaking.

3. Remove the stain and save. The staining solution can be used many times (20–40) before replacing.

4. Destain the gel by successive incubations in 25% methanol, 7.5% acetic acid at room temperature with shaking.

   Sensitivity is 0.1–0.5 μg per track.

## Notes

i. Staining and destaining time can be substantially reduced by using hot stain or destaining solutions. Heat the stain or destain in a microwave oven or a water bath (about 50–60°C). Staining times can be shortened to approximately 20 minutes, and destaining will take approximately 1–2 hours.

ii. Adding foam rubber, wool, or other components that will bind the dye will speed destaining times, particularly when destaining at room temperature.

## Coomassie Blue staining—Quick method

### Caution

Acetic acid, methanol, trichloroacetic acid, see Appendix IV.

1. Place the gel in a clean glass or plastic dish. Add approximately 5 gel volumes of 0.25% Coomassie Brilliant Blue R-250 in 50% trichloroacetic acid.

2. Incubate at room temperature for 20 minutes with shaking.

3. Drain the stain and save (it is good for numerous stainings). Wash the gel with water to remove the stain that has not penetrated the gel.

4. Add several gel volumes of destain (25% methanol, 7% acetic acid). Change as needed. Warming the gel will help speed destaining, as will including a sponge, a paper towel, or any material that will bind the stain in the destain solution.

   Sensitivity is 1.0 μg per track.

## Coomassie Blue staining—Maximal sensitivity

### Caution

Acetic acid, ammonium sulfate, trichloroacetic acid, see Appendix IV.

1. Prior to staining, the Coomassie Brilliant Blue G-250 (a dimethylated derivative of Coomassie Brilliant Blue R-250) must be purified. Commercial sources are contaminated with compounds that increase the background. Dissolve 4 g of dye in 250 ml of 7.5% acetic acid. Heat to 70°C. Add 44 g of ammonium sulfate. After the ammonium sulfate has dissolved, cool the mixture to room temperature. Recover the dye by filtration or centrifugation at 3000*g* for 10 minutes. Remove the supernatant and allow the dye to dry.

2. To prepare the staining solution, dissolve 30 g of ammonium sulfate in 500 ml of 2% phosphoric acid. After the ammonium sulfate has dissolved *completely*, add 0.5 g of the purified Coomassie Brilliant Blue G-250 dissolved in 10 ml of water. Store at room temperature.

3. After electrophoresis, transfer the gel to a clean glass or plastic container. Add 5 gel volumes of 12.5% trichloroacetic acid.

4. Incubate for 1 hour or longer at room temperature with shaking.

5. Drain well. Shake the Coomassie Brilliant Blue G-250 stain to disperse large colloids. Add to the gel.

6. Incubate overnight at room temperature with shaking.

7. Pour the stain back into the stock bottle. The stain solution can be used for multiple stainings. Wash the gel with water or standard destain solution and observe.

8. To fix the colloidal stain to the proteins, add 5 gel volumes of 20% ammonium sulfate and incubate overnight at room temperature with shaking. After fixing the gel, it can be stained again for added sensitivity. Repeat the staining from step 5.

   Sensitivity is 0.05–0.1 μg per track.

## Silver staining of gels—Ammoniacal silver staining

### Caution

Acetic acid, ammonia, ammonium hydroxide, ethanol, formaldehyde, glutaraldehyde, hydrochloric acid, silver nitrate, sodium hydroxide, see Appendix IV.

1. Wear gloves and use only clean glassware. Fingerprints will stain, and dirty glassware will affect the sensitivity of these reactions.

2. After running a standard gel, place in 5 gel volumes of 50% ethanol, 10% acetic acid for 30 minutes to overnight with shaking.

3. Remove the 50% ethanol, 10% acetic acid and rinse the gel in deionized water. Add 5 gel volumes of 20% ethanol and incubate for 30 minutes with shaking.

4. Remove the ethanol and add 5 gel volumes of 20% ethanol. Incubate for 30 minutes with shaking.

5. Remove the ethanol and move to a fume hood. Add 5 gel volumes of 5% glutaraldehyde prepared in deionized water. Incubate at room temperature for 30 minutes with shaking in a fume hood.

6. Remove the glutaraldehyde and rinse the gel with deionized water. Add 5 gel volumes of 20% ethanol. Incubate for 20 minutes at room temperature with shaking. This step and the following steps do not need to be performed in the fume hood.

7. Remove the 20% ethanol and repeat the ethanol wash twice (step 6).

8. After the last ethanol wash, rinse the gel with deionized water and add 5 gel volumes of deionized water. Incubate for 10 minutes at room temperature with shaking.

9. Remove the water wash and add 4 gel volumes of a freshly prepared ammonia/silver solution. For 100 ml: Add 1.4 ml of 14.8 M ammonium hydroxide to 100 ml of water. Add 190 µl of 10 N sodium hydroxide. Place this on a vortex and slowly add 1 ml of a freshly prepared solution of silver nitrate (0.8 g of silver nitrate in 1 ml of water). Add the silver nitrate dropwise. A precipitate will appear but will dissolve quickly.

   Incubate for 30 minutes at room temperature with shaking.

10. Remove the ammonia/silver solution, and wash the gel with several changes of deionized water over 20 minutes. Precipitate the silver in the used ammonia/silver solution by adding hydrochloric acid.

11. Remove the water and add 5 gel volumes of freshly prepared 0.005% citric acid, 0.019% formaldehyde (diluted from a commercial 37% solution). Mix gently. The bands will start to develop within a few minutes. As the background begins to change, pour off the developer and wash the gel with water. A little practice will tell you when to stop this step. Stop the reaction by incubating the gel in 10% acetic acid, 20% ethanol.

    Sensitivity is about 1–10 ng per band.

## Note

Several companies supply good silver staining kits.

## Silver staining of gels—Neutral silver staining

### Caution

Acetic acid, ethanol, formaldehyde, silver nitrate, see Appendix IV.

1. Wear gloves and use only clean glassware. Fingerprints will stain, and dirty glassware will affect the sensitivity of these reactions.

2. After running a standard gel, place in 5 gel volumes of 30% ethanol, 10% acetic acid for 3 hours to overnight with shaking.

3. Remove the ethanol/acetic acid solution, and add 5 gel volumes of 30% ethanol. Incubate for 30 minutes at room temperature with shaking. Repeat the 30% ethanol wash.

4. Remove the ethanol solution and add 10 gel volumes of deionized water. Incubate for 10 minutes at room temperature with shaking. Repeat the water wash twice.

5. Remove the water and add 5 gel volumes of 0.1% silver nitrate solution (diluted from a 20% stock stored in a brown bottle at room temperature). Incubate for 30 minutes at room temperature with shaking.

6. Remove the silver nitrate solution and wash the gel for 20 seconds under a stream of deionized water.

7. Add 5 gel volumes of 2.5% sodium carbonate, 0.02% formaldehyde (pH > 4.0). Incubate at room temperature with shaking. Bands should begin to appear after several minutes. Incubate until the background begins to darken.

8. Stop the reaction by washing in 1% acetic acid. Wash with several changes of deionized water of 10 minutes each. **Optional:** A thin film of gray may develop on the gel surface. This can be removed by a short wash in a photographic reducer such as Farmer's (0.5% for 30 seconds).

   Sensitivity is 1–10 ng per band.

## Notes

i. To intensify the silver staining, repeat steps 5–8.
ii. Several companies supply good silver staining kits.

## Copper staining of gels*

A useful alternative to the more traditional staining methods using Coomassie Brilliant Blue or silver is copper staining. Incubating gels in a solution of copper chloride ($CuCl_2$) allows the formation of a white opaque precipitate apparently involving both Tris and SDS. Protein bands remain clear, leaving a negative image of the polypeptide separation pattern. The proteins are not fixed in the gel and can be eluted by simple removal of the Cu ions by chelation with EDTA. This method is particularly useful for the rapid localization of protein bands either for immunization or for further protein chemistry studies. The stained patterns are as easy to photograph as Coomassie or silver stained gels.

1. After electrophoresis, the gels should be washed briefly with distilled water, using several changes over 30 seconds. Longer washes will begin to allow the Tris or SDS to elute and should be avoided.

2. Place the gel in a glass or plastic tray. Add at least 5 gel volumes of 0.3 M $CuCl_2$.

3. Incubate at room temperature with agitation for 5 minutes. Longer incubation times may be suitable with thicker gels. As the $CuCl_2$ enters the

*Lee et al. (1987).

gel, a white precipitate will form in the regions of the gel that do not contain proteins.

4. Wash the gel for several minutes with distilled water. Observe against a dark background.

   Sensitivity is 10–100 ng per band for 0.5-mm gels and approximately 1 μg per band for 1-mm gels.

## Note

The staining can be reversed by incubating in 0.25 M EDTA, 0.25 M Tris (pH 9.0).

## Fixing gels

### Caution

Acetic acid, methanol, trichloroacetic acid, see Appendix IV.

For many purposes, proteins separated by electrophoresis need to be precipitated or bound within the gel. Collectively, these techniques are described as fixation. Gels of all percentages and widths can be fixed by washing with acids or alcohols. This is commonly done by soaking a gel at room temperature in 12.5% trichloroacetic acid or destain (7% acetic acid, 25% methanol). If bromophenol blue is used as a tracking dye, it can also act as a pH indicator to determine whether the acid has diffused into the gel. The bromophenol blue turns yellow below pH 5.0. Incubate for 10 minutes after the blue turns to yellow. If no tracking dye has been used or if it has been run off the bottom of the gel, fix for 30 minutes for gels up to 1 mm thick, 45 minutes for gels 1–1.5 mm, and 1 hour for gels over 1.5 mm.

## Drying gels

1. Wash the gel briefly in water.

2. Place the gel onto a piece of plastic wrap with the cut corner marking the number 1 lane in the lower right-hand side.

3. Carefully cut the plastic wrap to a size just larger than the gel. A sharp scalpel is useful, if the countertop resists cutting.

4. Place a piece of absorbent paper (Whatman 3MM or equivalent, cut larger than the gel, but smaller than the size of the gel dryer) onto the gel. If the paper is dry, the gel will stick to the paper, making handling easier.

5. Place the gel with the plastic wrap and paper on a second piece of absorbent paper in a gel dryer. The order should be plastic wrap, gel, paper, paper, and then the vacuum source. Apply a good vacuum and gentle heat.

   For most percentages of gels the vacuum produced from a water aspirator or a vacuum pump is sufficient for drying; however, house vacuums often are too slow for most applications. Heat can be applied from either the top or bottom, but higher-percentage gels crack less often when the heat is applied to the top (plastic wrap side).

6. Dry for 30 minutes to 2 hours (30 minutes for minigels, 2 hours for 2 mm or wider gels). Release the vacuum to the gel and remove.

   The gel is now ready for exposure to film or storage.

## Rehydrating dried polyacrylamide gels

### Caution

Methanol, see Appendix IV.

1. Peel the paper from the dried gel. Starting at one corner, peel the paper from the back of the gel, working toward the center. Some paper will remain on the gel and eventually the paper will tear. Switch to another corner and repeat. Continue until all of the surrounding paper and much of the backing paper is removed.

2. Submerge the gel completely in a large container of water. As the gel begins to rehydrate, it will pull away from the remaining backing paper.

3. As the gel rehydrates it will shrink severely. After several minutes the remaining backing paper can be removed from the gel.

4. After the paper has been removed, incubate at room temperature with gentle shaking for 30 minutes. The gel will begin to swell within a few minutes.

5. After the gel has reached its normal size, it can be transferred into any appropriate buffer. Continued incubation in water will cause the gel to swell to a size larger than the original starting size. Maintaining the gel in 25% methanol will hold the gel at approximately its normal size.

## Autoradiography and Fluorography

### Caution

Diphenyloxazole (PPO), radioactive substances, see Appendix IV.

### *Autoradiography*

1. Place the dried gel or blot in direct contact with the emulsion of an X-ray film. Kodak XAR or Fuji RX films are suitable. Blots with $^{14}C$ or $^{35}S$ markers or samples must be oriented in the proper direction with the correct side facing the film to ensure proper exposure.
2. Expose in a sealed, lightproof container for the appropriate length of time at room temperature.
3. Develop using the manufacturer's instructions.

### *Fluorography (PPO-impregnated gels)*

1. Place the gel or blot in direct contact with the emulsion of the X-ray film.
2. Expose in a sealed, lightproof container for the appropriate length of time at –70°C.
3. Develop using the manufacturer's instructions.

### *Exposure with intensifying screens ($^{32}P$ or $^{125}I$)**

1. Place a piece of X-ray film on a calcium tungstate intensifying screen. Place the gel or blot in direct contact with the emulsion of the film.
2. Expose in a sealed, lightproof container for the appropriate length of time at –70°C.

*Swanstrom and Shank (1978).

 Develop using the manufacturer's instructions.

*Sensitivities of autoradiography versus fluorography*

| Isotope[a] | Autoradiography cpm needed for overnight band | Fluorography method | Fluorography cpm needed for overnight band | Enhancement |
|---|---|---|---|---|
| $^{3}H$ | $>10^{7}$ | PPO[a]-impregnated gel –70°C | 3000 | 1000 |
| $^{14}C$ | 2000 | PPO-impregnated gels –70°C | 200 | 10 |
| $^{32}P$ | 50 | Screen, –70°C | 10 | 5 |
| $^{35}S$ | 1000 | PPO-impregnated gels –70°C | 100–200 | 5–10 |
| $^{125}I$ | 100 | Screen, –70°C | 10 | 10 |

[a] See Appendix IV for caution.

## References

Anker H.S. 1970. A solubilizable acrylamide gel for electrophoresis. *FEBS Lett.* **7:** 293.

Bonner W.M. and Laskey R.A. 1974. A film detection method for tritium-labelled proteins and nucleic acids in polyacrylamide gels. *Eur. J. Biochem.* **46:** 83–88.

Cleveland D.W., Fischer S.G., Kirschner M.W., and Laemmli U.K. 1977. Peptide mapping by limited proteolysis in sodium dodecylsulfate and analysis by gel electrofocusing. *J. Biol. Chem.* **252:** 1102–1106.

Davis B.J. 1964. Disc electrophoresis. II. Method and application to human serum proteins. *Ann. N.Y. Acad. Sci.* **121:** 404–427.

Fischer S.G. 1983. Peptide mapping in gels. *Methods Enzymol.* **100:** 424–430.

Hansen J.N. 1976. Electrophoresis of ribonucleic acid on a polyacrylamide gel which contains disulfide cross-linkages. *Anal. Biochem.* **76:** 37–44.

Hansen J.N., Pheiffer B.H., and Boehnert J.A. 1980. Chemical and electrophoretic properties of solubilizable disulfide gels. *Anal. Biochem.* **105:** 192–301.

Jovin T.M., Dante M.L., and Chrambach A. 1970. Multiphasic buffer systems output, PB 196085–19609, *National Tech. Info. Service.*

Knowles R.W. 1987. Two-dimensional gel analysis of transmembrane proteins. In *Histocompatibility testing* (ed. B. Dupont), pp. 1–45. Springer Verlag, New York.

Laemmli U.K. 1970. Cleavage of structural proteins during the assembly of the head of bacteriophage T4. *Nature* **227:** 680–685.

Laskey R.A. and Mills A.D. 1975. Quantitative detection of $^{3}H$ and $^{14}C$ in polyacrylamide gels by fluorography. *Eur. J. Biochem.* **56:** 335–341.

Lee C., Levin A., and Branton D. 1987. Copper staining: A five-minute protein stain for sodium dodecyl sulfate-polyacrylamide gels. *Anal. Biochem.* **166:** 308–312.

Ornstein L. 1964. Disc electrophoresis. I. Background and theory. *Ann. N.Y. Acad. Sci.* **121:** 321–349.

Raymond S. and Weintraub L. 1959. Acrylamide gel as a supporting medium for zone electrophoresis. *Science* **130:** 711.

Riordan J.F. and Vallee B.L. 1972. Reactions with *N*-ethylmaleimide and *p*-mercuribenzoate. *Methods Enzymol.* **25:** 449–456.

Schagger H. and von Jagow G. 1987. Tricine-sodium dodecyl sulfate-polyacrylamide gel electrophoresis for the separation of proteins in the range from 1 to 100 kDa. *Anal. Biochem.* **166:** 368–379.

Smithies O. 1955. Zone electrophoresis in starch gels: Group variations in the serum proteins of normal human adults. *Biochemistry* **61:** 629–641.

Sobieszek A. and Jertschin P. 1986. Urea-glycerol-acrylamide gel electrophoresis of acidic low molecular weight muscle proteins: Rapid determination of myosin light chain phosphorylation in myosin, actomyosin and whole muscle samples. *Electrophoresis* **7:** 417–425.

Summers D.F., Maizel J.V., Jr., and Darnell J.E., Jr. 1965. Evidence for virus-specific noncapsid proteins in poliovirus-infected HeLa cells. *Proc. Natl. Acad. Sci.* **54:** 505–513.

Swanstrom R. and Shank P.R. 1978. X-ray intensifying screens greatly enhance the detection by autoradiography of the radioactive isotopes $^{32}P$ and $^{125}I$. *Anal. Biochem.* **86:** 184–192.

Ward S., Wilson D.L., and Gilliam J.J. 1970. Methods for fractionation and scintillation counting of radioisotope-labeled polyacrylamide gels. *Anal. Biochem.* **38:** 90–97.

Weber K. and Osborn M. 1969. The reliability of molecular weight determinations by dodecyl sulfate-polyacrylamide gel electrophoresis. *J. Biol. Chem.* **244:** 4406–4412.

# Appendix II
# Protein Techniques

## *Ammonium sulfate[a] saturation tables*

| Starting concentration | Final concentration | | | | | | | | | | | | | |
|---|---|---|---|---|---|---|---|---|---|---|---|---|---|---|
| | **10%** | **20%** | **25%** | **30%** | **35%** | **40%** | **45%** | **50%** | **55%** | **60%** | **65%** | **70%** | **75%** | **80%** |
| 0% | 56 | 114 | 144 | 176 | 209 | 243 | 277 | 313 | 351 | 390 | 430 | 472 | 516 | 561 |
| 10% | — | 57 | 86 | 118 | 150 | 183 | 216 | 251 | 288 | 326 | 365 | 406 | 449 | 494 |
| 20% | | — | 29 | 59 | 91 | 123 | 155 | 189 | 225 | 262 | 300 | 340 | 382 | 424 |
| 25% | | | — | 30 | 61 | 93 | 125 | 158 | 193 | 230 | 267 | 307 | 348 | 390 |
| 30% | | | | — | 30 | 62 | 94 | 127 | 162 | 198 | 235 | 273 | 314 | 356 |
| 35% | | | | | — | 31 | 63 | 94 | 129 | 164 | 200 | 238 | 278 | 319 |
| 40% | | | | | | — | 31 | 63 | 97 | 132 | 168 | 205 | 245 | 285 |
| 45% | | | | | | | — | 32 | 65 | 99 | 134 | 171 | 210 | 250 |
| 50% | | | | | | | | — | 33 | 66 | 101 | 137 | 176 | 214 |
| 55% | | | | | | | | | — | 33 | 67 | 103 | 141 | 179 |
| 60% | | | | | | | | | | — | 34 | 69 | 105 | 143 |

Values given are the number of grams to be added to 1 liter of solution to change the ammonium sulfate concentration from the starting concentration to final concentration. All values are adjusted for changes in volume at room temperature. The saturation of ammonium sulfate does not vary significantly between 4°C and 25°C, so the values given here can normally be used at both temperatures. Saturated ammonium sulfate is 4.1 M at 25°C (add 761 g to 1 liter of distilled $H_2O$).

[a] See Appendix IV for caution.

## Preparing acetone powders

### Caution

Acetone, see Appendix IV.

1. Prepare a fine suspension of tissue or cells in saline (0.9% NaCl). If a tissue is used, either discard any fibrous material by teasing it away from the remainder of the tissue or homogenize the whole tissue by placing it in a blender. (One gram of tissue should be resuspended in approximately 1.0 ml of saline.)

2. Transfer the tissue/saline suspension to ice for 5 minutes.

3. Add 8 ml of acetone (–20°C) per 2 ml of cell suspension. Mix vigorously. Incubate at 0°C for 30 minutes with occasional vigorous mixing.

4. Collect the precipitate by centrifugation at 10,000*g* for 10 minutes. Remove and discard the supernatant.

5. Resuspend the pellet with fresh acetone (–20°C) and mix vigorously. Allow to sit at 0°C for 10 minutes.

6. Spin at 10,000*g* for 10 minutes. Transfer the pellet to a clean piece of filter paper. Spread the precipitate and allow to air-dry at room temperature. As it dries, continue to spread and disperse the pellet.

7. After the powder is dry, transfer it to an airtight container. Remove any large pieces that will not break into a fine powder.

   Yield is approximately 10–20% of the original wet weight.

   To use acetone powders, add to a final concentration of 1%. Incubate for 30 minutes at 4°C. Spin at 10,000*g* for 10 minutes. Use the supernatant as a source of antibodies for your assay.

*Amino acids*

| Amino acid | Single-letter code | Triple-letter code | Molecular weight (pH 7) | Side chain pK | α-$NH_2$ pK | α-COOH pK |
|---|---|---|---|---|---|---|
| Alanine | A | Ala | 89 | | 9.87 | 2.35 |
| Arginine | R | Arg | 174 | 13.2 | 9.09 | 2.18 |
| Asparagine | N | Asn | 132 | | 8.8 | 2.02 |
| Aspartic acid | D | Asp | 133 | 3.65 | 9.6 | 1.88 |
| Cysteine | C | Cys | 121 | 8.33 | 10.78 | 1.71 |
| Glutamic acid | E | Glu | 147 | 4.25 | 9.67 | 2.19 |
| Glutamine | Q | Gln | 146 | | 9.13 | 2.17 |
| Glycine | G | Gly | 75 | | 9.6 | 2.34 |
| Histidine | H | His | 155 | 6.0 | 8.97 | 1.78 |
| Isoleucine | I | Ile | 131 | | 9.76 | 2.32 |
| Leucine | L | Leu | 131 | | 9.6 | 2.36 |
| Lysine | K | Lys | 146 | 10.28 | 8.9 | 2.2 |
| Methionine | M | Met | 149 | | 9.21 | 2.28 |
| Phenylalanine | F | Phe | 165 | | 9.24 | 2.58 |
| Proline | P | Pro | 115 | | 10.6 | 1.99 |
| Serine | S | Ser | 105 | | 9.15 | 2.21 |
| Threonine | T | Thr | 119 | | 9.12 | 2.15 |
| Tryptophan | W | Trp | 204 | | 9.39 | 2.38 |
| Tyrosine | Y | Tyr | 181 | 10.1 | 9.11 | 2.2 |
| Valine | V | Val | 117 | | 9.72 | 2.29 |

| Hydropathy values | | | |
|---|---|---|---|
| Hopp and Woods[a] | Kyte and Doolittle[b] | Solubility (g/100 ml of $H_2O$) | Amino acid |
| –0.5 | –1.8 | 15.8 | Alanine |
| 3.0 | 4.5 | 71.8 | Arginine |
| 0.2 | 3.5 | 2.4 | Asparagine |
| 3.0 | 3.5 | 0.42 | Aspartic acid |
| –1.0 | –2.5 | Freely | Cysteine |
| 3.0 | 3.5 | 0.72 | Glutamic acid |
| 0.2 | 3.5 | 2.6 | Glutamine |
| 0.0 | 0.4 | 22.5 | Glycine |
| –0.5 | 3.2 | 4.19 | Histidine |
| –1.8 | –4.5 | 3.36 | Isoleucine |
| –1.8 | –3.8 | 2.37 | Leucine |
| 3.0 | 3.9 | 66.6 | Lysine |
| –1.3 | –1.9 | 5.14 | Methionine |
| –2.5 | –2.8 | 2.7 | Phenylalanine |
| 0.0 | 1.6 | 154 | Proline |
| 0.3 | 0.8 | 36.2 | Serine |
| –0.4 | 0.7 | Freely | Threonine |
| –3.4 | 0.9 | 1.06 | Tryptophan |
| –2.3 | –1.3 | 0.038 | Tyrosine |
| –1.5 | –4.2 | 5.6 | Valine |

[a] Hopp and Woods (1981).
[b] Kyte and Doolittle (1982).

*Proteins used as molecular weight standards*

| Protein | Relative molecular weight | Calculated molecular weight | Native molecular weight/S value |
|---|---|---|---|
| Thyroglobulin | 340,000 | | 660,000/19S |
| Myosin | 205,000 | | 470,000 |
| | 21,000 | | |
| | 19,000 | | |
| | 17,000 | | |
| $\alpha_2$-Macroglobulin | 170,000 | 160,798 | 820,000/19S |
| β-Galactosidase | 116,000 | 116,365 | 540,000 |
| Phosphorylase-b | 94,000 | | |
| Phosphorylase-a | 92,500 | | 370,000 |
| Transferrin, human | 80,000 | 75,190 | 80,000 |
| Serum albumin, bovine | 68,000 | 66,322 | 68,000 |
| Catalase, bovine liver | 60,000 | 57,592 | 230,000 |
| Pyruvate kinase, muscle | 57,000 | | 220,000 |
| IgG | | | |
| Heavy chain | 55,000 | | 150,000 |
| Light chain | 22,000 | | |
| Glutamate dehydrogenase | 53,000 | 55,567 | |
| Leucine aminopeptidase | 53,000 | 51,698 | 300,000 |
| Fumerase | 49,000 | | 200,000 |
| Ovalbumin | 45,000 | 42,755 | |
| Alcohol dehydrogenase, liver | 41,000 | 39,572 | 80,000 |
| Aldolase, rabbit muscle | 40,000 | 39,216 | 160,000 |
| Creatine kinase, rabbit muscle | 40,000 | 43,117 | 80,000 |
| Alcohol dehydrogenase, yeast | 36,000 | 36,735 | 140,000 |
| Glyceraldehyde phosphate dehydrogenase | 36,000 | 35,880 | |
| Lactate dehydrogenase, pig | 36,000 | 36,481 | 140,000 |
| Tropomyosin, rabbit | 36,000 | 32,840 | 65,000 |
| Pepsinogen, pig | 35,000 | 39,538 | |
| Carbonic anhydrase | 29,000 | 29,343 | 180,000 |
| Chymotrypsinogen a, bovine | 24,000 | 25,669 | |
| Trypsinogen, bovine | 24,000 | 23,996 | |
| Trypsin inhibitor, soybean | 20,100 | 20,097 | |
| Apoferritin | 18,500 | | 440,000 |
| β-Lactoglobulin, bovine | 18,000 | 18,283 | 35,000 |
| Myoglobin | 17,000 | 17,080 | |
| Hemoglobin | 16,000 | | 64,000 |
| Lysozyme, chicken | 14,300 | 14,296 | |
| α-Lactalbumin, bovine | 14,200 | 14,188 | |
| Cytochrome *c* | 12,400 | | |
| Aprotinin | 6,500 | | |

*Genetic code*

| First nucleotide | Second nucleotide: U | | C | | A | | G | | Third nucleotide |
|---|---|---|---|---|---|---|---|---|---|
| U | UUU | Phe | UCU | Ser | UAU | Tyr | UGU | Cys | U |
| | UUC | Phe | UCC | Ser | UAC | Tyr | UGC | Cys | C |
| | UUA | Leu | UCA | Ser | UAA | Stop[a] | UGA | Stop[c] | A |
| | UUG | Leu | UCG | Ser | UAG | Stop[b] | UGG | Trp | G |
| C | CUU | Leu | CCU | Pro | CAU | His | CGU | Arg | U |
| | CUC | Leu | CCC | Pro | CAC | His | CGC | Arg | C |
| | CUA | Leu | CCA | Pro | CAA | Gln | CGA | Arg | A |
| | CUG | Leu | CCG | Pro | CAG | Gln | CGG | Arg | G |
| A | AUU | Ile | ACU | Thr | AAU | Asn | AGU | Ser | U |
| | AUC | Ile | ACC | Thr | AAC | Asn | AGC | Ser | C |
| | AUA | Ile | ACA | Thr | AAA | Lys | AGA | Arg | A |
| | AUG | Met | ACG | Thr | AAG | Lys | AGG | Arg | G |
| G | GUU | Val | GCU | Ala | GAU | Asp | GGU | Gly | U |
| | GUC | Val | GCC | Ala | GAC | Asp | GGC | Gly | C |
| | GUA | Val | GCA | Ala | GAA | Glu | GGA | Gly | A |
| | GUG | Val | GCG | Ala | GAG | Glu | GGG | Gly | G |

[a] Ochre codon.
[b] Amber codon.
[c] Opal codon.
**Note:** Genetic codes for various organisms can be found at http:// www3.ncbi.nlm.nih.gov/htbin-post/ Taxonomy/wprintgc? mode = t/.

*Amino acid and codon usage*

| Amino acid usage[a] | | | Codon usage[b] | | |
|---|---|---|---|---|---|
| **Amino acid** | ***E. coli*[c]** | **human[d]** | **Codon** | ***E. coli*[e]** | **human[e]** |
| **Alanine** | 11.1 | 7.0 | GCT | 0.19 | 0.28 |
| | | | GCC | 0.25 | 0.40 |
| | | | GCA | 0.22 | 0.22 |
| | | | GCG | 0.34 | 0.10 |
| **Leucine** | 7.9 | 10.4 | TTA | 0.11 | 0.06 |
| | | | TTG | 0.11 | 0.12 |
| | | | CTT | 0.10 | 0.12 |
| | | | CTC | 0.10 | 0.20 |
| | | | CTA | 0.03 | 0.07 |
| | | | CTG | 0.55 | 0.43 |
| **Valine** | 7.5 | 6.2 | GTT | 0.29 | 0.17 |
| | | | GTC | 0.20 | 0.25 |
| | | | GTA | 0.17 | 0.10 |
| | | | GTG | 0.34 | 0.48 |
| **Glycine** | 7.2 | 5.7 | GGT | 0.38 | 0.18 |
| | | | GGC | 0.40 | 0.33 |
| | | | GGA | 0.09 | 0.26 |
| | | | GGG | 0.13 | 0.23 |
| **Arginine** | 6.5 | 5.0 | CGT | 0.42 | 0.09 |
| | | | CGC | 0.37 | 0.19 |
| | | | CGA | 0.05 | 0.10 |
| | | | CGG | 0.08 | 0.19 |
| | | | AGA | 0.04 | 0.21 |
| | | | AGG | 0.03 | 0.22 |
| **Lysine** | 6.4 | 7.0 | AAA | 0.76 | 0.40 |
| | | | AAG | 0.24 | 0.60 |
| **Serine** | 6.3 | 8.1 | TCT | 0.19 | 0.18 |
| | | | TCC | 0.17 | 0.23 |
| | | | TCA | 0.12 | 0.15 |
| | | | TCG | 0.13 | 0.06 |
| | | | AGT | 0.13 | 0.14 |
| | | | AGC | 0.27 | 0.25 |
| **Isoleucine** | 6.1 | 2.9 | ATT | 0.47 | 0.35 |
| | | | ATC | 0.46 | 0.52 |
| | | | ATA | 0.07 | 0.14 |

*Amino acid and codon usage (continued)*

| | Amino acid usage[a] | | | Codon usage[b] | |
|---|---|---|---|---|---|
| **Amino acid** | **E. coli[c]** | **human[d]** | **Codon** | **E. coli[e]** | **human[e]** |
| **Threonine** | 5.8 | 5.6 | ACT | 0.21 | 0.23 |
| | | | ACC | 0.43 | 0.38 |
| | | | ACA | 0.12 | 0.27 |
| | | | ACG | 0.23 | 0.12 |
| **Glutamic acid** | 5.5 | 7.3 | GAA | 0.70 | 0.41 |
| | | | GAG | 0.30 | 0.59 |
| **Aspartic acid** | 5.2 | 4.9 | GAT | 0.59 | 0.44 |
| | | | GAC | 0.41 | 0.56 |
| **Glutamine** | 4.2 | 4.5 | CAA | 0.31 | 0.27 |
| | | | CAG | 0.69 | 0.73 |
| **Asparagine** | 3.5 | 3.5 | AAT | 0.39 | 0.44 |
| | | | AAC | 0.61 | 0.56 |
| **Proline** | 3.5 | 4.9 | CCT | 0.16 | 0.29 |
| | | | CCC | 0.10 | 0.33 |
| | | | CCA | 0.20 | 0.27 |
| | | | CCG | 0.55 | 0.11 |
| **Methionine** | 2.2 | 1.8 | ATG | 1.00 | 1.00 |
| **Phenylalanine** | 3.6 | 4.5 | TTT | 0.51 | 0.43 |
| | | | TTC | 0.49 | 0.57 |
| **Tyrosine** | 2.6 | 3.6 | TAT | 0.53 | 0.42 |
| | | | TAC | 0.47 | 0.58 |
| **Histidine** | 2.5 | 2.5 | CAT | 0.52 | 0.41 |
| | | | CAC | 0.48 | 0.59 |
| **Tryptophan** | 1.2 | 1.3 | TGG | 1.00 | 1.00 |
| **Cysteine** | 1.1 | 3.4 | TGT | 0.43 | 0.42 |
| | | | TGC | 0.57 | 0.58 |

Note: Extensive codon usage tables for a wide variety of organisms can be found at http://www.dna.affrc.go.jp/nakamura/codon. html/.

[a] Amino acid usage given in percentage of the total amino acid composition.
[b] Fractional use of each codon for a particular amino acid.
[c] Grantham et al. (1981).
[d] Lathe (1985).
[e] Data from Gilbert (1989).

*Log odds matrix for relationships between protein sequences ($MDM_{78}$)*

| | A | R | N | D | C | Q | E | G | H | I | L | K | M | F | P | S | T | W | Y | V |
|---|---|---|---|---|---|---|---|---|---|---|---|---|---|---|---|---|---|---|---|---|
| A | 18 | | | | | | | | | | | | | | | | | | | |
| R | −15 | 61 | | | | | | | | | | | | | | | | | | |
| N | 2 | 0 | 20 | | | | | | | | | | | | | | | | | |
| D | −4 | −13 | 21 | 39 | | | | | | | | | | | | | | | | |
| C | −2 | −36 | −36 | −51 | 119 | | | | | | | | | | | | | | | |
| Q | −4 | 13 | 8 | 16 | −54 | 40 | | | | | | | | | | | | | | |
| E | 3 | −11 | 14 | 34 | −53 | 25 | 38 | | | | | | | | | | | | | |
| G | 13 | −26 | 3 | 6 | −34 | −12 | 2 | 48 | | | | | | | | | | | | |
| H | −14 | 16 | 16 | 7 | −34 | 29 | 7 | −21 | 65 | | | | | | | | | | | |
| I | −5 | −20 | −18 | −24 | −23 | −20 | −20 | −26 | −24 | 45 | | | | | | | | | | |
| L | −19 | −30 | −29 | −40 | −60 | −18 | −34 | −41 | −21 | 24 | 59 | | | | | | | | | |
| K | −12 | 34 | 10 | 1 | −54 | 7 | −1 | −17 | 0 | −19 | −29 | 47 | | | | | | | | |
| M | −11 | −4 | −17 | −26 | −52 | −10 | −21 | −28 | 22 | 37 | 4 | 64 | | | | | | | | |
| F | −35 | −45 | −35 | −56 | −43 | −47 | −54 | −48 | −18 | 10 | 18 | −53 | 2 | 91 | | | | | | |
| P | 11 | −2 | −5 | −10 | −28 | 2 | −6 | −5 | −2 | −20 | −25 | −11 | −21 | −46 | 59 | | | | | |
| S | 11 | −3 | 7 | 3 | 0 | −5 | 0 | 11 | −8 | −14 | −28 | −2 | −16 | −32 | 9 | 16 | | | | |
| T | 12 | −9 | 4 | −1 | −22 | −8 | −4 | 0 | −13 | 1 | −17 | 0 | −6 | −31 | 3 | 13 | 26 | | | |
| W | −58 | 22 | −42 | −68 | −78 | −48 | −70 | −70 | −28 | −51 | −18 | −35 | −42 | 4 | −56 | −25 | −52 | 173 | | |
| Y | −35 | −42 | −21 | −43 | 3 | −40 | −43 | −52 | −1 | −9 | −9 | −44 | −24 | 70 | −49 | −28 | −27 | −2 | 101 | |
| V | 2 | −25 | −17 | −21 | −19 | −19 | −18 | −14 | −22 | 37 | 19 | −24 | 18 | −12 | −12 | −10 | 3 | −62 | −25 | 43 |

Dayhoff (1978). Evolutionary relationship of amino acids. See Dayhoff for description of the calculations.

*Accepted amino acid substitutions*

| Second amino acid | First amino acid: A | R | N | D | C | Q | E | G | H | I | L | K | M | F | P | S | T | W | Y | V |
|---|---|---|---|---|---|---|---|---|---|---|---|---|---|---|---|---|---|---|---|---|
| A | — | 2.7 | 4.8 | 7.4 | 12 | 6.2 | 13 | 32 | 2.3 | 4.5 | 6.7 | 3 | 5 | 2.9 | 29 | 22 | 25 | 0 | 3.9 | 18 |
| R | 0.82 | — | 0.75 | 0 | 3.6 | 8.1 | 0 | 0.55 | 11 | 2.0 | 1.2 | 25 | 2.9 | 1 | 5.6 | 3.9 | 0.84 | 34 | 0.58 | 1 |
| N | 3.0 | 1.5 | — | 26 | 0 | 3.4 | 4.4 | 8.6 | 24 | 2.4 | 2.6 | 17 | 0 | 1 | 2.3 | 12 | 7.1 | 3.8 | 7 | 0.65 |
| D | 4.2 | 0 | 23 | — | 0 | 5.1 | 39 | 8.9 | 4.6 | 0.88 | 0 | 4.5 | 0 | 0 | 0.84 | 2.8 | 2.4 | 0 | 0 | 0.85 |
| C | 0.91 | 0.9 | 0 | 0 | — | 0 | 0 | 0.55 | 1.1 | 1.1 | 0 | 0 | 0 | 0 | 0.84 | 3.3 | 4.2 | 0 | 5.8 | 2.5 |
| Q | 2.6 | 11 | 2.2 | 3.7 | 0 | — | 20 | 1.7 | 26 | 0.54 | 5.2 | 7.8 | 3.4 | 0 | 7.8 | 1.3 | 1.6 | 0 | 0 | 1.3 |
| E | 7.3 | 0 | 4.1 | 40 | 0 | 28 | — | 6.2 | 2.5 | 2.4 | 1.1 | 5.5 | 1.2 | 0 | 3.4 | 2.5 | 1.3 | 0 | 1.9 | 1.8 |
| G | 16 | 0.9 | 6.9 | 7.8 | 3.6 | 2.0 | 5.3 | — | 1.1 | 0 | 1.2 | 3.2 | 1.2 | 2.5 | 4.1 | 13 | 2.1 | 0 | 0 | 4.8 |
| H | 0.58 | 9.3 | 10 | 2.1 | 3.6 | 1.6 | 1.1 | 0.55 | — | 0.2 | 2.8 | 1.2 | 0 | 2.9 | 4.2 | 0.7 | 0.59 | 3.8 | 7.8 | 1.5 |
| I | 1.8 | 2.7 | 1.6 | 0.63 | 6.1 | 0.54 | 1.7 | 0 | 3.2 | — | 18 | 2.3 | 9.8 | 13 | 0.59 | 0.57 | 5.4 | 0 | 2.5 | 33 |
| L | 2.6 | 1.5 | 1.6 | 0 | 0 | 5.0 | 0.7 | 0.94 | 4.3 | 17 | — | 2.1 | 36 | 24 | 3.6 | 0.9 | 2.2 | 16 | 4.5 | 15 |
| K | 1.6 | 43 | 14 | 4.1 | 0 | 9.9 | 4.9 | 3.3 | 2.4 | 20 | 2.7 | — | 16 | 0 | 3.6 | 4.8 | 8.4 | 0 | 1.9 | 0.85 |
| M | 0.80 | 1.5 | 0 | 0 | 0 | 1.3 | 0.33 | 3.9 | 0 | 3.8 | 14 | 4.8 | — | 2.5 | 0.34 | 0.57 | 1.2 | 0 | 0 | 3.8 |
| F | 0.55 | 0.63 | 0.31 | 0 | 0 | 0 | 0 | 0.94 | 2.2 | 6.1 | 12 | 0 | 2.9 | — | 0.59 | 1.1 | 0.42 | 13 | 51 | 0.5 |
| P | 9.5 | 6.0 | 1.2 | 0.48 | 3.6 | 6.2 | 1.9 | 2.7 | 5.4 | 0.49 | 3 | 2.3 | 0.69 | 1 | — | 7.7 | 3.1 | 0 | 0 | 2.5 |
| S | 21 | 12.3 | 19 | 4.7 | 42 | 3.1 | 4.1 | 25 | 2.8 | 1.4 | 2.2 | 8.9 | 3.4 | 5.9 | 23 | — | 29 | 22 | 4.3 | 2.1 |
| T | 16 | 1.8 | 7.5 | 2.7 | 3.6 | 2.5 | 1.7 | 2.8 | 1.5 | 8.7 | 3.6 | 11 | 8.3 | 1.5 | 6.1 | 20 | — | 0 | 4.5 | 9.3 |
| W | 0 | 2.4 | 0.13 | 0 | 0 | 0 | 0 | 0 | 0.32 | 0 | 0.91 | 0 | 0 | 1.5 | 0 | 0.49 | 0 | — | 1.2 | 0 |
| Y | 0.55 | 0.26 | 1.6 | 0 | 11 | 0 | 0.47 | 0 | 4.3 | 0.88 | 1.6 | 0.53 | 0 | 38 | 0 | 0.63 | 0.97 | 7.6 | — | 0.85 |
| V | 10 | 1.8 | 0.57 | 0.82 | 12 | 1.8 | 1.8 | 5.3 | 3.2 | 45 | 21 | 0.9 | 13 | 1.5 | 4.2 | 1.2 | 7.8 | 0 | 3.3 | — |
|  | 364[a] | 111 | 227 | 208 | 28 | 149 | 211 | 182 | 93 | 148 | 142 | 188 | 58 | 68 | 119 | 349 | 238 | 8 | 51 | 200 |

Calculated from Dayhoff (1978). Related proteins derived from 34 superfamilies and grouped into 71 evolutionary trees were compared for accepted mutations at a single site. A total of 1572 changes were used to assemble the database. The frequency for an amino acid to change to another amino acid is given as a percentage of the total changes detected for that amino acid. Also listed are the total changes used to determine the percentage.

[a] Total number of amino acids tested.

*David's life chart II*

| Molecular weight (daltons) | 1 μg | 1 nmole |
|---|---|---|
| 100 | 10 nmoles or $6 \times 10^{15}$ molecules | 0.1 μg |
| 1,000 | 1 nmole or $6 \times 10^{14}$ molecules | 1 μg |
| 10,000 | 100 pmoles or $6 \times 10^{13}$ molecules | 10 μg |
| 20,000 | 50 pmoles or $3 \times 10^{13}$ molecules | 20 μg |
| 30,000 | 33 pmoles or $2 \times 10^{13}$ molecules | 30 μg |
| 40,000 | 25 pmoles or $1.5 \times 10^{13}$ molecules | 40 μg |
| 50,000 | 20 pmoles or $1.2 \times 10^{13}$ molecules | 50 μg |
| 60,000 | 17 pmoles or $10^{13}$ molecules | 60 μg |
| 70,000 | 14 pmoles or $8.6 \times 10^{12}$ molecules | 70 μg |
| 80,000 | 12 pmoles or $7.5 \times 10^{12}$ molecules | 80 μg |
| 90,000 | 11 pmoles or $6.6 \times 10^{12}$ molecules | 90 μg |
| 100,000 | 10 pmoles or $6 \times 10^{12}$ molecules | 100 μg |
| 120,000 | 8.3 pmoles or $5 \times 10^{12}$ molecules | 120 μg |
| 140,000 | 7.1 pmoles or $4.3 \times 10^{12}$ molecules | 140 μg |
| 160,000 | 6.3 pmoles or $3.8 \times 10^{12}$ molecules | 160 μg |
| 180,000 | 5.6 pmoles or $3.3 \times 10^{12}$ molecules | 180 μg |
| 200,000 | 5 pmoles or $3 \times 10^{12}$ molecules | 200 μg |

## David's life chart III

### Some useful nucleotide dimensions

1 cm of DNA ≈ $3 \times 10^6$ nucleotides

| Organism | Base pairs/ haploid genome | Base pairs/ diploid genome | Length/cell | Mass |
|---|---|---|---|---|
| Human | $3 \times 10^9$ | $6 \times 10^9$ | 2 meters (diploid) | 6 pg |
| Fly | $1.65 \times 10^8$ | $3.3 \times 10^8$ | 100 cm (dipolid) | 0.3 pg |
| Yeast | $1.35 \times 10^7$ | $2.7 \times 10^7$ | 10 cm (diploid) | 0.03 pg |
| *E. coli* | $4.7 \times 10^6$ | — | 1.5 cm (haploid) | 0.0045 pg |
| SV40 | $5 \times 10^3$ | — | 1.7 nm | 0.000006 pg |

### Some useful cell dimensions

| Organism | Dimensions | Volume |
|---|---|---|
| *S. cerevisiae* | 5 μm | 66 $\mu m^3$ |
| *S. pombe* | 2 × 7 μm | 22 $\mu m^3$ |
| Mammalian cell | 10–20 μm | 500–4,000 $\mu m^3$ |
| *E. coli* | 1 × 3 μm | 2 $\mu m^3$ |
| Mammalian mitochondrion | 1 μm | 0.5 $\mu m^3$ |
| Mammalian nucleus | 5–10 μm | 66–500 $\mu m^3$ |
| Plant chloroplast | 1 × 4 μm | 3 $\mu m^3$ |
| Bacteriophage lambda | 50 nm (head only) | $6.6 \times 10^{-5}$ $\mu m^3$ |
| Ribosome | 30 nm diameter | $1.4 \times 10^{-5}$ $\mu m^3$ |
| Globular monomeric protein | 5 nm diameter | $6.6 \times 10^{-8}$ $\mu m^3$ |

### Some useful concentrations

| | |
|---|---|
| **Total cell protein concentration** | Detergent soluble protein = 1–2 mg/$10^7$ mammalian cells or 100–200 mg/ml for soluble proteins only |
| **Specific protein concentrations** | |
| **Nucleus (200 $\mu m^3$):** | |
| Abundant transcription factor | **1** nM (100,000 copies/nucleus) |
| Rare transcription factor | **10** pM (1,000 copies/nucleus) |
| **Serum** | 50–100 mg/ml |

## Protein quantitation—Bradford*

This assay is relatively accurate for most proteins, except for small basic polypeptides such as ribonuclease or lysozyme. It is also hampered by detergent concentrations over about 0.2% (e.g., Triton X-100, SDS, NP-40). (See also Spector et al. 1998, Table 56.1.)

### Caution

Ethanol, sodium dodecyl sulfate, see Appendix IV.

1. Prior to the assay, prepare the Bradford dye concentrate. Dissolve 100 mg of Coomassie Brilliant Blue G-250 in 50 ml of 95% ethanol. Add 100 ml of concentrated phosphoric acid. Add distilled water to a final volume of 200 ml. The dye is stable at 4°C for at least 6 months. This dye concentrate is also available commercially from Bio-Rad.

2. Prepare a series of protein samples for a standard curve. Use a protein as similar in its properties to your sample as possible (i.e., if doing antibody concentrations, use purified antibody). If your sample is unknown, use antibody. The standard curve will be linear between about 20 and 150 μg in 100 μl.

3. Prepare your test samples in 100 μl of the same buffer used for the standard curve (PBS is fine).

4. Dilute the concentrated dye binding solution 1 in 5 with distilled water. Filter if any precipitate develops.

5. Add 5 ml of diluted dye-binding solution to each sample. Allow the color to develop for at least 5 minutes but not longer than 30 minutes. The red dye will turn blue as it binds protein. Read the absorbance at 595 nm.

6. Calculate the concentration of the unknown sample by comparing with the standard curve.

### Note

BSA gives a value about twofold higher than its weight for Bradford dye-binding assays.

*Bradford (1976).

## Protein quantitation—Bradford spot test*

This assay is particularly useful for testing column fractions to locate the protein eluate (e.g., testing affinity column eluates).

### Caution

Ethanol, see Appendix IV.

1. Prior to the assay, prepare the Bradford dye concentrate. Dissolve 100 mg of Coomassie Brilliant Blue G-250 in 50 ml of 95% ethanol. Add 100 ml of concentrated phosphoric acid. Add distilled water to a final volume of 200 ml. The dye is stable at 4°C for at least 6 months. The dye concentrate is available commercially from Bio-Rad.

2. Remove 8 µl of each protein sample to be tested and transfer to a strip of Parafilm, Saran Wrap, or well of micro well tray. Be sure to include a sample of the elution buffer to give you a background reading.

3. Add 2 µl of concentrated Bradford dye solution to each sample. Mix by pipetting.

4. The samples that contain protein will turn blue within approximately 2 minutes. The sensitivity of this assay is about 10 µg/ml. The reaction is very sensitive to the presence of detergents at concentration over about 0.2%, but is not affected by potassium chloride, sodium chloride, magnesium chloride, or EDTA, and only slightly by Tris.

*Adapted from Bradford (1976).

## Protein quantitation—Coomassie spot test*

This assay is particularly useful for testing column fractions to locate the protein eluate (e.g., testing affinity column eluates).

### Caution

Acetic acid, methanol, see Appendix IV.

1. Rule Whatman 3MM paper or equivalent into 4-mm squares.
2. Spot 5 μl of sample on a square.
3. Dry the samples under a constant air flow. A hair dryer will dry the spots in approximately 1 minute or less.
4. Dip the paper in 0.25% Coomassie Brilliant Blue in 10% methanol, 7% acetic acid for 30 seconds.
5. Wash the paper 3–5 minutes in 10% methanol, 7% acetic acid. Dry.

*C. Anderson (pers. comm.).

## Protein quantitation—UV detection*

Absorbance of UV irradiation by proteins is the quickest of all methods for quantitating protein solutions. Readings are most often performed at 280 nm. The absorbance maximum at 280 nm is due primarily to the presence of tyrosine and tryptophan. Absorbance at 205 nm is also used. Absorbance at 205 nm is due primarily to the peptide bond, although other amino acids also contribute. In addition to the speed with which absorbance readings can be made, one major advantage of UV quantitation is that none of the sample is destroyed in determining the concentration.

### *Pure protein solutions*

1. Read the absorbance versus a suitable control at 280 nm.

2. For antibodies and BSA, use the table to calculate the concentration. A very rough approximation for other proteins is 1 absorbance unit is equal to 1 mg/ml.

| Protein | $A_{280}$ (for 1 mg/ml) |
|---|---|
| IgG | 1.35 |
| IgM | 1.2 |
| BSA | 0.7 |

### *Protein solutions contaminated with nucleic acids*

1. Read the absorbance versus a suitable control at 280 nm and 260 nm or 280 nm and 205 nm.

2. Calculate the approximate concentration using one of the equations below:
Protein concentration (in mg/ml) $= (1.55 \times A_{280}) - (0.76 \times A_{260})$
Protein concentration (in mg/ml) $= A_{205}/(27 + 120\ A_{280}/A_{205})$

*Layne (1957) and Peterson (1983).

## Protein quantitation—Bicinchoninic acid*

### Caution

Bicinchoninic acid, see Appendix IV.

1. The two reagents needed for the bicinchoninic acid assays are available from Pierce Chemical. Mix 50 volumes of reagent A to 1 volume of reagent B.

2. Adjust the protein samples to 100 μl. Prepare standard of BSA at 100, 50, 25, and 12.5 μg/100 μl.

3. Add 2 ml of the combined reagent to each sample. Incubate at room temperature for 2 hours or 37°C for 30 minutes.

4. Read the samples versus an appropriate blank at 562 nm.

*Smith et al. (1985).

## Protein quantitation—Lowry*

### Caution

Phenol, SDS, sodium hydroxide, see Appendix IV.

1. Prior to the assay dissolve 20 g of sodium carbonate in 500 ml of distilled water. Dissolve 1 g of $CuSO_4 \cdot 5H_2O$ and 2 g of sodium tartrate in 500 ml of distilled water. Place the copper/tartrate solution on a magnetic stirrer and slowly add the carbonate. Store with refrigeration. This solution is stable for over 1 year.

2. The Folin–Ciocalteu phenol reagent can be prepared in the laboratory, but it can be purchased economically from numerous suppliers.

3. Combine 1 volume of the copper/tartrate/carbonate solution to 2 volumes of 5% SDS and 1 volume of 0.8 M sodium hydroxide. Stable at room temperature for 2 weeks. Label as Reagent A.

4. Combine 1 volume of the 2 N Folin–Ciocalteu phenol reagent with 5 volumes of distilled water. Store in an amber bottle at room temperature. Stable for months. Label as Reagent B.

5. Samples (of 5–100 µg) should be adjusted to 1 ml by adding water. Prepare standards of BSA containing 100, 50, 25, and 12.5 µg/ml.

6. Add 1.0 ml of Reagent A to each protein sample. Mix and incubate for 10 minutes at room temperature.

7. Add 0.5 ml of Reagent B and mix immediately. Incubate at room temperature for 30 minutes.

8. Read the absorbance at 750 nm. Prepare a standard curve and compute the protein concentration.

*Lowry et al. (1951); Peterson (1983).

*Proteases*

| Protease | Class | Cleavage site | Known inhibitors |
|---|---|---|---|
| **Aminopeptidase M** | Metalloprotease | Amino-terminal L-amino acids with free amino groups. Not X-Pro, not D or Q | 2,2′ Bipyridine, 1,10-phenanthroline |
| **Bromelain** | Thiolprotease | No specificity | $\alpha_2$-Macroglobulin, TPCK, TLCK, alkylation |
| **Carboxypeptidase A** | Zinc metalloprotease | Carboxy-terminal L-amino acids with free amino groups. Not R, P, or hydroxyproline. | EDTA, EGTA |
| **Carboxypeptidase B** | Zinc metalloprotease | Carboxy-terminal K, R | EDTA, EGTA, basic amino acids |
| **Carboxypeptidase Y** | Serine carboxypeptidase | Carboxy-terminal amino acids | PMSF |
| **Cathepsin C** | Thiolprotease | Amino-terminal dipeptides, blocked by amino-terminal K or R, or P as 2nd or 3rd amino acid | Iodoacetate, formaldehyde |
| **Chymotrypsin** | Serine protease | After F, T, or Y | Aprotinin, PMSF, TPCK, $\alpha_2$-macroglobulin |
| **Collagenase** | Metalloprotease | After X in P-X-G-P | EDTA, EGTA, reducing agents, but not serum. |
| **Dispase** | Metalloprotease | No specificity | EDTA, EGTA, $Hg^{++}$, and heavy metals |
| **Endoproteinase Arg-C** | Serine protease | After R | $\alpha_2$-Macroglobulin, TLCK |
| **Endoproteinase Asp-N** | Metalloprotease | Before D and cysteic acid | EDTA, $\alpha$-phenanthroline |
| **Endoproteinase Glu-C (*S. aureus* V8)** | Serine protease | After E, or after D or E | $\alpha_2$-Macroglobulin, TLCK |
| **Endoproteinase Lys-C** | Serine protease | After K | TLCK, aprotinin, leupeptin |
| **Enterokinase** | Serine protease | After K in D-D-D-D-K- (used to remove FLAG tag) | |
| **Factor Xa** | Serine protease | After R | PMSF, APMSF, soybean trypsin inhibitor |
| **Ficin** | Thiolprotease | No specificity | TPCK, TLCK, $\alpha_2$-macroglobulin |
| **Kallikrein** | Serine protease | After some R | Leupeptin, aprotinin |
| **Papain** | Thiolprotease | On long incubation, broad specificity | TPCK, TLCK, leupeptin, $\alpha_2$-macroglobulin, alkylating agents |
| **Pepsin** | Acid protease | Broad specificity | Pepstatin |
| **Plasmin** | Serine protease | After K or R | PMSF, TLCK, aprotinin, $\alpha_2$-macroglobulin |
| **Pronase** | Mixture | No specificity | B.M. Complete Tablets |
| **Proteinase K** | Serine protease | Broad specificity | PMSF, Pefabloc SC |
| **Subtilisin** | Serine protease | Broad specificity | PMSF, $\alpha_2$-macroglobulin, benzamidine |
| **Thermolysin** | Zinc-metalloprotease | Before nonpolar residues | EDTA |
| **Thrombin** | Serine protease | After R | TLCK, PMSF, leupeptin, aprotinin, $\alpha_2$-macroglobulin, benzamidine |
| **Trypsin** | Serine protease | After K or R | TLCK, PMSF, leupeptin, aprotinin, $\alpha_2$-macroglobulin |

Most of the information in this table is derived from Boehringer Mannheim (1998) and Calbiochem (1996/1997).

*Protease inhibitors*

| Inhibitor | Protease target | Effective concentrations | Stock solution | Comments |
|---|---|---|---|---|
| **Antipain** | Papain and trypsin | 50 μg/ml | 1 mg/ml in $H_2O$ | Chymotrypsin, pepsin, plasmin unaffected |
| APMSF | Trypsin-like serine proteases | 10–40 μg/ml, or 10–20 μM | 100 mM in $H_2O$ | Less toxic than PMSF. Doesn't inhibit chymotrypsin or acetylcholinesterases |
| Aprotinin | Serine proteases | 0.06–2 μg/ml | 10 mg/ml in PBS | Avoid repeated freezing |
| Bestatin | Aminopeptidases | 40 μg/ml | Make in methanol[a] | Doesn't inhibit carboxypeptidases |
| Calpain inhibitors I and II | Calpain (calcium-dependent cysteine proteases) | I: 17 μg/ml<br>II: 7 μg/ml | Make in ethanol[a] | Membrane permeable |
| Chymostatin | Chymotrypsin | 6–60 μg/ml | Make in DMSO[a] | |
| Complete Tablets (Boehringer Mannheim) | Serine, cysteine, and metalloproteases | 1 tablet per 10–50 ml cell extract | | Contain no EDTA |
| EDTA | Metalloproteases | 0.2–0.5 mg/ml or 0.5–1.3 μM | 500 mM in $H_2O$, pH 8.0 | |
| Leupeptin | Serine and thiolproteases | 0.5–2 μg/ml | 10 mg/ml in $H_2O$ | |
| $\alpha_2$-Macroglobulin | Broad spectrum | 1 unit/ml | 100 units/ml in PBS | Avoid reducing agents |
| Pefabloc SC (Boehringer Mannheim) | Serine proteases | 0.1–1.0 mg/ml or 0.4–4 mM | 100 mM in $H_2O$ | Nontoxic, more stable at neutral pH than PMSF |
| Pepstatin | Acid proteases | 0.7 μg/ml | 1 mg/ml in methanol | |
| PMSF | Serine proteases | 17–170 μg/ml | 10 mg/ml in isopropanol | Add fresh at each step |
| TLCK | Trypsin | 37–50 μg/ml | 1 mg/ml in 50 mM acetate, pH 5.0 | Chymotrypsin unaffected |
| TPCK | Chymotrypsin | 70–100 μg/ml | 3 mg/ml in ethanol | Trypsin unaffected |

Most of the information in this table is derived from Boehringer Mannheim (1998) and Calbiochem (1996/1997)

[a] DMSO, ethanol, methanol, see Appendix IV for caution.

## Preparing dialysis tubing

Some tubing does not require this preparation. Check with the manufacturer's instructions to make this determination.

1. Cut the dialysis tubing to appropriate lengths. For most work, lengths of 10, 20, and 30 cm are useful.

2. Place the tubing in a large volume of 5 mM EDTA, 200 mM sodium bicarbonate.

3. Boil for 5 minutes. Pour off the EDTA/bicarbonate wash. Rinse briefly with deionized water. Add a large volume of 5 mM EDTA, 200 mM sodium bicarbonate and boil for 5 minutes. Make sure the tubing remains submerged during this step.

4. Discard the second wash. Rinse the tubing thoroughly with deionized water. Add a large volume of deionized water and cover (aluminum foil is fine).

5. Autoclave for 10 minutes on liquid cycle. Store at 4°C. For most purposes, the addition of 0.02% sodium azide will not interfere with the dialysis, and this will eliminate the chances of microbial growth.

   To use, wear gloves and remove an appropriate length of tubing. Wash the tubing extensively, both inside and out, in a stream of deionized or distilled water.

## TCA precipitation—Filtration

### Caution

Ethanol, radioactive substances, trichloroacetic acid, see Appendix IV.

1. To measure the amount of incorporation of a radiolabeled precursor into protein, transfer a standard volume of each sample (normally 5 µl) to 100 µl of 1 mg/ml of BSA in a 1.5-ml conical tube.

2. Add 1 ml of ice-cold 10% trichloroacetic acid (TCA) to each tube. Mix.

3. Incubate on ice for 30 minutes.

4. Place glass fiber filters into a suitable filtration device. Apply a gentle vacuum and prewet by passing a few milliliters of 10% TCA through the filter.

5. Add the sample dropwise to the filter using the center of the filter as a target for adding the drops. The precipitated proteins will be trapped by the filter, but the unincorporated precursors will pass through.

6. Wash the filter twice with 10% TCA using a few milliliters for each wash.

7. Wash the filter twice with 95% ethanol using a few milliliters for each wash.

8. Remove the filters and allow to dry. Placing the filters on a sheet of aluminum foil under an infrared light will speed drying.

   Add the dry filters to counting vials, add scintillant, and count.

## Note

i. Adding a nonradioactive form of the labeled molecule to the TCA solution will lower the background. For example, add cold methionine to TCA to lower background of [$^{35}$S]methionine.

## TCA precipitation—Spotting

### Caution

Ethanol, radioactive substances, trichloroacetic acid, see Appendix IV.

1. To measure the amount of incorporation of a radiolabeled precursor into protein, mix a standard volume of each sample (normally 5 μl) with 5 μl of 10 mg/ml BSA.

2. Apply the mixed sample to the center of a dry glass fiber filter. Place the filters in a shallow tray or petri dish. Filters should be marked prior to use.

3. Carefully flood the disk with ice-cold 10% trichloroacetic acid (TCA).

4. Incubate on ice or at 4°C for 30 minutes.

5. Drain the TCA from the dish and add fresh 10% TCA. Incubate for 5 minutes with shaking at room temperature. Drain the TCA and repeat twice.

6. Drain the TCA and add 95% ethanol. Incubate for 5 minutes with shaking at room temperature.

7. Remove the filters and allow to dry. Placing the filters on a sheet of aluminum foil under an infrared light will speed drying.

   Add the dry filters to counting vials, add scintillant, and count.

## Note

i. Adding a nonradioactive form of the labeled molecule to the TCA solution will lower the background. For example, add cold methionine to TCA to lower background of [$^{35}$S]methionine.

*Chromogenic substrates yielding water-soluble products*

| Enzyme | Substrate | Abbreviation | Starting color | Final color | Absorbance peak (in nm) |
|---|---|---|---|---|---|
| **Horseradish peroxidase** | 2,2′-Azinodi[ethylbenzthiazoline] sulfonate[a] | ABTS | Clear | Green | 410<br>650 |
| | *o*-Phenylenediamine[b] | OPD | Clear | Brown | 492 |
| | 3,3′,5,5′-Tetramethylbenzidine[c] | TMB | Clear | Yellow | 450 |
| **Alkaline phosphatase** | *p*-Nitrophenol phosphate[d] | PNPP | Clear | Yellow | 405 |
| **β-Galactosidase** | *o*-Nitrophenyl-β-*d*-galactopyranoside[e] | ONPG | Clear | Yellow | 410 |

[a] Porstmann et al. (1981).
[b] Voller et al. (1979).
[c] Holland et al. (1974); Hardy and Heimer (1977).
[d] Snyder et al. (1972).
[e] Craven et al. (1965).

*Chromogenic substrates yielding water-insoluble product*

| Enzyme | Substrate | Abbreviation | Starting color | Final color | Soluble in alcohol? |
|---|---|---|---|---|---|
| **Horseradish peroxidase** | Diaminobenzidene[a,b] | DAB | Clear | Brown | No |
| | Diaminobenzidene with nickel enhancement[c] | DAB/nickel | Clear | Gray/black | No |
| | 3-Amino-9-ethylcarbazole[d] | AEC | Clear | Red | Yes |
| | 4-Chloro-1-naphthol[a,e] | — | Clear | Blue | Yes |
| **Alkaline phosphatase** | Naphthol-AS-B1-phosphate/fast red TR[f] | NABP/FR | Clear | Red | Yes |
| | Naphthol-AS-MX-phosphate/fast red TRg | NAMP/FR | Clear | Red | No |
| | Naphthol-AS-BI-phosphate/new fuchsin[h] | NABP/NF | Clear | Red | No |
| | Bromochloroindolyl phosphate/ nitroblue tetrazolium[i] | BCIP/NBT | Clear | Purple | — |
| **β-Galactosidase** | 5-Bromo-4-chloro-3-indolyl-β-*d*-galactopyranoside[j] | BCIG | Clear | Blue | No |
| | Naphthol AS-BI-β-*d*-galactopyranoside[k] | NABG | Clear | Red | No |

[a] See Appendix IV for caution.
[b] Graham and Karnovsky (1966).
[c] Hsu and Soban (1982).
[d] Graham et al. (1965).
[e] Nakane (1968).
[f] Pearse (1968); Ponder and Wilkinson (1981).
[g] Amersham handbook.
[h] Stutte (1967); Malik and Daymon (1982).
[i] McGadey (1970); Leary et al. (1983).
[j] Bondi et al. (1982).
[k] Gossrau (1973).

# Substrates for chemiluminescence detection

##  Caution

DMSO, hydrogen peroxide, see Appendix IV.

### Stock solutions

| | |
|---|---|
| 30% $H_2O_2$ | (store at 4°C) |
| 250 mM Luminol in DMSO | (store at room temperature wrapped in foil) |
| 90 mM *p*-Coumaric acid in DMSO | (store at room temperature wrapped in foil) |
| 100 mM Tris-HCl (pH 8.5) | |

### Working solution*

To make up 12 ml of working solution (enough for a large blot)

| | |
|---|---|
| 12 ml | Tris-HCl (pH 8.5) |
| 3.8 µl | 30% $H_2O_2$ |
| 60 µl | 250 mM luminol |
| 26.6 µl | 90 mM *p*-coumaric acid |

*Always make up fresh just before you wish to develop the blot.

Incubate on the blot for 1 minute, then expose the blot to film.

## References


Bondi A., Chieregatti G., Eusebi V., Fulcheri E., and Bussolati G. 1982. The use of β-galactosidase as a tracer in immunocytochemistry. *Histochemistry* **76:** 153–158.

Bradford M.M. 1976. A rapid and sensitive method for the quantitation of microgram quantities of protein utilizing the principle of protein-dye binding. *Anal. Biochem.* **72:** 248–254.

Craven G.R., Steers E., Jr., and Anfinsen C.B. 1965. Purification, composition, and molecular weight of the β-galactosidase of *Escherichia coli* K12. *J. Biol. Chem.* **240:** 2468–2477.

Dayhoff M.O. 1978. *Atlas of protein sequence and structure*, vol. 5 (suppl. 3). National Biomedical Research Foundation, Washington, D.C.

Gilbert D.G. 1989. IUBio archive of molecular and general biology software and data. An Internet resource available at ftp,gopher,http://iubio.bio.indiana.edu.

Gossrau R. 1973. Splitting of naphthol AS-BI β-galactopyranoside by acid β-galactosidase. *Histochemie* **37:** 89–91.

Graham R.C., Jr. and Karnovsky M.J. 1966. The early stages of absorption of injected horseradish peroxidase in the proximal tubules of mouse kidney ultrastructural cytochemistry by a new technology. *J. Histochem. Cytochem.* **14:** 291–302.

Graham R.C., Jr., Lundholm U., and Karnovsky M.J. 1965. Cytochemical demonstration of peroxidase activity with 3-amino-9-ethylcarbazole. *J. Histochem. Cytochem.* **13:** 150–152.

Grantham R., Gautier C., Gouy M., Jacobzone M., and Mercier R. 1981. Codon catalog usage is a genome strategy modulated for gene expressivity. *Nucleic Acids Res.* **9:** R43–R74.

Hardy H. and Heimer L. 1977. A safer and more sensitive substitute for diamino-benzidine in the light microscopic demonstration of retrograde and anterograde axonal transport of HRP. *Neurosci. Lett.* **5:** 235–240.

Holland V.R., Saunders B.C., Rose F.L., and Walpole A.L. 1974. Safer substitute for benzidine in detection of blood. *Tetrahedron* **30:** 3299.

Hopp T.P. and Woods K.R. 1981. Prediction of protein antigenic determinants from amino acid sequences. *Proc. Natl. Acad. Sci.* **78:** 3824–3828.

Hsu S.-M. and Soban E. 1982. Color modification of diaminobenzidine (DAB) precipitation by metallic ions and its application for double immunohistochemistry. *J. Histochem. Cytochem.* **30:** 1079–1082.

Kyte J. and Doolittle R.F. 1982. A simple method for displaying the hydropathic character of a protein. *J. Mol. Biol.* **157:** 105–132.

Lathe R. 1985. Synthetic oligonucleotide probes deduced from amino acid sequence data. Theoretical and practical considerations. *J. Mol. Biol.* **183:** 1–12.

Layne E. 1957. Spectrophotometric and turbidimetric methods for measuring proteins. *Methods Enzymol.* **3:** 447–454.

Leary J.J., Brigati D.J., and Ward D.C. 1983. Rapid and sensitive colorimetric method for visualizing biotin-labeled DNA probes hybridized to DNA or RNA immobilized on nitrocellulose: Bio-blots. *Proc. Natl. Acad. Sci.* **80:** 4045–4049.

Lowry O.H., Rosebrough N.J., Farr A.L., and Randall R.J. 1951. Protein measurement with the Folin phenol reagent. *J. Biol. Chem.* **193:** 265–275.

Malik N.J. and Daymon M.E. 1982. Improved double immunoenzyme labeling using alkaline phosphatase and horseradish peroxidase. *J. Clin. Pathol.* **35:** 1092–1094.

McGadey J. 1970. A tetrazolium method for nonspecific alkaline phosphatase. *Histochemie* **23:** 180–184.

Nakane P.K. 1968. Simultaneous localization of multiple tissue antigens using the peroxidase-labeled antibody method: A study of pituitary glands of the rat. *J. Histochem. Cytochem.* **16:** 557–560.

Pearse A.G.E. 1968. Alkaline phosphatases. In *Histochemistry: Theoretical and applied*, 3rd edition, vol. 1, pp. 517–521. Churchill Livingstone, Edinburgh, United Kingdom.

Peterson G.L. 1983. Determination of total protein. *Methods Enzymol.* **91:** 95–119.

Ponder B.A. and Wilkinson M.M. 1981. Inhibition of endogenous tissue alkaline phosphatase with the use of alkaline phosphatase conjugates in immunohistochemistry. *J. Histochem. Cytochem.* **29:** 981–984.

Porstmann B., Porstmann T., and Nugel E. 1981. Comparison of chromogens for the determination of horseradish peroxidase as a marker for enzyme immunoassay. *J. Clin. Chem. Clin. Biochem.* **19:** 435–439.

Smith P.K., Krohn R.I., Hermanson G.T., Mallia A.K., Gartner F.H., Provenzano M.D., Fujimoto E.K., Goeke N.M., Olson B.J., and Klenk D.C. 1985. Measurement of protein using bicinchoninic acid. *Anal. Biochem.* **150:** 76–85.

Snyder S.L., Wilson I., and Bauer W. 1972. The subunit composition of *Escherichia coli* alkaline phosphatase in 1 M tris. *Biochim. Biophys. Acta* **258:** 178–187.

Spector D.L., Goldman R.D., and Leinwand L.A. 1998. *Cells: A laboratory manual*, vols. 1–3. Cold Spring Harbor Laboratory Press, Cold Spring Harbor, New York.

Stutte H.J. 1967. Hexazotiertes triamino-tritolylmethanchlorid (Neufuchsin) als Kupplungssalz in der fermenthistochemie. *Histochemie* **8:** 327–331.

Voller A., Bidwell D.E., and Bartlett A. 1979. *The enzyme linked immunosorbent assay (ELISA): A guide with abstracts of microplate applications.* Dynatech Laboratories, Alexandria, Virginia.

# Appendix III
# General Information

*Commonly used buffers*

| Buffer | Synonyms | pK | Molecular weight |
|---|---|---|---|
| **Phosphate ($pK_1$)** | | 2.12 | 98.0, free acid |
| **Glycine-HCl**[a] | | 2.34 | 111.53 |
| **Citrate ($pK_1$)** | | 3.14 | 192.1, free acid |
| **Formate** | | 3.75 | 68.0, Na salt |
| **Carbonate ($pK_1$)** | | 3.76 | 106.0 |
| **Succinate ($pK_1$)** | | 4.19 | 118.1, free acid |
| **Acetate** | | 4.75 | 82.0, Na salt |
| **Citrate ($pK_2$)** | | 4.76 | 214.1, Na salt |
| **Succinate ($pK_2$)** | | 5.57 | 162.1, diNa salt |
| **MES** | | 6.15 | 195.2, hydrate |
| **Carbonate ($pK_2$)** | Bicarbonate | 6.36 | 84.0, bicarbonate |
| **Citrate ($pK_3$)** | | 6.39 | 294.1, triNa salt, dihydrate |
| **PIPES** | | 6.8 | 302.4 |
| **ACES** | | 6.9 | 182.2 |
| **MOPS**[a] | | 7.2 | 209.7 |
| **HEPES** | | 7.55 | 238.3 |
| **Phosphate ($PK_2$)** | | 7.21 | 120.0, Na salt, monobasic |
| **TES** | | 7.7 | 229.2 |
| **Barbital** | Barbitone Veronal | 7.78 | 128.1, barbituric acid |
| **Triethanolamine**[a] | | 7.8 | 149.2 |
| **TRICINE** | | 8.15 | 179.2 |
| **TRIS** | | 8.3 | 121.1 |
| **BICINE** | | 8.35 | 163.2 |
| **Glycylglycine** | | 8.4 | 132.1 |
| **Borate** | | 9.24 | 201.2, Na tetraborate |
| **CHES** | | 9.5 | 207.3 |
| **Ethanolamine**[a] | | 9.5 | 61.1 |
| **Glycine-NaOH**[a] | | 9.6 | 97.1, Na salt hydrate |
| **CAPS** | | 10.4 | 221.3 |
| **Triethylamine**[a] | | 10.7 | 101.2 |
| **Phosphate ($pK_3$)** | | 12.3 | 141.9, Na salt, dibasic |

[a] See Appendix IV for caution.

*Concentrations of commercial liquids*

| Compound | Molecula weight | Molarity | pH of dilute solutions | | |
|---|---|---|---|---|---|
| | | | 1 M | 0.1 M | 0.01 M |
| **Acetic acid, glacial**[a] | 60.05 | 17.4 | 2.4 | 2.9 | 3.4 |
| **Formic acid**[a] | 46.02 | 23.4 | | | |
| **Hydrochloric acid,**[a] **38%** | 36.47 | 11.6 | 0.1 | 1.1 | 2.02 |
| **Nitric acid,**[a] **70%** | 63.02 | 16 | | | |
| **Phosphoric acid** | 98.0 | 18.1 | | 1.5 | |
| **Sulfuric acid**[a] | 98.08 | 18 | | | |
| **Ammonium hydroxide**[a] | 35.0 | 14.8 | | | |
| **Ethanolamine,**[a] **99%** | 61.08 | 16.5 | | | |
| **Triethylamine**[a] | 101.19 | 7.16 | | | |
| **Formaldehyde,**[a] **37%** | 30.3 | 12.2 | | | |
| **Hydrogen peroxide,**[a] **30%** | 34.02 | 8.8 | | | |
| **β-Mercaptoethanol**[a] | 78.13 | 14.4 | | | |
| **Formamide**[a] | 45.04 | 25.1 | | | |
| **Proprionic acid** | 74.08 | 13.4 | | | |
| **Ethylene glycol**[a] | 62.07 | 17.9 | | | |

[a] See Appendix IV for caution.

*Strains of laboratory mice*

| Strain | Abbreviation | Coat color | Class II haplotype[a] | Comments |
|---|---|---|---|---|
| **A/J** | A | White (Albino) | k | |
| **AKR** | AK | White(Albino) | k | |
| **BALB/c** | C | White (Albino) | d | Isogenic for most myeloma parents |
| **CBA** | CB | Agouti | k | |
| **C3H** | C3 | Agouti | k | |
| **C57BL/6** | B6 | Black | b | Common parent for transgenic $F_2$ |
| **C57BL/10** | B10 | Black | b | Many H2 congenics on this background |
| **DBA/2** | D2 | Dilute brown | d | Common parent for transgenic $F_2$ |
| **NZB** | | Black | d | Good for anti-"self" antibodies |
| **SJL** | | White (Albino) | s | Common parent for transgenic $F_2$ |
| **129** | - | White or light chinchilla | b | Parent of many teratocarcinomas |

The standard method to describe an $F_1$ cross is to list the two mice used for the mating followed by the designation "$F_1$." The female is always given first, followed by the male. Therefore, a B6D2$F_1$ is a C57BL/6 female crossed with a DBA/2 male.

[a] Klein et al. (1983).

*Preparation of stock solutions*

| Solution | Method of preparation | Comments |
|---|---|---|
| **Phosphate-buffered saline (PBS)** | Dissolve 8.0 g of NaCl, 0.2 g of KCl, 1.44 g of $Na_2HPO_4$, and 0.24 g of $KH_2PO_4$ in 800 ml of distilled $H_2O$. Adjust the pH to 7.4. Adjust the volume to 1 liter. Dispense in convenient volumes and sterilize by autoclaving. Store at room temperature. | Can be made as a 10× stock |
| **Tris-buffered saline (TBS) (25 mM Tris)** | Dissolve 8.0 g of NaCl, 0.2 g of KCl, and 3 g of Tris base in 800 ml of distilled $H_2O$. Adjust the pH to 8.0 with 1 M HCl. Adjust the volume to 1 liter. Dispense in convenient volumes and sterilize by autoclaving. Store at room temperature. | |
| **10% Sodium azide[a]** | Dissolve 10 g of sodium azide in 100 ml of distilled $H_2O$. Store at room temperature. | Do not use sodium azide for experiments using live organisms or for reactions that use horseradish peroxidase. |
| **3% Bovine serum albumin in phosphate-buffered saline (3% BSA/PBS)** | Add 3 g of BSA (Fraction V) to 100 ml of PBS. Allow to dissolve. Add 0.2 ml of 10% sodium azide. Store at 4°C. | |
| **1 M Tris** | Dissolve 121 g of Tris base in 800 ml of distilled $H_2O$. Adjust to the desired pH by adding concentrated HCl. Adjust the volume to 1000 ml with distilled $H_2O$. Dispense in convenient volumes and sterilize by autoclaving. Store at room temperature. | |
| **500 mM EDTA** | Add 186 g of disodium ethylene diamine tetraacetate · $2H_2O$ to 400 ml of distilled $H_2O$. Add NaOH to adjust the pH to 8.0 and to allow the EDTA to dissolve. Bring volume to 500 ml with distilled $H_2O$. Dispense in convenient volumes and sterilize by autoclaving. Store at room temperature. | |
| **100% (wt/vol) Trichloroacetic acetic acid (TCA)[a]** | Add 227 ml of distilled $H_2O$ to a 500-g bottle of TCA. | |
| **30% Acrylamide mix[a]** | Dissolve 29.2 g of acrylamide (electrophoresis grade) and 0.8 g of *N*, *N'*-methylene-bisacrylamide (electrophoresis grade) in 80 ml of distilled $H_2O$. Adjust the volume to 100 ml. Store at room temperature. | |

|  |  |  |
|---|---|---|
| **1.5 M Tris (pH 8.8)** | Dissolve 181.5 g of Tris base in 800 ml of distilled $H_2O$. Adjust the pH to 8.8 with concentrated HCl. Adjust the volume to 1 liter. Dispense in convenient volumes and sterilize by autoclaving. Store at room temperature. | |
| **1.0 M Tris (pH 6.8)** | Dissolve 12.1 g of Tris base in 80 ml of distilled $H_2O$. Adjust the pH to 6.8 with concentrated HCl. Adjust the volume to 100 ml. Sterilize by autoclaving. Store at room temperature. | |
| **10% Sodium dodecyl sulfate (SDS)[a]** | Dissolve 10 g of SDS in 100 ml of distilled $H_2O$. Store at room temperature. | |
| **10% Ammonium persulfate (APS)[a]** | Dissolve 0.5 g of ammonium persulfate (electrophoresis grade) in 5 ml of distilled $H_2O$. Store at 4°C. | Make fresh solution weekly. |
| **2× Laemmli sample buffer[a]** | Add 4 ml of 10% SDS, 2 ml of glycerol, and 1.2 ml of 1 M Tris (pH 6.8) to 2.8 ml of distilled $H_2O$. Add 0.01% bromophenol blue as a tracking dye. Store at room temperature. | To prepare 1× sample buffer, mix 5 parts 2 ×, 4 parts water, and 1 part 1 M DTT. |
| **1 M Dithiothreitol[a]** | Dissolve 5 g of DTT in 32 ml of distilled $H_2O$. Dispense in 1-ml aliquots. Store at –20°C. | |
| **10× Laemmli running buffer[a]** | To a 10-liter carboy, add 8 liters of distilled $H_2O$, 303 g of Tris base, 1442 g of glycine, and 100 g of SDS. After all the chemicals have dissolved, adjust the pH to 8.3. Adjust the volume to 10 liters with $H_2O$. Store at room temperature. | To prepare 1× running buffer, dilute the 10× stock 1 in 10 with distilled $H_2O$. |
| **Destain[a]** | To a 10-liter carboy add 2.5 liters of methanol and 700 ml of glacial acetic acid. Adjust the volume to 10 liters with $H_2O$. Store at room temperature. | |
| **4% Paraformaldehyde[a,b]** | Dissolve EM grade paraformaldehyde in PBS in Pyrex container with stir bar (4 g to 100 ml). Add a few drops of NaOH and heat in a hood (keep bottle cap loose) at 60°C to dissolve. Cool to room temperature and adjust pH to 7.4. Make fresh prior to use. | |

*Preparation of stock solutions (continued)*

| Solution | Method of preparation | Comments |
|---|---|---|
| **Gelvatol**[a,b] | Dissolve 0.35 g of Gelvatol in 3 ml of deionized $H_2O$ and 1.5 ml of glycerol. (PBS can be substituted for water.) Heat the solution with stirring in a boiling water bath until the Gelvatol is completely dissolved. Add anti-fade agents as desired. Store at 4°C (can be stored for months). | |
| **Glycerol anti-fade mounting medium**[a,b] | Dissolve in 100 ml of glycerol: 5 g of *n*-propyl gallate, 0.25 g of DABCO, 2.5 mg of *p*-phenylenediamine. Add several pellets of NaOH to bring pH above neutral. Stir thoroughly (>1 day). Store aliquots at –20°C wrapped in foil. | |
| **1 M NaCl/0.05 M sodium phosphate (pH 7.5)** | For liter: Combine 200 ml of 5 M NaCl, 500 ml of 0.1 M sodium phosphate (pH 7.5), and 300 ml of $H_2O$. | |
| **NP-40 lysis buffer** | For 1 liter: Combine 30 ml of 5 M NaCl, 100 ml of 10% NP-40, 50 ml of 1 M Tris (pH 8.0), and 820 ml of $H_2O$. Store at 4°C. | |
| **RIPA buffer**[a] | For 1 liter: Combine 30 ml of 5 M NaCl, 100 ml of 10% NP-40, 50 ml of DOC, 100 ml of 10% SDS, 50 ml of 1 M Tris (pH 8.0), and 670 ml of $H_2O$. Store at 4°C. | |

[a] See Appendix IV for caution.
[b] Adapted from Spector et al. (1998).

## Detergents

Detergents* form one class of polar lipids, characterized by their solubility in water. They have a bipartite structure with one hydrophobic portion and one hydrophilic portion. The presence of these two groups makes detergents useful for lysis of lipid membranes, solubilization of antigens, and washing of immune complexes.

A wide variety of chemicals can be classified as detergents. Of these, the most useful for biological studies fall into two groups based on the structure of their hydrophobic regions. Most biologically important detergents have hydrophobic regions with an 8- to 16-member alkyl chain (either with or without a phenolic moiety) or a structure that resembles the aromatic hydrophobic group of bile salts. The hydrophobic region leads to the solubilization of lipid bilayers, and only hydrophobic regions that are effective in this dissolution are useful for most biological applications.

Detergents are classified further by the type of hydrophilic group. These groups can be anionic, cationic, amphoteric, or nonionic. Examples of useful members of each of the four classes are shown on p. 464. In general, nonionic and amphoteric detergents are less denaturing to protein antigens than ionic detergents. Of the ionic detergents, sodium cholate and sodium deoxycholate are less denaturing than other ionic detergents.

Many of the properties of detergents can be described by three values: the critical micelle concentration, the micelle molecular weight, and the hydrophile–lipophile balance.

- **Critical micelle concentration** (CMC). The CMC is the concentration at which monomeric detergent molecules join to form micelles. Below this concentration, detergent molecules are found predominately as monomers; above the CMC, the detergent molecules form micelles.
- **Micelle molecular weight**. Micelles formed by a particular detergent will have a characteristic molecular weight. Detergents with large micelle molecular weights, such as the nonionic detergents, are difficult to dialyze.
- **Hydrophile–lipophile balance** (HLB). The HLB gives a numerical value to the overall hydrophilic properties of the detergent. Values above 7 indicate that the detergent is more soluble in water than in oils. For most biological applications, values of 12.5 and higher are needed. Although there are many exceptions, the HLB values can be used to give a general view of how denaturing a detergent will be. Values between 12 and 16 are relatively nondenaturing, whereas values above 20 indicate increasing denaturing possibilities. However, this correlation often does not apply outside of the detergents considered here, and differs from one protein to another.

Both the CMC and the micelle molecular weight vary in different buffers. All of the values given in the table on p. 464 will vary with the addition of salts or changes in temperature or pH. In general, adding salt lowers the CMC and raises the micelle size. The addition of as little as 100 mM sodium chloride may induce dramatic changes in these values. The extent of change in CMC or micelle molecular weight caused by varying the temperature or pH depends on the various detergents, but two detergents that are

*For reviews see Helenius and Simons (1975); Helenius et al. (1979); Furth (1980).

drastically affected by temperature or pH are SDS (temperatures below 20°C often lead to crystallization) and DOC (insoluble below about pH 7.5).

## Detergent removal

The ease with which detergents can be removed from protein solutions depends on a number of variables, including (1) the properties of the detergent itself, (2) the hydrophobic/hydrophilic characteristics of the protein, and (3) the other components of the buffer.

- **Ionic detergents with relatively low micelle size and high CMC.** Dilute as much as possible and dialyze. Add mixed bed resin to dialysis buffer to increase exchange rate.
- **Ionic detergents.** Add urea to 8 M, then bind detergent to an ion-exchange column. Protein flows through in 8 M urea. Dialyze to remove urea.
- **Ionic detergents.** Gel filtration on G25 column. For some proteins, equilibrate column in another detergent below its CMC.
- **Amphoteric detergents.** Dilute if possible, dialyze.
- **Nonionic detergents.** Gel filtration on G200 column. For some proteins, equilibrate column in another detergent below the CMC.
- **Nonionic detergents.** Dilute if possible, dialyze extensively against DOC, then slowly remove DOC by dialysis.
- **Nonionic detergents.** Velocity sedimentation into sucrose without detergent.
- **Nonionic detergent.** Bind protein to affinity matrix or ion-exchange column, wash extensively to remove detergent, then elute protein. For some proteins, equilibrate column in another detergent below the CMC.

*Properties of many commonly used detergents*

| Detergent | Abbreviation | Commercial name | Molecular weight | Relative purity | CMC (g/100 ml) | Micelle molecular weight | HLB number | Comments |
|---|---|---|---|---|---|---|---|---|
| **Anionic** | | | | | | | | |
| **Sodium dodecylsulfate**[a] | SDS | | 288 | Homogeneous | 0.24 | 18,000 | 40 | Excellent solubilization, highly denaturing |
| **Sodium dodecyl-*N*-sarcosinate** | | | 293 | Homogeneous | | | 24.7 | Excellent solubilization, strong denaturant |
| **Sodium cholate** | | | 431 | Homogeneous | 0.57 | 1,800 | 18 | Keep pH above 8.0, moderately denaturing |
| **Sodium deoxycholate**[a] | DOC | | 433 | Homogeneous | 0.2 | 4,200 | 16 | Keep pH above 8.0, avoid divalent cations moderately denaturing |
| **Cationic** | | | | | | | | |
| **Cetyltrimethylammonium bromide** | CTAB | | 364 | Homogeneous | 0.033 | 62,000 | | Highly denaturing |
| **Amphoteric** | | | | | | | | |
| **3-[(Cholamidopropyl)-dimethyl ammonio]-1-propanesulfonate** | CHAPS | | 651 | Homogeneous | 0.5 | | | Fair solubilization, weakly denaturing, easily dialyzed |
| **Zwittergent 3–12** | | | 305 | Homogeneous | 0.12 (calculated from 3.6 mM) | | | Good for gentle extraction |
| **Nonionic** | | | | | | | | |
| **Polyoxyethylene (10) cetyl alcohol** | | Brij 56 | 683 | Heterogeneous | 0.00014 | 130,000 | 12.9 | |
| **Polyoxyethylene (20) cetyl alcohol** | | Brij 58 | 1120 | Heterogeneous | 0.008 | 82,000 | 15.7 | Good solubilization |
| **Polyoxyethylene (23) lauryl alcohol** | | Brij 35 | 1200 | Heterogeneous | 0.58 | 49,000 | | |
| **Polyoxyethylene (4–5) *p-t*-octyl phenol** | | Triton X-45 | 405 | Heterogeneous | 0.0044 | | 10.4 | Selective extraction |
| **Polyoxyethylene (7–8) *p-t*-octyl phenol** | | Triton X-114 | 537 | Heterogeneous | 0.011 | | 12.4 | Selective extraction |
| **Polyoxyethylene (9) *p-t*-octyl phenol** | | Nonidet P-40 | 603 | Heterogeneous | 0.017 | 90,000 | 13.1 | Good solubilization, weakly denaturing |
| **Polyoxyethylene (9–10) *p-t*-octyl phenol** | | Triton X-100 | 625 | Heterogeneous | 0.016 | 90,000 | 13.5 | |
| **Polyoxyethylene (9–10) nonylphenol** | | Triton N-101 | 642 | Heterogeneous | 0.005 | 66,000 | 13.4 | Good solubilization, weekly denaturing |
| **Polyoxyethylene (20) sorbitol mololaurate** | | Tween 20 | 1230 | Heterogeneous | 0.006 | | 16.7 | Good solubilization, mildly denaturing good washing |
| **Polyoxyethylene (20) sorbitol monopalmitate** | | Tween 40 | 1280 | Heterogeneous | 0.003 | | 15.6 | |
| **Polyoxyethylene (20) sorbitol monoleate** | | Tween 80 | 1310 | Heterogeneous | 0.0013 | | 15.0 | |
| **Octyl-β-glucoside** | | | 292 | Homogeneous | 0.7 | | | Fair solubilization, easily dialyzed |
| **Digitonin**[a] | | | 1229 (monomer) | Heterogeneous | 0.022 (calculated from 0.18 mM) | | | |
| **Dodecyl-β-D-maltoside** | | | 606 | Homogeneous | 0.011 (calculated from 0.18 mM) | | | |

[a] See Appendix IV for caution.

## References


Furth A.J. 1980. Removing unbound detergent from hydrophobic proteins (review). *Anal. Biochem.* **109:** 207–215.

Helenius A. and Simons K. 1975. Solubilization of membranes by detergents. *Biochim. Biophys. Acta* **415:** 29–79.

Helenius A., McCaslin D.R., Fries E., and Tanford C. 1979. Properties of detergents. *Methods Enzymol.* **56:** 734–749.

Klein J., Figueroa F., and David C.S. 1983. H-2 haplotypes, genes and antigens: Second listing. II. The H-2 complex. *Immunogenetics* **17:** 553–596.

Spector D.L., Goldman R.D., and Leinwand L.A. 1998. *Cells: A laboratory manual*, vols. 1–3. Cold Spring Harbor Laboratory Press, Cold Spring Harbor, New York.

# Appendix IV
# Cautions

The following general cautions should always be observed.

- **The absence of a warning** does not necessarily mean that the material is safe, since information may not always be complete or available.
- **Proper disposal procedures** must be used for all chemical, biological, and radioactive waste.
- Consult your local safety office for specific guidelines on **appropriate gloves.**
- **Acids and bases** that are concentrated should be handled with great care. Wear goggles and appropriate gloves. A face shield should be worn when handling large quantities.

  Strong acids should not be mixed with organic solvents as they may react. Especially, sulfuric acid and nitric acid may react highly exothermically and cause fires and explosions.

  Strong bases should not be mixed with halogenated solvent as they may form reactive carbenes which can lead to explosions.

  For proper disposal of strong acids and bases, dilute them by placing the acid or base onto ice and neutralizing them. **Do not pour water into them.** If the solution does not contain any other toxic compound, the salts can be flushed down the drain.
- Never **pipet** solutions using mouth suction. This method is not sterile and can be dangerous. Always use a pipet aid or bulb.
- **Halogenated and nonhalogenated** solvents should be kept separately (e.g., mixing chloroform and acetone can cause unexpected reactions in the presence of bases).
- **Photographic fixatives and developers** also contain chemicals that can be harmful. Handle them with care and follow manufacturer's directions.
- **Power supplies and electrophoresis equipment** pose serious fire hazard and electrical shock hazards if not used properly.
- The use of **microwave ovens and autoclaves** in the lab requires certain precautions. Accidents have occurred involving their use (e.g., to melt agar or bactoagar stored in bottles or to sterilize). Often the screw top is not completely removed and there is not enough space for the steam to vent. When the containers are removed from the microwave or autoclave, they can explode and cause severe injury. Always completely remove bottle caps before microwaving or autoclaving. An alternative method for routine agarose gels that do not require sterile agar is to weigh out the agar and place the solution in a flask.

# Hazardous materials

**Acetic acid, concentrated,** must be handled with great care. It is harmful by inhalation, ingestion, or skin absorption. Wear appropriate gloves and goggles and use in a chemical fume hood.

**Acetone** causes eye and skin irritation and is irritating to mucous membranes and upper respiratory tract. Do not breathe the vapors. It is also extremely flammable. Wear appropriate gloves and safety glasses.

**Acrylamide** (unpolymerized) is a potent neurotoxin and is absorbed through the skin (the effects are cumulative). Avoid breathing the dust. Wear appropriate gloves and a face mask when weighing powdered acrylamide and methylene-bisacrylamide. Use in a chemical fume hood. Polyacrylamide is considered to be nontoxic, but it should be handled with care because it might contain small quantities of unpolymerized acrylamide.

AEC, see **Aminoethylcarbazole**

**Aminoethylcarbazole (AEC)** may be harmful by inhalation, ingestion, and skin absorption. Wear appropriate gloves and safety glasses.

**3-Amino-1,2,4-triazole (ATA)** is a carcinogen. Wear appropriate gloves, safety glasses, and other protective clothing. Avoid breathing vapors. Use only in a chemical fume hood.

**Ammonia, concentrated,** is corrosive, toxic, and can be explosive. It is harmful by inhalation, ingestion, and skin absorption. Use only with mechanical exhaust. Wear appropriate gloves and safety glasses.

**Ammonium chloride ($NH_4Cl$), concentrated,** may be harmful by inhalation, ingestion, or skin absorption. Wear appropriate gloves and safety glasses. Use in a chemical fume hood.

**Ammonium hydroxide** is a solution of ammonia in water. It is caustic and should be handled with great care. As ammonia vapors escape from the solution, they are corrosive, toxic, and can be explosive. Use only with mechanical exhaust. Wear appropriate gloves and use only in a chemical fume hood.

**Ammonium persulfate** is extremely destructive to tissue of the mucous membranes and upper respiratory tract, eyes, and skin. Inhalation may be fatal. Wear appropriate gloves, safety glasses, and protective clothing. Use only in a chemical fume hood. Wash thoroughly after handling.

**Animal treatment:** Procedures for the humane treatment of animals must be observed at all times. Consult your local animal facility for guidelines.

**Aprotinin** may be harmful by ingestion, inhalation, or skin absorption. It may also cause allergic reactions. Exposure may cause gastrointestinal effects, muscle pain, blood pressure changes, or bronchospasm. Wear appropriate gloves and safety glasses. Do not breathe the dust. Use only in a chemical fume hood.

**Bromochloroindolyl-β-D-galactopyranoside** (BCIG) is hazardous. Handle with care.

**BCIG,** see **Bromochloroindolyl-β-D-galactopyranoside**

**BCIP,** see **5-Bromo-4-chloro-3-indolyl-phosphate**

**Bicinchoninic acid** is an irritant. Wear appropriate gloves and goggles. Avoid contact with the eyes and skin and do not breathe the vapors. Use in a chemical fume hood.

**Biotin** may be harmful by inhalation, ingestion, or skin absorption. Wear appropriate gloves and safety glasses. Use in a chemical fume hood.

**Bisacrylamide** is a potent neurotoxin and is absorbed through the skin (the effects are cumulative). Avoid breathing the dust. Wear appropriate gloves and a face mask when weighing powdered acrylamide and methylene-bisacrylamide.

**Bleach** is poisonous, can be explosive, and may react with organic solvents. It is also harmful by ingestion and destructive to the skin. Wear appropriate gloves and safety glasses.

**BrdU,** see **5-Bromo-2′-deoxyuridine**

**Bromochloroindolyl-β-D-galactopyranoside** (BCIG) is hazardous. Handle with care.

**5-Bromo-4-chloro-3-indolyl-phosphate** (BCIP) is hazardous. Handle with care.

**5-Bromo-2′-deoxyuridine (BrdU)** is a mutagen. It may be harmful by inhalation, ingestion, or skin absorption. It may cause irritation. Avoid breathing the dust. Wear appropriate gloves and safety glasses and always use in a chemical fume hood.

**Chloroform** is irritating to the skin, eyes, mucous membranes, and respiratory tract. It is a carcinogen and may damage the liver and kidneys. Wear appropriate gloves and safety glasses and always use in a chemical fume hood.

**4-Chloro-1-naphthol** is irritating to the eyes, skin, mucous membranes, and respiratory tract. Handle with care. Wear appropriate gloves and safety glasses.

**Copper chloride** (**$CuCl_2$**) is toxic and an irritant. It may be harmful by inhalation, ingestion, or skin absorption. Wear appropriate gloves and safety glasses. Do not breathe the dust. Use in a chemical fume hood.

**$CuCl_2$,** see **Copper chloride**

**Cyanogen bromide** is extremely toxic and is volatile. It may be fatal by inhalation, ingestion, or skin absorption. Do not breathe the vapors. Wear appropriate gloves and always use in a chemical fume hood. Keep away from acids.

**DAB,** see **3,3′-Diaminobenzidine tetrahydrochloride**

**DABCO,** see **1,4-Diazabicyclo-[2,2,2]-octane**

**DAPI,** see **4′,6-Diamidine-2′ phenylindole dihydrochloride**

**Deoxycholate (DOC)** may be harmful by inhalation, ingestion, or skin absorption. Do not breathe the dust. Wear appropriate gloves and safety glasses.

**4′,6-Diamidine-2′ phenylindole dihydrochloride (DAPI)** is a possible carcinogen. It may be harmful by inhalation, ingestion, or skin absorption. It may also cause irritation. Avoid breathing the dust and vapors. Wear appropriate gloves and safety glasses and use in a chemical fume hood.

**3,3′-Diaminobenzidine tetrahydrochloride (DAB)** is a carcinogen. Handle with extreme care. Avoid breathing vapors. Wear appropriate gloves and safety glasses and use in a chemical fume hood.

**1,4-Diazabicyclo-[2,2,2]-octane (DABCO)** is harmful by inhalation, ingestion, or skin absorption. Wear appropriate gloves and safety glasses. Use in a chemical fume hood.

**Dibutyl phthalate** is harmful by inhalation, ingestion, or skin absorption. Wear appropriate gloves and safety glasses. Do not breathe the vapors.

**Digitonin** may be fatal if inhaled, ingested, or absorbed through the skin. Wear appropriate gloves and safety glasses. Use in a chemical fume hood.

**Dimethyl benzyl ammonium chloride** may be harmful by inhalation, ingestion, or skin absorption. Wear appropriate gloves and safety glasses and work in a chemical fume hood.

***N,N*-Dimethylformamide (DMF)** is irritating to the eyes, skin, and mucous membranes. It can exert its toxic effects through inhalation, ingestion, or skin absorption. Chronic inhalation can cause liver and kidney damage. Wear appropriate gloves and safety glasses. Use in a chemical fume hood.

**Dimethyl pimelimidate (DMP)** is irritating to the eyes, skin, mucous membranes, and upper respiratory tract. It can exert harmful effects by inhalation, ingestion, or skin absorption. Avoid breathing the vapors. Wear appropriate gloves, face mask, and safety glasses and do not inhale.

**Dimethyl sulfoxide (DMSO)** is harmful by inhalation or skin absorption. Wear appropriate gloves and safety glasses. Use in a chemical fume hood. DMSO is also combustible. Store in a tightly closed container. Keep away from heat, sparks, and open flame.

**Diphenyloxazole (PPO)** may be carcinogenic. Wear appropriate gloves. Consult the local institutional safety officer for specific handling and disposal procedures.

**Dithiothreitol (DTT)** is a strong reducing agent that emits a foul odor. Wear lab coat and safety glasses and use in a chemical fume hood when working with the solid form or highly concentrated stocks.

**DMF,** see ***N,N*-Dimethylformamide**

**DMP,** see **Dimethyl pimelimidate**

**DMSO,** see **Dimethyl sulfoxide**

**DOC,** see **Deoxycholate**

**DPX** is composed of Distyrene, a plasticizer, and xylene and is commercially available. Follow the manufacturer's guidelines for handling DPX.

**DTT,** see **Dithiothreitol**

**Ethanol** may be harmful by inhalation, ingestion, or skin absorption. Wear appropriate gloves and safety glasses.

**Ethanolamine** is toxic and harmful by inhalation, ingestion, or skin absorption. Handle with care and avoid any contact with the skin. Wear appropriate gloves and goggles and use in a chemical fume hood. Ethanolamine is highly corrosive and reacts violently with acids.

**Ethylene glycol** may be harmful by inhalation, ingestion, or skin absorption. Wear appropriate gloves and safety glasses. Use in a chemical fume hood.

***N*-Ethylmaleimide (NEM)** is harmful by inhalation, ingestion, or skin absorption. Wear appropriate gloves and safety glasses. Always use in a chemical fume hood.

**FITC,** see **Fluorescein isothiocyanate**

**Fluorescein** is harmful by inhalation, ingestion, or skin absorption. Wear appropriate gloves and safety glasses. Use in a chemical fume hood.

**Fluorescein isothiocyanate (FITC)** may be harmful by inhalation, ingestion, or skin absorption. Wear appropriate gloves and safety glasses.

**Formaldehyde** is highly toxic and volatile. It is also a carcinogen. It is readily absorbed through the skin and is irritating or destructive to the skin, eyes, mucous membranes, and upper respiratory tract. Avoid breathing the vapors. Wear appropriate gloves and safety glasses. Always use in a chemical fume hood. Keep away from heat, sparks, and open flame.

**Formalin** is a solution of formaldehyde in water. See **Formaldehyde**

**Formamide** is teratogenic. The vapor is irritating to the eyes, skin, mucous membranes, and upper respiratory tract. It may be harmful by inhalation, ingestion, or skin absorption. Wear appropriate gloves and safety glasses. Always use in a chemical fume hood when working with concentrated solutions of formamide. Keep working solutions covered as much as possible.

**Glacial acetic acid,** see **Acetic acid**

**β-Glucuronidase** may be harmful by inhalation, ingestion, or skin absorption. Wear respirator, appropriate gloves, and safety glasses.

**Glutaraldehyde** is toxic. It is readily absorbed through the skin and is irritating or destructive to the skin, eyes, mucous membranes, and upper respiratory tract. Wear appropriate gloves and safety glasses. Always use in a chemical fume hood.

**Guanidine hydrochloride** is irritating to the mucous membranes, upper respiratory tract, skin, and eyes. Wear appropriate gloves and safety glasses. Avoid breathing the dust.

**HCl,** see **Hydrochloric acid**

**Heptane** is harmful by inhalation, ingestion, or skin absorption. Wear appropriate gloves and safety glasses. It is extremely flammable. Keep away from heat, sparks, and open flame.

**$H_2O_2$,** see **Hydrogen peroxide**

**$H_3PO_4$,** see **Phosphoric acid**

**Hydrochloric acid (HCl)** is volatile and may be fatal if inhaled, ingested, or absorbed through the skin. It is extremely destructive to mucous membranes, upper respiratory tract, eyes, and skin. Wear appropriate gloves and safety glasses and use with great care in a chemical fume hood. Wear goggles when handling large quantities.

**Hydrogen peroxide ($H_2O_2$)** is corrosive, toxic, and extremely damaging to the skin. It is harmful by inhalation, ingestion, and skin absorption. Wear appropriate gloves and safety glasses.

***N*-Hydroxysuccinimide** is an irritant and may be harmful by inhalation, ingestion, or skin absorption. Wear appropriate gloves and safety glasses.

**Isobutanol,** see **Isobutyl alcohol**

**Isobutyl alcohol (Isobutanol)** is extremely flammable and my be harmful by inhalation or ingestion. Wear appropriate gloves and safety glasses. Keep away from heat, sparks, and open flame.

**Isopentane (2-methylbutane)** is extremely flammable. Keep away from heat, sparks, and open flame. It may be harmful by inhalation, ingestion, or skin absorption. Wear appropriate gloves and safety glasses.

**Isotope $^{125}$I** accumulates in the thyroid and is a potential health hazard. Consult the local radiation safety office for further guidance in the appropriate use and disposal of radioactive materials. Wear appropriate gloves when handling radioactive substances. The $^{125}I_2$ formed during oxidation of $Na^{125}I$ is volatile. Work in an approved chemical fume hood with a charcoal filter when exposing the $Na^{125}I$ to oxidizing reagents such as chloramine-T, IODO-GEN, or acids. Because the oxidation proceeds very rapidly and releases large amounts of volatile $^{125}I_2$ when chloramine-T is used, it is important to be well prepared for each step of the reaction, so that the danger of contamination from volatile radiation can be minimized. Shield all forms of the isotope by lead. When handling the isotope, wear one or two pairs of appropriate gloves, depending on the amount of isotope being used and the difficulty of the manipulation required.

**Leupeptin** (or **its hemisulfate**) may be harmful by inhalation, ingestion, or skin absorption. Wear appropriate gloves and safety glasses. Use in a chemical fume hood.

**LiCl,** see **Lithium chloride**

**Lithium chloride (LiCl)** is an irritant to the eyes, skin, mucous membranes, and upper respiratory tract. It may be harmful by inhalation, ingestion, or skin absorption. Wear appropriate gloves, safety goggles, and use in a chemical fume hood. Do not breathe the dust.

**Maleimide** is extremely harmful and may be fatal by inhalation, ingestion, or skin absorption. Do not breathe the dust. Wear appropriate gloves and safety goggles and work in a chemical fume hood.

**β-Mercaptoethanol (2-Mercaptoethanol)** may be fatal if inhaled or absorbed through the skin and is harmful if ingested. High concentrations are extremely destructive to the mucous membranes, upper respiratory tract, skin, and eyes. Wear appropriate gloves and safety glasses. Always use in a chemical fume hood.

**Merthiolate®,** see **Thimerosal**

**Methanol** is poisonous and can cause blindness. It is harmful by inhalation, ingestion, or skin absorption. Adequate ventilation is necessary to limit exposure to vapors. Avoid inhaling these vapors. Wear appropriate gloves and goggles. Use only in a chemical fume hood.

**2-Methylbutane,** see **Isopentane**

**Methyl salicylate** is volatile and may be harmful by inhalation, ingestion, or skin absorption. Do not breathe the dust. Wear appropriate gloves and safety glasses and work in a chemical fume hood.

**NaOH,** see **Sodium hydroxide**

**NBT,** see **4-Nitro blue tetrazolium chloride**

**NEM,** see ***N*-Ethylmaleimide**

**$NH_4Cl$,** see **Ammonium chloride**

**Nickel chloride** (**$NiCl_2$**) is toxic and may be harmful by inhalation, ingestion, or skin absorption. Do not breathe the dust. Wear appropriate gloves and safety glasses.

**$NiCl_2$,** see **Nickel chloride.**

**4-Nitro blue tetrazolium chloride** (**NBT**) is hazardous. Handle with care.

**OCT** is composed of polyvinyl alcohol, polyethylene glycol, and dimethyl benzyl ammonium chloride. Follow the manufacturer's guidelines for handling OCT.

**Paraformaldehyde** is highly toxic. It is readily absorbed through the skin and is extremely destructive to the skin, eyes, mucous membranes, and upper respiratory tract. Avoid breathing the dust. Wear appropriate gloves and safety glasses, and use in a chemical fume hood. Paraformaldehyde is the undissolved form of formaldehyde.

**Pepstatin A** may be harmful by inhalation, ingestion, or skin absorption. Wear appropriate gloves and safety glasses. Use in a chemical fume hood.

**Phenol** is extremely toxic, highly corrosive, and can cause severe burns. Wear appropriate gloves, goggles, and protective clothing. Always use in a chemical fume hood. Rinse any areas of skin that come in contact with phenol with a large volume of water and wash with soap and water; do not use ethanol!

***p*-Phenylenediamine** is harmful by inhalation, ingestion, or skin absorption. Wear appropriate gloves and safety glasses. Use in a chemical fume hood.

**Phenyl hydrazine (or its hydrochloride)** is highly toxic and is a carcinogen. It is harmful by inhalation, ingestion, or skin absorption. Wear appropriate gloves and safety glasses and work in a chemical fume hood.

**Phosphoric acid** (**$H_3PO_4$**)**, concentrated,** is corrosive and an irritant and may be harmful by inhalation, ingestion, or skin absorption. Wear appropriate gloves and safety glasses.

**Picric acid powder** is caustic and potentially explosive if it is dissolved and then allowed to dry out. Care must be taken to ensure that stored solutions do not dry out. Handle all concentrated acids with great care. It is also highly toxic and may be harmful by inhalation, ingestion, or skin absorption. Wear appropriate gloves and goggles.

**Polyacrylamide** is considered to be nontoxic, but it should be treated with care because it may contain small quantities of unpolymerized material (see **Acrylamide**).

**Potassium ferrocyanide** may be fatal if inhaled, ingested, or absorbed through the skin. Wear appropriate gloves and safety glasses and always use with extreme care in a chemical fume hood. Keep away from strong acids.

**Potassium thiocyanate** causes eye and skin irritation. It may be harmful by inhalation, ingestion, or skin absorption. Wear appropriate gloves and safety goggles. Do not breathe the dust.

**PPO,** see **Diphenyloxazole**

**Propidium iodide** is harmful by inhalation, ingestion, or skin absorption. It is irritating to the eyes, skin, mucous membranes, and upper respiratory tract. It is mutagenic and possibly carcinogenic. Wear appropriate gloves, safety glasses, and protective clothing, and always use with extreme care in a chemical fume hood.

**Radioactive substances:** Wear appropriate gloves when handling. Consult the local safety office for further guidance in the appropriate use and disposal of radioactive materials. Always monitor thoroughly after using radioisotopes.

**SDS,** see **Sodium dodecyl sulfate**

**Silver lactate** may be harmful by inhalation, ingestion, or skin absorption. Wear appropriate gloves and safety glasses. Do not breathe the dust or mist.

**Silver nitrate** is a strong oxidizing agent and should be handled with care. It may be harmful by inhalation, ingestion, or skin absorption. Avoid contact with skin. Wear appropriate gloves and safety glasses. It can cause explosions upon contact with other materials.

**Sodium acetate,** see **Acetic acid**

**Sodium azide** is highly poisonous. It blocks the cytochrome electron transport system. Solutions containing sodium azide should be clearly marked. Wear appropriate gloves and handle sodium azide with great care.

**Sodium deoxycholate** is irritating to mucous membranes and the respiratory tract and is harmful if ingested. Wear appropriate gloves and safety glasses when handling the powder and do not inhale the dust.

**Sodium dodecyl sulfate (SDS)** is harmful if inhaled. Wear a face mask when weighing SDS.

**Sodium ethylmercurithiosalicylate,** see **Thimerosal**

**Sodium hydroxide (NaOH), concentrated, and solutions containing NaOH** are highly toxic and caustic and should be handled with great care. Wear appropriate gloves and a face mask. All other concentrated bases should be handled in a similar manner.

**Sulfosalicylic acid (dihydrate)** is extremely destructive to the mucous membranes and respiratory system. Do not breathe the dust. Wear appropriate gloves and safety glasses and work only in a chemical fume hood.

**Sulfuric acid** is highly toxic and extremely destructive to tissue of the mucous membranes and upper respiratory tract, eyes, and skin. It causes burns, and contact with other materials (e.g., paper) may cause fire. Wear appropriate gloves, safety glasses, and lab coat and use in a chemical fume hood.

**TCA,** see **Trichloroacetic acid**

**TEMED,** see ***N,N,N′,N′*-Tetramethylethylenediamine**

***N,N,N′,N′*-Tetramethylethylenediamine (TEMED)** is extremely destructive to tissue of the mucous membranes and upper respiratory tract, eyes, and skin. Inhalation may be fatal. Prolonged contact can cause severe irritation or burns. Wear appropriate gloves, safety glasses, and other protective clothing and use in a chemical fume hood. Wash thoroughly after handling. Flammable: Vapor may travel a considerable distance to source of ignition and flash back. Keep away from heat, sparks, and open flame.

**Tetramethylrhodamine isothiocyanate (TRITC)** may be harmful by inhalation, ingestion, or skin absorption. Wear appropriate gloves and safety glasses.

**Thimerosal** is highly toxic and harmful by inhalation, ingestion, or skin absorption. Do not breathe the dust. Wear appropriate gloves and safety glasses.

**Toluene** vapors are irritating to the eyes, skin, mucous membranes, and upper respiratory tract. Toluene can exert harmful effects by inhalation, ingestion, or skin absorption. Wear appropriate gloves and safety glasses and do not inhale. Use in a chemical fume hood. Toluene is extremely flammable. Keep away from heat, sparks, and open flame.

**Tresyl chloride (2,2,2-Trifluoroethanesulfonyl chloride)** is corrosive and may be harmful by inhalation, ingestion, or skin absorption. Do not breathe the vapors. Wear appropriate gloves and safety glasses and work in a chemical fume hood. Keep away from heat, sparks, and open flame.

**Trichloroacetic acid (TCA)** is highly caustic. Always wear appropriate gloves and goggles.

**Triethylamine** is highly toxic and flammable. It is extremely corrosive to the mucous membranes, upper respiratory tract, eyes, and skin. It may be harmful by inhalation, ingestion, or skin absorption. Wear appropriate gloves and safety glasses. Use in a chemical fume hood. Keep away from heat, sparks, and open flame.

**2,2,2-Trifluoroethanesulfonyl chloride,** see **Tresyl chloride**

**TRITC,** see **Tetramethylrhodamine isothiocyanate**

**UV light** and/or **UV radiation** is dangerous and can damage the retina of the eyes. Never look at an unshielded UV light source with naked eyes. View only through a filter or safety glasses that absorb harmful wavelengths. UV radiation is also mutagenic and carcinogenic. To minimize exposure, make sure that the UV light source is adequately shielded. Wear protective appropriate gloves when holding materials under the UV light source.

**Xylene** must always be used in a chemical fume hood. It is flammable and may be narcotic at high concentrations. Keep away from heat, sparks, and open flame.

## Appendix V

# Trademarks

The following trademarks and registered trademarks are accurate to the best of our knowledge at the time of printing. Please consult individual manufacturers and other resources for specific information.

| | |
|---|---|
| Affigel 10 | Bio-Rad |
| Affinica Tresyl | Schleicher & Schuell Inc. |
| AffiPrep 10 | Bio-Rad |
| AminoLink | Pierce Chemical Co. |
| Anti-FLAG | Immunology Ventures |
| Brij 35 | ICI America |
| Brij 56 | ICI America |
| Brij 58 | ICI America |
| CM Bio-Gel A Gel | Bio-Rad |
| CNBr-activated Sepharose | Pharmacia |
| Complete Tablets | Boehringer Mannheim GmbH |
| Coomassie Blue | Imperial Chemical Industries, Ltd. |
| Coomassie Brilliant Blue G-250 | Imperial Chemical Industries, Ltd. |
| Coomassie Brilliant Blue R-250 | Imperial Chemical Industries, Ltd. |
| ECH Sepharose 4B | Pharmacia |
| ECL | Amersham International plc |
| EGFP | CLONTECH Laboratories Inc. |
| FLAG tag | Immunology Ventures |
| His·Tag | Novagen Inc. |
| HiTrap NHS-Activated | Pharmacia |
| HSV·Tag | Novagen Inc. |
| IODO-GEN | Pierce Chemical Co. |
| Kodak XAR | Eastman Kodak Co. |
| Levamisole | Vector Laboratories Inc. |
| Lipshaw Number 1 | Shandon Lipshaw |
| Mowiol | Hoechst AG |
| Nonidet P-40 | Shell International Petroleum Co. Ltd. UK |
| Novatope | Novagen Inc. |
| Parafilm | American National Can Co. |
| PCR | Hoffman-LaRoche |
| Pefabloc | Pentapharm Ltd. |
| Pelikan Fount India drawing ink | Pelikan |
| PhosphorImager | Molecular Dynamics |
| Plexiglas | Rohm & Haas Co. |
| Pronase | Calbiochem-Novabiochem Corp. |

| | |
|---|---|
| PYREX | Corning Inc. |
| Reacti-Gel 6X | Pierce Chemical Co. |
| Reacti-Gel GF-2000 | Pierce Chemical Co. |
| Saran Wrap | Dow Chemical Company |
| 3M Scotch epoxy 2216 B/A | 3M Company |
| S·Tag (S peptide tag) | Novagen Inc. |
| SulfoLink | Pierce Chemical Co. |
| T7·Tag | Novagen Inc. |
| Teflon | E.I. DuPont deNemours and Co., Inc. |
| Texas Red | Molecular Probes Inc. |
| Thimerosal p1057 | Sigma-Aldrich |
| Triton X-45 | Rohm & Haas Co. |
| Triton X-100 | Rohm & Haas Co. |
| Triton N-101 | Rohm & Haas Co. |
| Triton X-114 | Rohm & Haas Co. |
| Tween 20 | ICI America |
| Tween 40 | ICI America |
| Tween 80 | ICI America |
| UltraLink | Pierce Chemical Co. |
| UltraLink Iodoacetyl | Pierce Chemical Co. |
| Vectabond | Vector Laboratories Inc. |
| Whatman 3 MM | Whatman Inc. |
| ZWITTERGENT | Calbiochem-Novabiochem Corp. |
| Zymolyase | Seikagaku America Inc. |

# Appendix VI
# Suppliers

With the exception of those suppliers listed in the text with their addresses, all suppliers mentioned in this manual can be found in the BioSupplyNet Source Book and on the Web site at:

http: //www.biosupplynet.com

If a copy of BioSupplyNet Source Book was not included with this manual, a free copy can be ordered by using any of the following methods:

- Complete the Free Source Book Request Form found at the Web site at:

http: //www.biosupplynet.com

- E-mail a request to info@biosupplynet.com
- Fax a request to 516-349-5598

# Index*



*t and f indicate that the information can be found in the tables and figures, respectively.